NEUROSCIENCE RESEARCH PROGRESS

# NEURORESTORATOLOGY

## VOLUME 1

## THEORIES AND TECHNIQUES OF NEURORESTORATOLOGY

# NEUROSCIENCE RESEARCH PROGRESS

NEUROSCIENCE RESEARCH PROGRESS

# NEURORESTORATOLOGY

## VOLUME 1

## THEORIES AND TECHNIQUES OF NEURORESTORATOLOGY

HONGYUN HUANG
GEOFFREY RAISMAN
PAUL R. SANBERG
AND
HARI S. SHARMA
EDITORS
LIN CHEN
ASSOCIATE EDITOR

NOVA BIOMEDICAL

*New York*

**Library of Congress Cataloging-in-Publication Data**

ISBN: 978-1-63463-599-8

*Published by Nova Science Publishers, Inc. † New York*

# Contents

# Preface

> Faith is the "eternal elixir" which gives life, power, and action to the impulse of thought! Faith is the starting point of all accumulation of riches! Faith is the basis of all "miracles", and all mysteries, which cannot be analyzed by the rules of science! Faith is the only known antidote for failure! Faith is the element, the "chemical" which, when mixed with prayer, gives one direct communication with Infinite Intelligence. Faith is the element which transforms the ordinary vibration of thought, created by the finite mind of man, into the spiritual equivalent. Faith is the only agency through which the cosmic force of Infinite Intelligence can be harnessed and used by man.
>
> — Napoleon Hill

Neurorestoratology is a discipline which studies neural regeneration, repair and replacement of damaged components of the nervous system, neuroplasticity, neuroprotection and neuromodulation, vasculogenesis and recovery mechanisms of immune regulation [11]. Its aim is to restore, promote and maintain the integrity of impaired or lost neuronal functions and/or structures, using novel cell-based comprehensive neurorestorative strategies [5, 6, 9, 12-14]. Although it is a new discipline, it is one of the most important disciplines in modern medicine [11]. Arguably, it is also the most important discipline in neuroscience [4, 6, 9]. The central nervous system (CNS) neurorestorable theory has influenced considerably or altered the thinking of many clinicians and healthcare providers who subsequently adopted new approaches to treat patients with CNS damages or neurodegenerative diseases. This has opened new doors to treat what were once considered incurable CNS damages or degenerative disorders, including some that have been believed as untreatable for thousands of years.

The neurorestorative process, i.e., the neural insults together with whatever has caused the restoration, has been generalized as a whole and reveals the dynamic interaction between neural insults and restorative mechanisms. Currently, more and more clinicians, researchers and societies [3] in neuroscience have collaborated to actively explore neurorestorative strategies and to study the mechanisms that are translated now in clinical practice as effective therapeutic methods to improve patients' quality of life or prolong their lifespan. Although some of them are still wondering about the scientific potential of neurorestoratology and its efficacy in clinical settings, they have committed themselves to neurorestoratology, either intentionally or by accident. This is further evident from the fact that newly proposed large brain research projects, such as the American Brain Project (BRAIN Initiative) and the

European "Human Brain Project, aim at exploring and solving the puzzles of brain functions. Excitingly, adopting *CNS neurorestorative theory, neurorestorative process* and *neurorestorative law,* the discipline of neurorestoratology has already moved in this direction and is able to provide original knowledge to this new area in neuroscience [9].

"Rome was not build in a day," and the discipline of neurorestoratology will also require more time to evolve as a distinct branch of medicine. In the last two centuries, pioneers in this field have explored several neurorestorative strategies and their possible mechanisms, but, unfortunately, most of their achievements have been ignored, likely due to the assumption that the sequelae of CNS damages or diseases could not be restored.

We believe the time has come to challenge these assumptions and demonstrate, through research and clinical practices in neurorestoratology, that CNS damages and diseases are restorable. As gold or diamonds must be excavated from mines in order to create jewels, in the same way major achievements in neurorestoratology that could change the face of modern neuroscience and related clinical practices must be rescued from oblivion and widely publicized. To establish neurorestoratology as a major discipline in the medical curriculum and practices requires collecting, classifying, and presenting novel research and clinical data in the field, and, ultimately, evolving from what are currently disorganized and scattered neurorestorative strategies and mechanisms into a recognized and indispensable discipline.

This book, "Neurorestoratology," is the first book that systematically expounds the main aspects of neurorestoratology. It includes three sections with 22 chapters in two volumes. It systematically elaborates *CNS neurorestorable theory* and neurorestorative mechanisms, comprehends the *neurorestorative process* as a whole and *neurorestorative law,* and fully describes all neurorestorative strategies and their continuing clinical progresses and achievements, especially the cell-based comprehensive neurorestorative strategies.

Section One provides an overview of neurorestoratology, including the origin and development of the discipline and each neurorestorative strategy. The pioneers' unyielding exploration and development of this discipline is recorded and reproduced. The *CNS neurorestorable theory, neurorestorative process, neurorestorative law* and their mechanisms are presented and discussed in detail to help readers easily understand the basics of neurorestoratology and the dynamic changes of neural degeneration or damages, along with neurorestorative mechanisms at the physiological and pathophysiological levels.

Section Two is devoted to the techniques and effects of CNS neurorestorative strategies, including cell therapy, neuromodulation, medicine and factors, bio- and tissue-engineering, neurorestorative surgery and alternative therapies. In addition, neurorehabilitation as a complementary neurorestorative strategy is described.

Section Three presents neurorestorative strategies to treat trauma or neurodegenerative diseases in the nervous system. Neurorestorative therapy for spinal cord injury (SCI), traumatic brain injury (TBI), stroke, multiple sclerosis (MS), amyotrophic lateral sclerosis (ALS), Parkinson's disease (PD), Alzheimer's disease (AD), cerebral palsy (CP), autism, optic neuropathy, and peripheral nerve injury are presented in great detail. Recent advancements and scientific progress in these areas suggest that standing or walking is not a just dream for some patients with complete chronic spinal cord injury [5- 7, 10]. Likewise, patients with ALS, Parkinson's disease, dementia and other neurodegenerative diseases can also be stabilized or have their functions improved for a period of time [5, 6, 8]. Similarly, with the help of such treatments, patients with chronic stroke can improve their quality of life

[2, 5, 6] and children with cerebral palsy can have their intelligence and self-care abilities improved significantly [1, 5, 6].

Improving the quality of life and prolonging lifespan has been a desire of human beings since time immemorial. The ethical stance presented in the World Medical Association's Declaration of Helsinki requires physicians to try their best to help patients with new medical methods. We hope this book will accelerate a change in thinking among clinicians and healthcare providers and encourage more of them to utilize neurorestorative strategies with their patients. It is also our hope that this book will further advance the concept of neurorestoratology and its implementation in translational medicine.

We are deeply indebted to all of the pioneers who dedicated themselves to neurorestoratology and its foundational work. We appreciate all of the authors and the editorial team who contributed their wisdom, efforts and enthusiasm to this maiden volume of "Neurorestoratology." We honestly thank the Secretary of Editors, Miss Jiangfeng Guo for her utmost professional work. We hope this is only the beginning and, in near future, that more and more research will contribute to this newly developed field and further expand the scope of this book.

We appreciate the dedication, hard work and professional support of the NOVA publishers to make this volume a reality, and hope the book will be of value to students, researchers and clinicians around the world.

*Hongyun Huang, M.D., Ph.D., Beijing, China*
*Geoffrey Raisman, Ph.D., London, UK*
*Paul R. Sanberg, Ph.D., D.Sc., Tampa, FL, USA*
*Hari Sharma, Ph.D., D. Med.Sci., Uppsala, Sweden*
*Chen Lin, M.D., Beijing, China*

## References

[1] Chen L, Huang H, Xi H, Xie Z, Liu R, Jiang Z, Zhang F, Liu Y, Chen D, Wang Q, Wang H, Ren Y, Zhou C. Intracranial transplant of olfactory ensheathing cells in children and adolescents with cerebral palsy: a randomized controlled clinical trial. *Cell Transplant.* 2010;19(2):185-191.

[2] Chen L, Xi H, Huang H, Zhang F, Liu Y, Chen D, Xiao J. Multiple cell transplantation based on an intraparenchymal approach for patients with chronic phase stroke. *Cell Transplant.* 2013;22 Suppl 1:S83-91.

[3] Chinese Branch of the International Association of Neurorestoratology, Preparatory Committee of Chinese Association of Neurorestoratology. Standard recommendations for the application of Chinese clinical cell therapy for neurorestoration. *Cell Transplant.* 2013;22 Suppl 1:S5-10.

[4] Huang H. Neurorestoratology, a distinct discipline and a new era: A brief introduction to the first IANR section. *Cell Transplant.* 2010;19(2):129-131.

[5] Huang H, Chen L, Sanberg P. Cell therapy from bench to bedside translation in CNS Neurorestoratology era. *Cell Medicine, Part B of Cell Transplant.* 2010;1(1):15-46.

[6] Huang H, Chen L, Sanberg P. Clinical achievements, obstacles, falsehoods, and future directions of cell-based neurorestoratology. *Cell Transplant.* 2012;21(S1):S3-S11.

[7] Huang H, Chen L, Wang H, Xiu B, Li B, Wang R, Zhang J, Zhang F, Gu Z, Li Y, Song Y, Hao W, Pang S, Sun J. Influence of patients' age on functional recovery after transplantation of olfactory ensheathing cells into injured spinal cord injury. *Chin Med J.* 2003;116(10):1488-1491.

[8] Huang H, Chen L, Xi H, Wang H, Zhang J, Zhang F, Liu Y. Fetal olfactory ensheathing cells transplantation in amyotrophic lateral sclerosis patients: a controlled pilot study. *Clin Transplant* 2008;22:710-718.

[9] Huang H, Sharma HS. Editorial. Neurorestoratology: one of the most promising new disciplines at the forefront of neuroscience and medicine. *Journal of Neurorestoratology* 2013;1:37-41.

[10] Huang H, Xi H, Chen L, Zhang F, Liu Y. Long-term outcome of olfactory ensheathing cell therapy for patients with complete chronic spinal cord injury. *Cell Transplant.* 2012;21:S23-S31.

[11] International Association of Neurorestoratology. Beijing Declaration of International Association of Neurorestoratology (IANR). *Cell Transplant.* 2009;18(4):487.

[12] Sharma HS, Muresanu DF, Sharma A. Novel therapeutic strategies using nanodrug delivery, stem cells *Expert Rev Neurother.* 2013;13(10):1085-8.

[13] Sharma HS, Sharma A. New strategies for CNS *Expert Rev Neurother.* 2011;11(8):1121-4.

[14] Sharma HS, Sharma A. New therapeutic advances in CNS *Expert Rev Neurother.* 2012;12(8):901-5.

# About the Editors

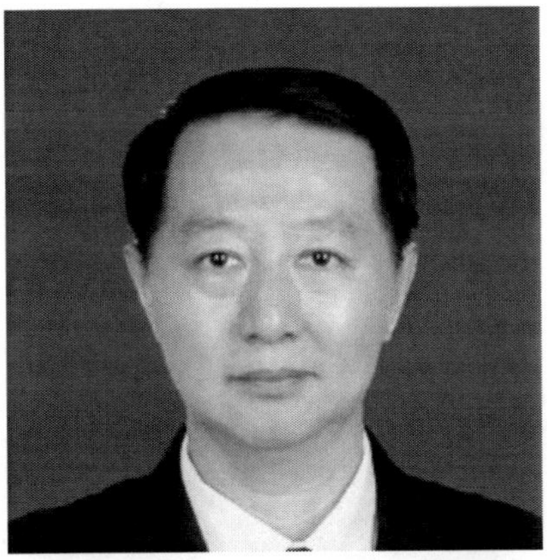

**Hongyun Huang M.D., Ph.D.**

**Hongyun Huang**, Honorary Director, Institute of Neurorestoratology, General Hospital of Armed Police Forces, China; Neurosurgeon in Chief, Neurorestoratology Center, Beijing Rehabilitation Hospital of Capital Medical University; President, Beijing Hongtianji Neuroscience Academy.

Founding President, International Association of Neurorestoratology; Guest Editor, *Cell Transplantation;* Editor in Chief, *Journal of Neurorestoratology*; Associate Editor, *American Journal of Neuroprotection and neuroregeneration*

Dr. Huang specializes in Spinal Neurosurgery, Stereotactic and Functional Neurosurgery, Tumor Neurosurgery and Neurorestoratology. He has initiated clinical neurorestorative innovation through cell therapy since 2001 for treating diseases and damages involving central nervous system (CNS), such as: spinal cord injury, sequela of brain damage and stroke (cerebral infarction and hemorrhage), amyotrophic lateral sclerosis (ALS) or motor neuron disease (MND), cerebral palsy, Alzheimer's disease (AD), Parkinson's disease (PD), multiple sclerosis (MS), Friedreich's ataxia, multiple system atrophy and related disorders. His intervention with cell therapy produced encouraging results. Patients with these incurable CNS diseases thus could achieve partial neurological function recovery and improve their quality of life. Basing on this success story, Dr. Huang put forward the CNS neurorestorable theory and neurorestorative processes that generalize the entire insults and restoring mechanisms as a whole, revealed the *Neurorestorative Law* and validated cell-based comprehensive neurorestorative therapy.

This therapy refers to multiple-cell types, multiple-routes, multiple-processes and /or in combination with other strategies including neurostimulation/ neuromodulation and neurorehabilitation.

So far Dr. Huang has successfully treated over 2000 patients with incurable neurological diseases or damages from about 100 countries and regions using cell-based comprehensive neurorestorative therapy.

Dr. Huang was the first to put forward and establish the discipline of Neurorestoratology as a separate entity. In collaboration with top experts worldwide in this field, he founded the International Association of Neurorestoratology (IANR) in 2007. He has published over 100 scientific papers in peer-reviewed journals in the field of neurorestoration and edited two books *OEC Transplantation* and *CNS Neurorestoratology.*

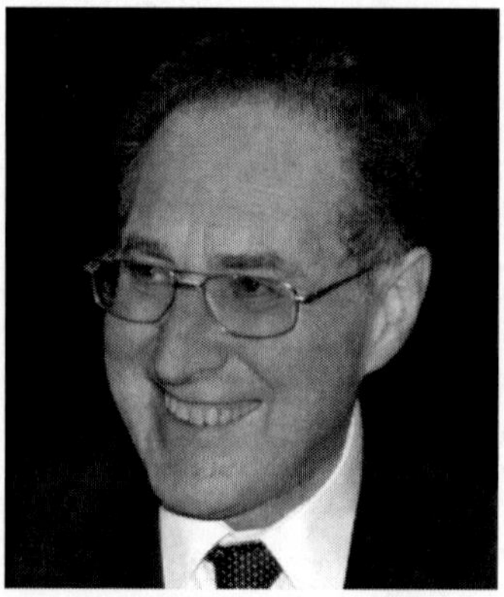

**Geoffrey Raisman, M.D., Ph.D., FRS**

**Professor Geoffrey Raisman** is Chair of Neural Regeneration and Director of the Spinal Repair Unit at the UCL Institute of Neurology, Queen Square, London. He was awarded the Wakeman Award for Research in Neurosciences, and the Reeve-Irvine Medal 2005 for critical contributions to promoting repair of the damaged spinal cord and recovery of function.

His training was at Oxford University, Harvard Medical School, and he was Head of the Division of Neurobiology, MRC National Institute for Medical Research, 1974-2004 and is Life Honorary President of the International Association of Neurorestoratology. His original work was the demonstration of the formation of new connections after CNS injury, for which he introduced the term 'plasticity' in 1969. He has described the repair of spinal cord lesions by transplantation of olfactory ensheathing cells, and more recently, the role of the fortified astrocytes in the pathogenesis of glaucoma.

Key awards: Wakeman Award for Research in Neurosciences,Duke University, North Carolina, 1980; Elected Fellow of the Academy of Medical Sciences (FMedSci), 1999; Elected Fellow of the Royal Society, 2001; Fellow of the Royal Society of Arts, 2002; British Neuroscience Association Award, Outstanding Contribution to British Neuroscience, 2004; Reeve-Irvine Medal for critical contributions to promoting repair of the damaged spinal cord and recovery of function, 2005; Life Honorary President, International Association of Neurorestoratology, 2010.

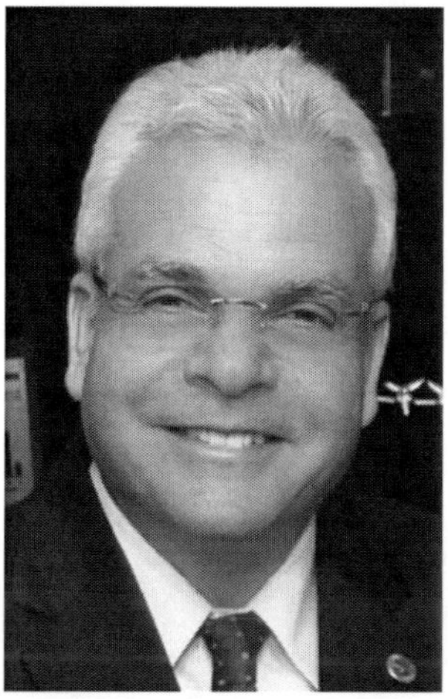

**Paul R. Sanberg, Ph.D., D.Sc.**

**Dr. Paul R. Sanberg** is Senior Vice President for Research & Innovation, Distinguished University Professor, and Executive Director of the Center of Excellence for Aging and Brain Repair at the University of South Florida, in Tampa, Florida, USA. He is a member of the Board of Scientific Counselors for the National Institute of Drug Abuse at the National Institutes of Health and has served on numerous scientific advisory boards for health-related foundations and companies.

He is an inventor on 39 U.S. and over 70 foreign patents. His work has been instrumental in translating new pharmaceutical and cellular therapeutics to clinical trials and commercialization for Tourette syndrome, stroke, amyotrophic lateral sclerosis (ALS), Alzheimer's, Huntington's, and Parkinson's disease, and he has significant biotech and pharmaceutical industry experience in these areas. He is the author of more than 600 scientific publications and is considered a highly cited scientist, with more than 22,000 citations to his published work.

He is editor-in-chief of *Technology and Innovation* and serves on editorial boards for more than 30 scientific journals. Dr. Sanberg is president and Charter Fellow of the National Academy of Inventors, chair of the Florida Inventors Hall of Fame Advisory Board, and has served as president of a number of professional societies, including the American Society for Neural Transplantation and Repair, Cell Transplant Society, and International Behavioral Neuroscience Society. He is a Fellow of the American Association for the Advancement of Science (AAAS), AAAS-Lemelson Invention Ambassador, and serves on the evaluation committee of the United States National Medal of Technology and Innovation.

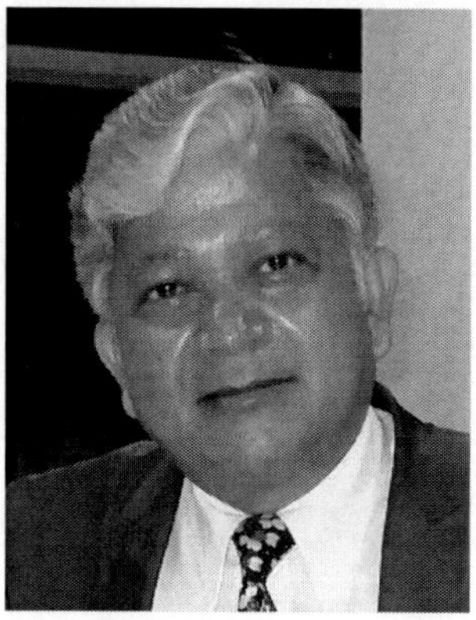

**Hari Shanker Sharma, Ph.D. (BHU), Dr. Med Sci (UU)**

**Hari Shanker Sharma**, *Director of Research (International Experimental Central Nervous System Injury & Repair, IECNSIR)*, University Hospital, Uppsala University is Professor of Neurobiology (MRC), Docent in Neuroanatomy (UU) and is currently affiliated with Department of Surgical Sciences, Division of Anesthesiology and Intensive Care Medicine, Uppsala University, Sweden. Hari Sharma is a qualified Neuroanatomist and experimental neurpathologist trained in Germany, Switzerland, Sweden and in USA. His main research is currently focused on neurotoxicity of nanoparticle and nanowired drug delivery of agents for enhanced neuroprotection in a variety of CNS insults or neurodegenerative diseases in relation to the blood-brain barrier (BBB) function supported by European Aerospace Research and Development (EOARD), London, UK and US Air Force Research Laboratory, Wright Patterson Air Force Base, Dayton, Oh, USA. He is the recipient of Prestigious US TechConnect Global Innovation Award 2013 at the National Innovation Summit & Innovation Showcase, Washington DC May 12-16, 2013 on his work on Nanowired cerebrolysin in Neuropathic Pain. His contribution on the role of the BBB on brain edema development (1989-2011) was recognized by the Executive Council of Brain Edema Society for the 1$^{st}$ US Neurosurgeon Anthony Marmarou Award in Tokyo, Japan October 22-26, 2011. On his accomplishment on nanomedicine and nanoneurotoxicity he was decorated with Mahatma Gandhi Pravasi Gold Medal 2012 in the House of Lords, London UK. He is also the recipient of "Hind Rattan Award" (Jewel of India) by Govt. of India in 2012, New Delhi on the eve or republic day of India followed by "Navrattan Award" (Nine jewels of India) on Jan 25$^{th}$, 2013 and "Bharat Jyoti Award" (Glory fo India), New Delhi Jan 12, 2013. Some other key awards include "Certificate of Excellence" by US Food & Drug Administration (FDA) by National Centre for Toxicological Research (NCTR), Jefferson, AR, USA (2005); Distinguished International Scientists Collaboration Award (DISCA) of National Institute of Health (NIH) at National Institute on Drug Abuse (NIDA), Baltimore, MS, USA for the year 2006 and 2007; Rönnows Award for best medical researcher in Neuroanatomy, Faculty of Medicine, Uppsala University, (1996); and Hwassers Prize for the Best Thesis of the year in the Basic Medical Research from Faculty of Medicine, Uppsala University (1999). Hari Sharma is Founding President of the Global College of Neuroprotection & Neuroregeneration (2004-); current President of International Association of Neurorestoratology; and elected Senior Expert of Asia-Pacific CEO Association, Worldwide (APCEO) (2012-) for his contribution to uplift scientific research in many countries Globally that may have better economic and social benefit for the mankind. Dr

Sharma has published over 400 research papers, and edited 18 book volumes. He is the Editor-in-Chief of American Journal of Neuroproetction and Neuroregeneration, and the European Editor of Central Nervous system-Neurological Disorders Drug Target (2013-). Dr. Sharma is on board of various International Journals in *Neuroscience, Neuropharmacology and Nanotechnology* disciplines and is the designated Ambassador of the City of Uppsala, Sweden.

**ASSOCIATE EDITOR:**

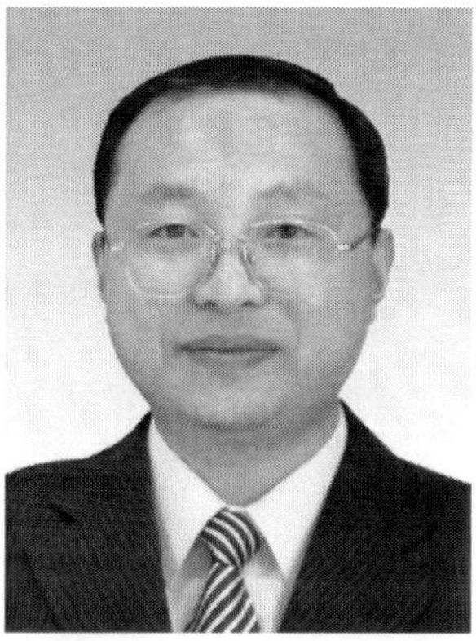

**Lin Chen, MD., Ph.D**

**Dr. Lin Chen, MD. & Ph.D.** Associate chief physician, Department of Neurosurgery, Tsinghua University Yuquan Hospital.

He serves as the Secretary-General of International Association of Neurorestoratology (IANR), Secretary-General of the Chinese Medical Association Professional Committee Neurorestoratology Committee, Deputy Director General of China Association of young Neurosurgery Peripheral Nerve Surgery Group of the First Committee, the member of China Rehabilitation Medicine professional Committee will spinal basic research study groups, the member of the China Rehabilitation Medicine professional Committee of nerve regeneration, editorial director of the journal of *Translational Neuroscience and Clinics*, the member of editorial board of *American Journal of Neuroprotection and Neuroregeneration*, the member of editorial board of *Journal of Neurorestoratology*.

He studied at Shandong Jining College of Medicine, Second Military Medical University of PLA, and Tsinghua University. Dr. Chen has nearly 20 years of clinical experience. In 1998 he began to study and work in the PLA Neurosurgery Center of PLA Navy General Hospital. Then he moved to Beijing Rehabilitation Hospital affiliated to Capital Medical University since 2006. In 2013, he started to work at the Second Affiliated Hospital of Tsinghua University (Yuquan Hospital).

In 1998, he first carried out the experimental study of subthalamic nucleus of stereotactic surgery for Parkinson's disease (PD). His earlier research included the α-Synuclein protein, amino acid γ- pathogenesis of PD and to explore the early diagnosis, magnetic resonance spectroscopy, clinical gene therapy, repetitive transcranial magnetic stimulation therapy, cell transplantation, nerve repair treatment. In 2001, he participated in the world's first clinic trial of olfactory ensheathing cell transplantation for complete spinal cord injured patients by Prof.

Hongyun Huang. Then he researched the long-term safety and effectiveness of cell-based treatment for a variety of intractable neurological diseases, and then, he participated in the creation of "neurorestoratology" new discipline and the establishment of the IANR leaded by Prof. Huang and improving discipline system.

So far, Dr. Chen has published 280 scientific articles and edited 11 academic monographs. Now he focus on the his research to neurorestorative and comprehensive treatments for spinal cord injury, early pediatric orthopedic repair of skull defects, restorative treatment of motor neuron disease, neuropathic pain, neurodegenerative diseases.

# Section 1: Neurorestoratology Overview

In: Neurorestoratology, volume 1
Editors: H. Huang, G. Raisman, P. R. Sanberg et al.
ISBN: 978-1-63463-599-8


*Chapter 1*

# Establishing Processes of Neurorestoratology

***Hongyun Huang[1,2,*], Paul R. Sanberg[3] and Lin Chen[4,5]***
[1]Beijing Rehabilitation Hospital of Capital Medical University, China
[2]Beijing Hongtianji Neuroscience Academy, China
[3]University of South Florida College of Medicine, US
[4]Tsinghua University Yuquan Hospital, Beijing, China
[5]Medical Center, Tsinghua University, Beijing, China

## 1. Background and Process of Establishing Neurorestoratology

Thousands of years ago (approx 2500 B.C.), spinal cord injuries were described as "crushed vertebra in his neck," as were symptoms of neurological deterioration without treatment, in the ancient Egyptian medical papyrus known as the Edwin Smith Surgical Papyrus, by the physician and architect of the Sakkara pyramids Imhotep (Anderberg L et al., 2007).

Nearly 90 years ago Ramon y Cajal stated with certainty: "Once the development was ended, the founts of growth and regeneration of the axons and dendrites dry up irrevocably. In the adult centers, the nerve paths are something fixed, ended, and immutable. Everything may die, nothing may be regenerated. It is for the science of the future to change, if possible, this harsh decree" (Cajal SRY., 1928).

However, it is the eternal desire for humans to prolong and improve their quality of life which, without doubt, should be the instinct and responsibility for physicians and neuroscientists to search for effective methods of neurorestoration. Obviously, it is inappropriate and overly pessimistic for physicians to always say that there is no way to help patients with the sequelae of diseases and damages in the central nervous system (CNS). So, although neuroregeneration and neurorestoration of CNS was thought to be almost impossible

* E-mail: hongyunh@gmail.com.

at that time and later on, scientists still tried to study the special mystery of human life through electrical stimulation (Aldini J., 1804; Sironi VA, 2011), transplanting brain tissues by Thompson in 1890 (Björklund A, 1991), nerve growth factor (NGF) administration (Levi-Montalcini R et al., 1951), gene therapy (Blomer U et al., 1996), and other means.

On the other hand, as depicted in Figure 1 (Huang H et al., 2010), physicians of traditional clinical disciplines have believed that the sequelae of stroke, CNS trauma, neurodegenerative diseases, and damage lack effective treatments. The majority of the medical community now still states: "Our knowledge of the pathophysiological processes, both the primary as well as the secondary, has increased tremendously. However all this knowledge has only led to improved medical care, but not to any therapeutic methods to restore, even partially, the neurological function" (Anderberg L et al., 2007). It means that there are no really effective interventions available for the restorative treatment of many CNS functional impairments and structural damages or their sequelae in the clinical practice of neurology, neurosurgery, neurorehabilitation, and all related clinical disciplines. We can see clearly that there is a question mark in Figure 1, which is similar to the original Dmitri Mendeleev periodic table where there are a number of blank boxes which remained to be filled later with newly–discovered elements. According to the inexorable law of neuroscientific and medical innovation, a new discipline (we propose the term "neurorestoratology" as this cross-disciplinary term) must arise to fill the question mark in Figure 1 in suitable time.

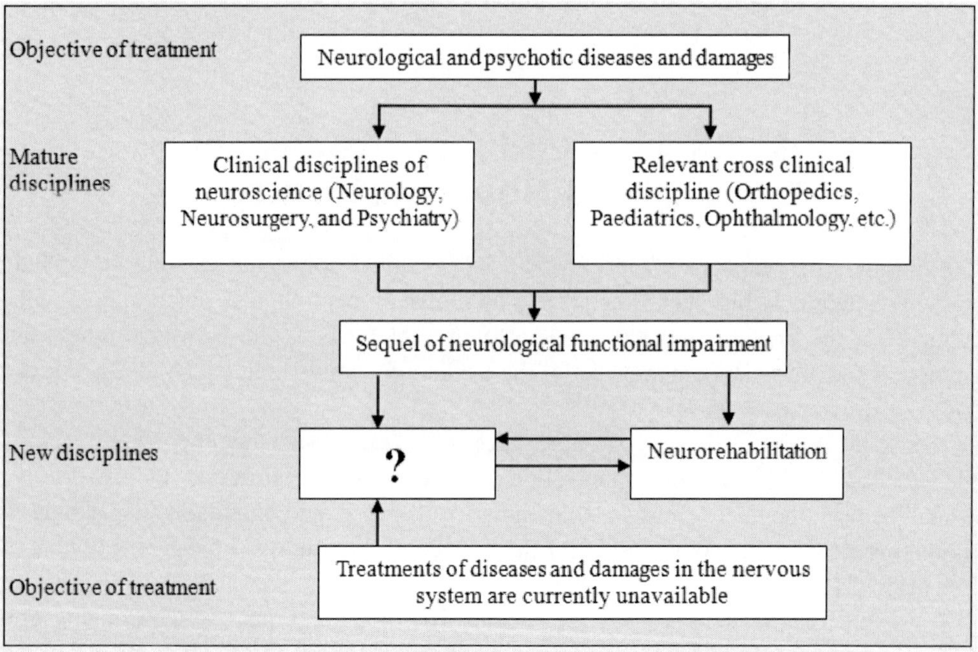


Modified from Cell Medicine 1(1), Huang H, Chen L, Sanberg P. Cell therapy from bench to bedside translation in CNS Neurorestoratology era. 15-46 (Figure 1), Copyright (2010), with permission from Cognizant Comm. Corp.

Figure1. Distribution of disease treated by clinical disciplines of neuroscience and relevant cross disciplines.

Over the past thirty years, evidence from basic research and/or from clinical application showed that diseases and damages in the CNS could be structurally and functionally restored by cell therapy, neuromodulation, medicine and bioengineering or tissue engineering strategies, especially over the last ten years (Huang H et al., 2010). It is important not to exaggerate its benefit. The far-reaching significance of these achievements is to start changing the traditional clinical misperception, that it is impossible to restore damaged CNS structures and functions. Many neurorestorative scientists and physicians are convinced that they are witnessing the birth of an important new discipline, neurorestoratology, for the treatment of CNS diseases and damages. Therefore, establishing neurorestoratology as a discipline, on the basis of CNS neurorestorable theory (Huang H et al., 2003), is necessary for the rapid development of this advanced realm, and the term "neurorestoratology" deserves to replace the question mark in Figure 1.

Neurorestoratology has been developing rapidly and has made great progress, especially in cell-based neurorestorative therapy, from bench to bedside. The most important pioneers listed below and also many others should be remembered forever, such as, Milan Dinitrijevic, Mark Tusznynski, Anders Björklund, Jeffrey Kordower, etc., as they dedicated themselves and made great contributions to neurorestoration or neurorestoratology.

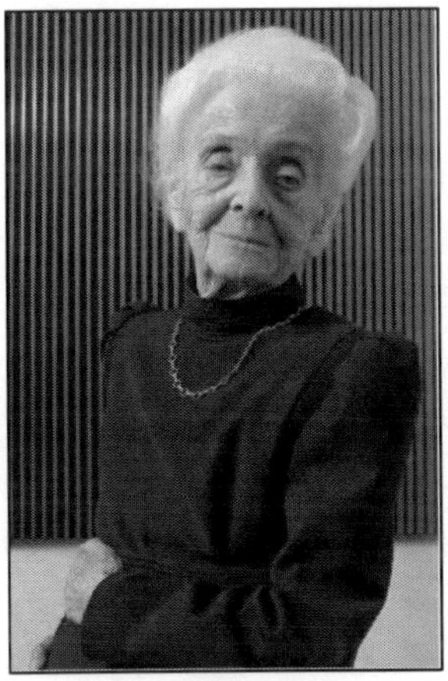

Rita Levi-Montalcini: the discoverer of nerve growth factor.

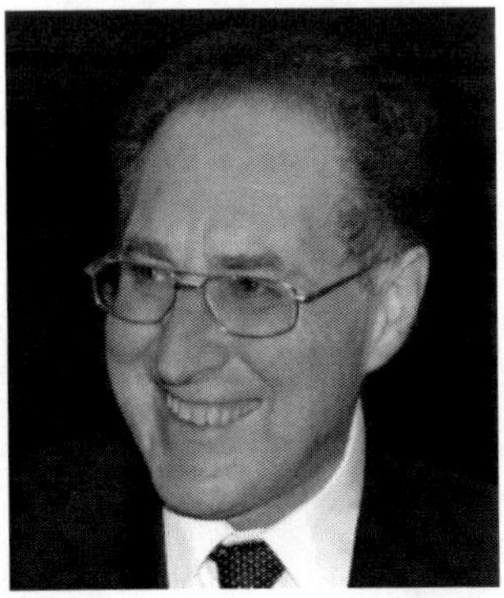

Geoffrey Raisman: the founder of neural plasticity theory in CNS and one of founders of Neurorestoratology.

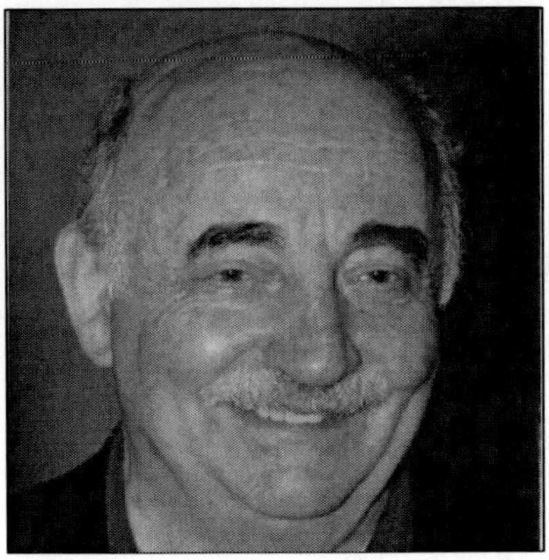

Albert Aguayo: the discoverer of neuroregeneration in CNS.

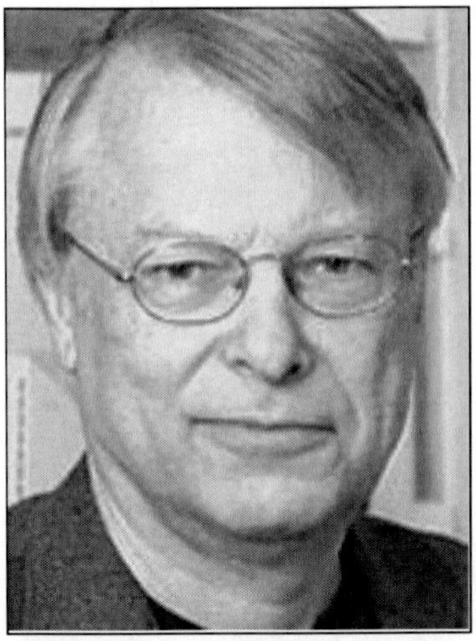

Lars Olson: the pioneer of clinical trial of nerve growth factor and neural tissue transplantation in CNS.

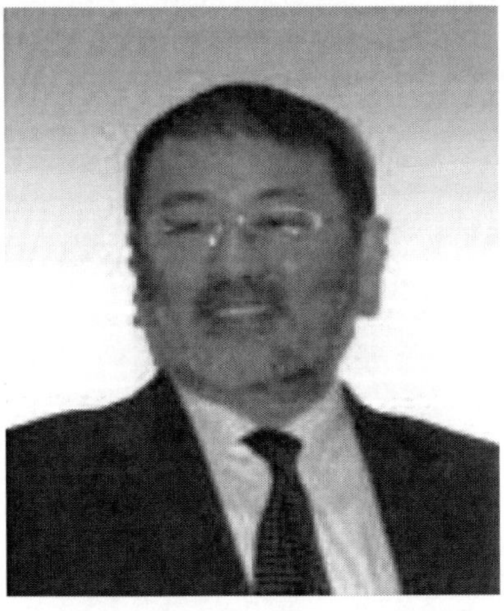

Wise Young: the pioneer of clinical neuroprotective drug treatment for spinal cord injury.

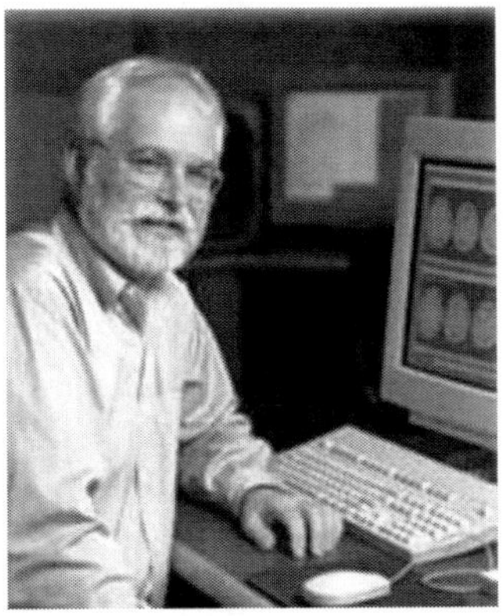

John Donoghue: the pioneer of clinical applying brain-computer interface.

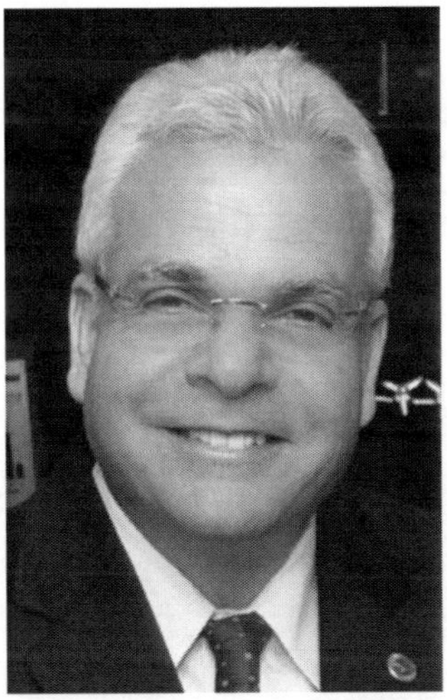

Paul R. Sanberg: the pioneer of cell-based medicine for neural repair and one of founders of Neurorestoratology.

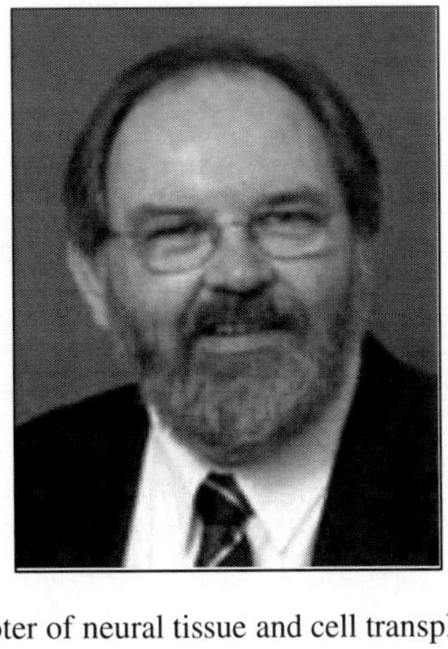

Stephen Dunnett: the active promoter of neural tissue and cell transplantation for neurorestoration.

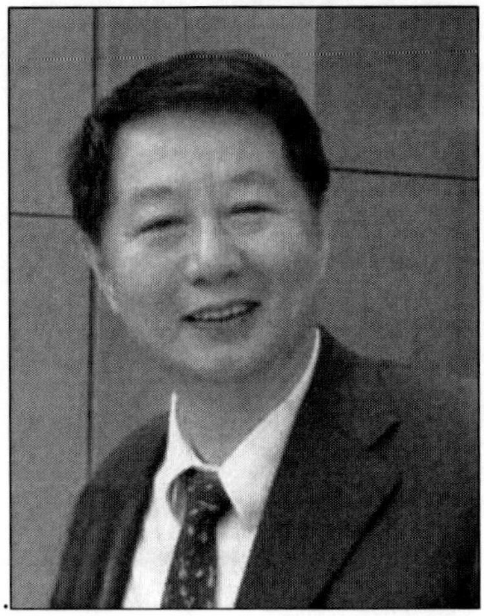

Hongyun Huang: the pioneer of clinical cell-based comprehensive neurorestorative strategies and the main founder of Neurorestoratology.

## 2. Evolution of the Name "Neurorestoratology"

Several scientific terms related to neurorestoration have been forwarded, such as restorative neurology, restorative neurosurgery, and neurorestorative surgery (Huang H et al., 2010). A description of their names and connotations is given below.

*Restorative Neurology.* Dimitrijevic put forward this term in 1985. It was defined as the branch of the neurological sciences that applied active procedures to improve the functioning of the impaired nervous system through selective structural and functional modification of abnormal neurocontrol according to underlying mechanisms and clinically unrecognized residual functions; its intervention strategies included neurostimulation, neuromodulation, and neurectomies (Dimitrijevic MR, 1985), cell transplants (Luque JM, 2004), and drugs (Liepert J, 2008).

*Restorative Neurosurgery.* This term was put forward by Liberson (Liberson WT, 1987). Then, restorative neurosurgery, as the frontier of neurosurgery, provided the potential to restore lost function. Intervention strategies include gene therapy, neurotrophic factors, and cell transplantation (Langmoen IA et al., 2003; Marquez YD et al., 2005; Richardson R M et al., 2009; Thompson TP et al.,1999), tissue engineering (Yamamoto M et al., 2009), and neurostimulation (Katayama Y, 2000; Taira T et al., 2003).

*Neural Repair.* Nicholls first introduced neural repair in 1987 (Nicholls JG, 1987).

*Neurorestorative Therapy or Surgery.* Intervention strategies include neural grafts and genic therapies (Fernández CI et al., 1995; Jiménez-Jiménez FJ, Molina JA, 1997) or pharmacotherapy (Zhang ZG et al., 2009) and electrostimulation (Taylor SM, 2008).

*Restorative Neuroscience.* Intervention strategies include cell transplantation, stimulation, and medicine (Andres RH et al., 2008).

*Neuroprosthetics.* This term developed from cochlear implant in 1957, then neural prosthesis through functional electrical stimulation in 1976 (Reswick JB, 1976) or neuroprosthesis through brain–computer interface to be controlled by "thought" (Muller-Putz GR et al., 2009).

Together, all of the medical terms mentioned above were not considered as distinct disciplines, but instead as branches or specific kinds of therapy of neurology, neurosurgery or some other discipline. More importantly, these branches or therapies share similar interventions that include cell and/or tissue transplantation, neurostimulation and/or neuromodulation, bioengineering and/or tissue-engineering, and drugs. Given that each is not sufficient by itself to represent the whole neurorestoration field, the term "neurorestoratology" was logically created and is more suitable for this discipline than any other term. It fully reflects the connotation of neurorestoration and this name can be more easily recognized as a discipline in parallel with neurology, neurosurgery and neurorehabilitation as a member of neuroscience or medicine.

In fact, neurorestoration is an integral part of many disciplines as shown in Figure 2, and is the natural meeting point for all. However, isolation in different disciplines had deprived scientists working in this arena of a common platform for scientific exchange until the independent discipline of Neurorestoratology was established (Huang H et al., 2012). From then on, Neurorestoratology has successfully provided a consolidated neurorestoration platform for effectively communicating to all basic scientists and clinicians (see Figure 3, Huang H et al., 2013). Meanwhile, the majority of these scientists continue to work in their original disciplines and some have become specialized physicians in Neurorestoratology.

# 3. Definition of Neurorestoratology

As a new discipline, the concept of neurorestoratology was clearly defined by *the Beijing Declaration of IANR,* which was adopted at the 2nd IANR Annual Conference in 2009 (IANR, 2009). The draft of the declaration was endorsed by 32 leading experts in neurorestoratology from 18 countries and regions.

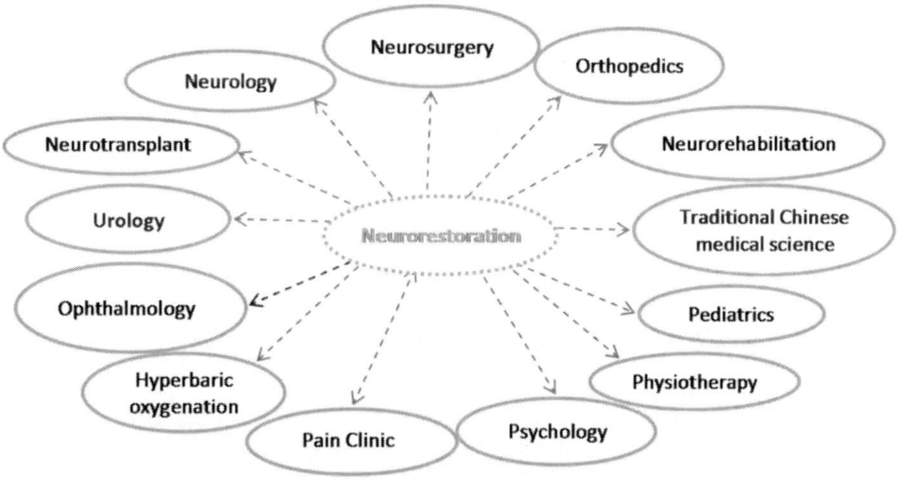


Modified from Cell Transplantation 21 Supplement 1, Hongyun Huang, Lin Chen and Paul R. Sanberg. Clinical Achievements, Obstacles, Falsehoods, and Future Directions of Cell-Based Neurorestoratology, S5 (Figure 2), Copyright (2012), with permission from Cognizant Comm. Corp.

Figure 2. Neurorestoration is the cross-point of all related disciplines.

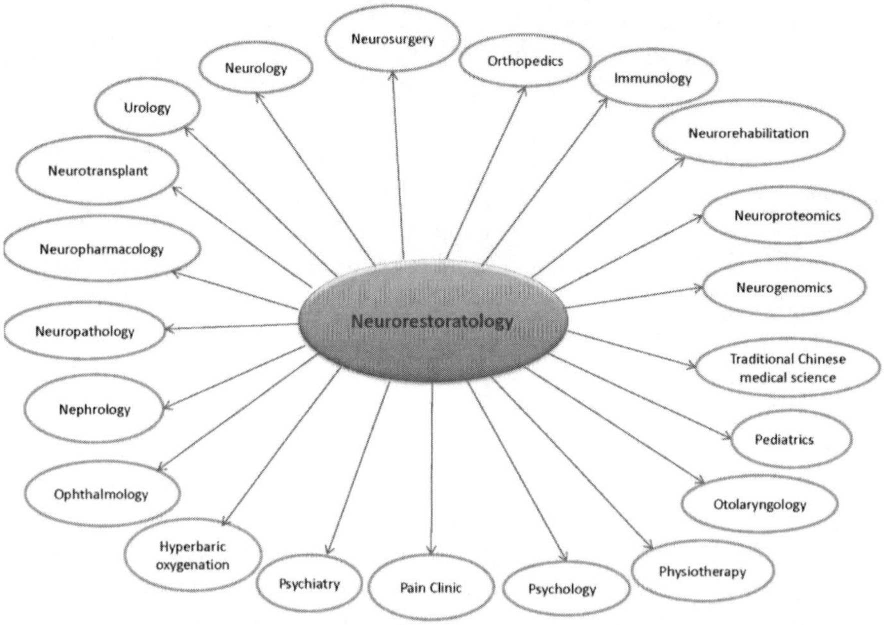


Modified from Cell Transplantation 21 Supplement 1, Hongyun Huang, Lin Chen and Paul R. Sanberg. Clinical Achievements, Obstacles, Falsehoods, and Future Directions of Cell-Based Neurorestoratology, S5 (Figure 3), Copyright (2012), with permission from Cognizant Comm. Corp.

Figure 3. Neurorestoratology provides a core platform and bridge for related disciplines with neurorestoration.

Neurorestoratology is a new and distinct discipline of medicine or the sub-discipline of neuroscience (Huang H et al., 2008; Chen L et al., 2009; IANR, 2009).

Neurorestoratology is the discipline that studies neural regeneration, repair and replacement of damaged components of the nervous system, neuroplasticity, neuroprotection, neuromodulation, neurogenesis, angiogenesis, immunomodulation and their mechanisms to cause improvement or recovery.

The goal of neurorestoratology is partially or completely to restore or maintain integrity of neurological functions and/or structures by neurorestorative strategies in humans, as far as possible; that is, to ensure that patients obtain increasing benefits through enhanced translation between basic research and clinical application. Current cell-based combination or comprehensive therapeutic strategies in neurorestoratology highlight the view of translational medicine (Huang H et al., 2010) and the principle of the Declaration of Helsinki, such as: "In the treatment of a patient, where proven prophylactic, diagnostic and therapeutic methods do not exist or have been ineffective, the physician, with informed consent from the patient, must be free to use unproven or new prophylactic, diagnostic and therapeutic measures, if in the physician's judgment it offers hope of saving life, re–establishing health or alleviating suffering. Where possible, these measures should be made the object of research, designed to evaluate their safety and efficacy.

In all cases, new information should be recorded and, where appropriate, published" (WMA General Assembly, http://www.wma.net/en/30publications/10policies/b3/ index. html).

Innovative intervention strategies of neurorestoratology include cell or tissue transplantation, tissue engineering or bioengineering, neuromodulation by electro-magnetic stimulation, pharmaceutical or chemical therapies, traditional neurorehabilitation, neurorestorative surgery (cordotomy or myelotomy and neurotisation or nerve bridging), and psychological methods, as well as all the necessary means (IANR, 2009). All of those neurorestorative methods are scattered in different disciplines, neurorestoratology integrates them together, into comprehensive therapeutic strategies.

The scope of study and treatment in neurorestoratology includes neurotrauma, neurodegeneration, cerebrovascular anoxia or ischemia, edema, demyelination, sensory and motor disorders, and neuropathic pain, as well as neural damage resulting from toxic physical and chemical factors, immune, infectious, inflammatory, hereditary, congenital, developmental, and other neural injuries (IANR, 2009).

# 4. Theory Basis or Mechanisms of Neurorestoratology in CNS

CNS neurorestorative theory was proposed by Huang et al., based on clinical achievements obtained from cell-based neurorestorative therapy (Huang H et al., 2003), which is the underlying basis of neurorestoratology. The theory also relies on basic research findings (below) which are mechanisms of neurorestoration. Liu found that intraspinal sprouting of dorsal root axons in cats (Liu CN; Chambers WW, 1958). Bechtereva found the relationship between certain forms of potentials and the variations in brain excitability (Bechtereva NP;Zontov VV, 1962). Raisman found neuronal plasticity in the septal nuclei of the adult rat (Raisman G, 1969). David reported that, when peripheral nerve segments were used as “bridges” between the medulla and spinal cord, axons from neurons at both these levels grew approximately 30 millimeters (David S, 1981). The regenerative potential of these central neurons seems to be expressed when the CNS glial environment is changed to that of the peripheral nervous system. Bornstein reported remyelination in CNS tissue (Bornstein MB;Raine CS, 1969), Altman found autoradiographic and histological evidence of postnatal hippocampal neurogenesis in rats (Altman J;Das GD, 1965). Young reported the beneficial effects or neuroprotection of high-dose corticosteroid treatment on both functional recovery and histopathological appearance of injured spinal cords (Young W;Flamm ES, 1982). Later, it was found that axonal sprouting, signal modulation, immunomodulation, neuronal plasticity, axonal remyelination and neurogenesis were mechanisms of CNS ability to achieve functional neurological restoration following damage (Bechtereva NP et al., 1975; Bendel O et al., 2005; Croll RP et al., 1990; Honmou O et al., 1996; Naftchi NE, 1982; Palladini G et al., 1996).

# 5. Characteristics of Neurorestoratology

There are a great many of mysteries in the brain still. The American “Brain Project (the BRAIN Initiative, http://blogs) and European “Human Brain Project” (D'Angelo E, 2012) were initiated to improve understanding of CNS function. However, the direction and principal aims of these two enormous projects remain unclear. While these two projects may focus on a technological understanding of brain function, essentially, they plan do what neurorestoratology has already been doing. However, there are five key characteristics or advantages of neurorestoratology over the U.S. Brain Project and European Human Brain Project.

First, neurorestoratology has a foundation of CNS neurorestorable theory as its guideline.

Second, neurorestoratology has clear goals and directions. As we know, any kind of damage or loss of neuronal function has a pathological basis, either at the gross microscopic level or gene and molecular levels, as well as at the electrophysiological levels. Theoretically, neurorestorative methods could be found for those pathological lesions; practically, some neurorestorative methods have already been able to restore those pathological lesions to some extent. Thus, the best way to restore or promote the recovery of damaged or lost neuronal function is by using neurorestorative approaches in an orderly manner in each phase, as shown by the neurorestorative roadmap in Figure 4 (Huang H et al., 2013). (See detailed explanation in part 10 of this chapter “Developing phases and directions of Neurorestoratology”.)

Third, there is a clear schematic diagram for implementing neurorestoration as shown in Figure 5 (Huang H et al., 2013). Accordingly, more functional recovery will result from new strategies than from current neurorestorative approaches. New strategies can further be explained by new mechanisms of current neurorestorative principles. Moreover, as any new neurorestorative strategy or mechanism that promotes functional recovery or offers a new explanation for functional recovery is introduced to meet the current need and enrich the current store of neurorestorative knowledge, the community of neurorestoratology actively encourages and favors such efforts to discover effective novel therapeutic strategies and their initial clinical pioneering results.

Fourth, more emphasis on translational medicine is needed to encourage and translate any new methods that promote patients’ neurorestorative effects in the shortest time; simultaneously any key clinical problems should be explored further by new research projects at the experimental level. Thus, a virtuous circle of bench and bedside would optimize the wisdom of physician and scientist through making full use of available scientific, social, economic, and government resources.

Finally, neurorestoratology is a discipline that aims to prolong or improve human health and quality of life – an eternal desire of clinicians and their patients that greatly need to be fulfilled. We firmly believe that the ongoing improvement of the neurorestorative ability should be a permanent process toward better human health care. Thus will neurorestoratology coexist with human beings forever (Huang H et al., 2013).

# 6. Structural Basis and Limitation of Neurorestoration

Even though CNS neurorestoration is valid according to the CNS neurorestorable theory, the potential ability for structural repair is quite limited and the improved functions are easy to lose. The reasons are:

1) There are ten billion neurons in the human brain. As soon as its damages cause functional impairment, it is hard to restore the whole lesion structure. It may only restore part of it.
2) Young children learn to walk through large numerous practices even if their CNS structure is normal. Even after CNS damage can be partially repaired, reconstruction requires it learning again how to work.
3) Generally, if a rat maintains 10% of its spinal cord structure, the animal still can stand up. Less than this and the animal will lose its ability to stand up. Conversely, reconstruction is only one aspect; reserve must also be conserved. So, restored functions by neurorestorative treatment need to be maintained by sustained exercise or neurorehabilitation throughout life, if patients want to have better quality of life.

# 7. Obstacles Met in the Development of Neurorestoratology

Even though cell-based comprehensive neurorestorative strategies have been developing rapidly around world, they have met and faced many obstacles in the past. These obstacles still exist and will continue to exist in the future. A great deal of promising neurorestorative strategies are often difficult to translate from the bench to the bedside. In the last 20 years, more than a thousand basic research papers have been published, demonstrating some degree of functional neurorestoration for CNS impairments in animal models, case studies and small clinical trials.

Simultaneously, thousands of review papers about these therapies, which were forecasted to be promising in the clinic, have been published, but most practical applications of these therapies existed only in these papers at that time (Huang H et al., 2012).

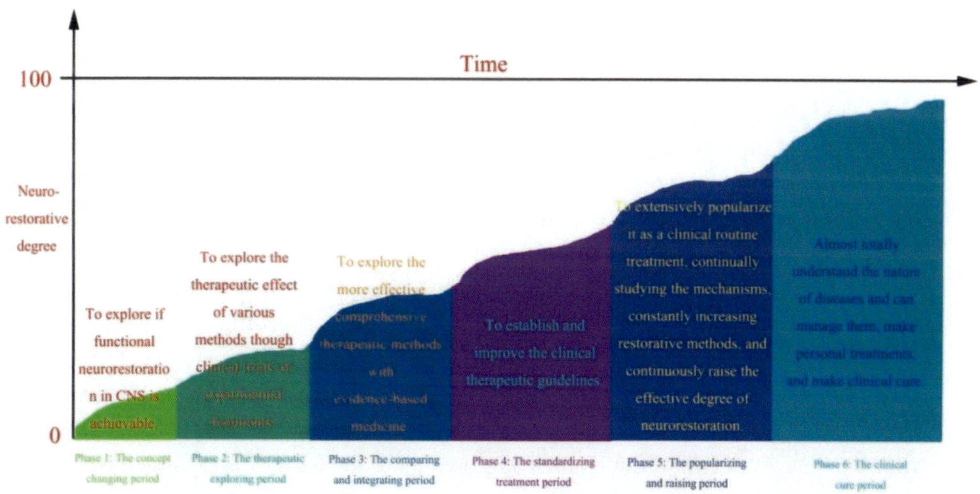


Reprinted from Journal of Neurorestoratology 1, Hongyun Huang, Hari Shanker Sharma. Neurorestoratology: one of the most promising new disciplines at the forefront of neuroscience and medicine, 39 (Figure 3), Copyright (2013), with permission from Dove Medical Press Limited.

Figure 4. Neurorestorative roadmap in central nervous system.

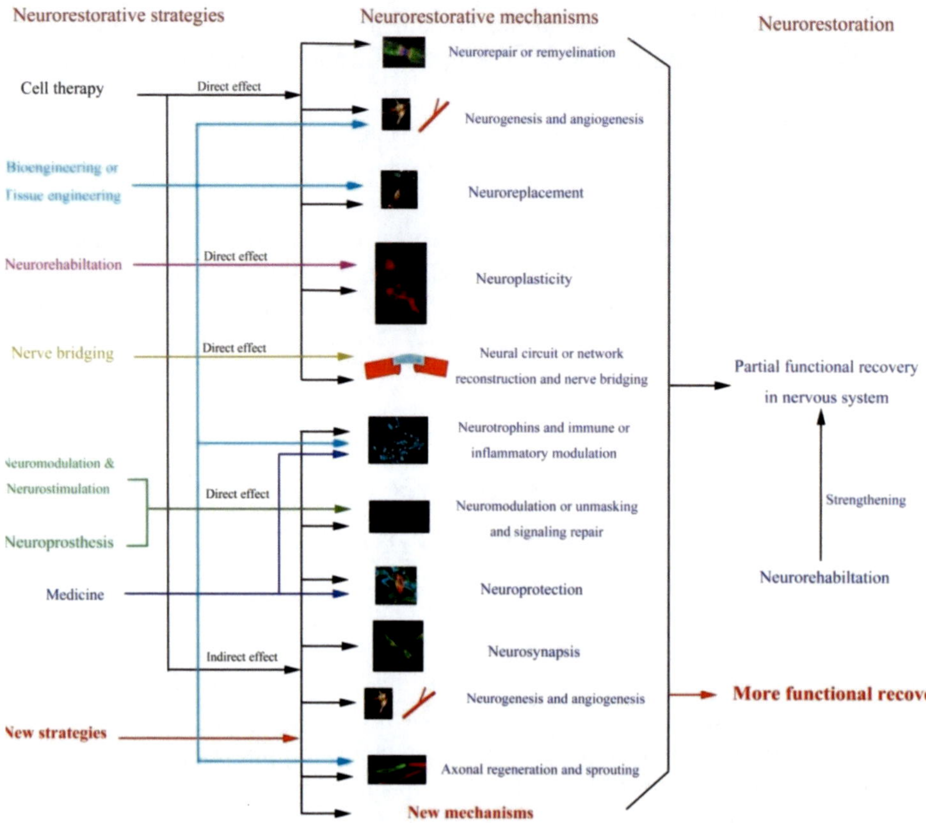


Reprinted from Journal of Neurorestoratology 1, Hongyun Huang, Hari Shanker Sharma. Neurorestoratology: one of the most promising new disciplines at the forefront of neuroscience and medicine, 39 (Figure 4), Copyright (2013), with permission from Dove Medical Press Limited.

Figure 5. Neurorestorative schematic diagram for implementation.

What are the obstacles that hinder the translation of neurorestorative strategies?

1. *Politics:* laws or governmental regulatory rules, or politicians' viewpoints: all can greatly affect the developing direction of this field. The best example of this occurred in the United States, where President George W. Bush and his successor, President Barack Obama, have different opinions about cell therapy, especially embryonic stem cell research. The cell-based comprehensive neurorestorative strategies in the U.S. could have a different fate between the two presidents. While President Bush supported laws and governmental rules to limit embryonic stem cell research, President Obama has re-addressed these limitations. Obviously the direction or developing speed of cell-based comprehensive neurorestorative strategies in the U.S. has been influenced by those laws or governmental rules (Sanberg P, 2005).
2. *Religion:* we understand that some religions reject the idea of allowing abortions. But no matter whether people are willing or not, abortions (or, rather, miscarriages) can spontaneously occur. The core issue is whether humans should use the aborted or miscarried tissue, especially when people know that the tissue could potentially help others to improve their function and quality of life. Regardless of religious beliefs,

logically, many individuals' answer to the question of using the tissue, once it becomes available, is positive, rather than discarding the tissue (Sanberg P, 1990).

3. *Ethics:* this is very complicated issue. It is currently believed that new clinical trials or experimental treatments should not start until they have been approved by a scientific and ethics committee (Borlongan CV et al., 2010). When donating, patients (or their representatives) should sign a consent document which informs them of potential benefits and risks. These are the core ethical issues to which attention should be paid. Unfortunately, some confuse political, legal, or religious issues with ethical issues. The most extreme view would be that aborted or miscarried tissue should be rejected outright for ethical reasons. According to this view, it doesn't matter whether the tissue is discarded, it could be argued that it is ethical to use the tissue, since the potential exists to help restore functions to other patients or improve their quality of life, an opinion shared by many. Once an abortion or miscarriage has occurred, the tissue is no longer viable to develop into an embryo.
4. *Economy:* while money is not everything, without financial support the study of cell-based comprehensive neurorestorative strategies cannot be carried out. Fortunately, attention is now being paid and support is being received from the governments of developed countries and rapidly developing countries, charitable organizations, and personal philanthropy.
5. *Scientific factors:* some scientists or physicians reject translation of some promising methods because they state that those methods are still immature. In fact, clinical practice is the primary way to check whether those methods are going to be effective or not for patients (Huang H et al., 2012).

# 8. Falsehoods of Recognition for Neurorestoratology

Neurorestoratology is a very new discipline, so it is not surprising that there are misconceptions about it. Three misconceptions or falsehoods are summarized below.

1) One side, hoping for an immediate cure. Patients who suffer severe spinal cord injury, traumatic brain injury, and progressive CNS degenerative disorders can come to believe that they are going to be cured almost immediately because of exaggerations by some companies or the media that purposely overstate that stem cells can easily and very soon solve all problems. Patients with devastating illnesses who have dreamed of a cure naturally tend to accept the higher expectation. These unrealistic hopes for a cure have driven people away from real world medical treatment and made them neglect functional recoveries already available with current neurorestorative strategies. Each specialist in this field knows that any progress may not be implemented easily but a little improvement is better than none, because small recoveries may be extremely important for a patient's survival and health. Another side is too pessimistic, that is, there are currently no known therapeutic methods to restore, even partially, neurological function (Anderberg L et al., 2007). To

counteract those misconceptions, we should inform patients with CNS lesions to value highly practical neurorestoration, which can be obtained today.

2) Paying too much attention to structural neuroregeneration or neuroreplacement which sometimes is one of the neurorestorative mechanisms. People should beware that overemphasizing neuroregeneration may lead in a less effective direction. There are many alternative mechanisms for functional neurorestoration (as listed above), especially signal modulation or plasticity, some of which may be mechanisms of currently achievable neurorestoration. Many people misunderstand and believe that neuroregeneration will bring neurological functional recovery or be equal to functional recovery, when in fact, neurorestoration means neurological functional recovery. It is more accurate to elucidate and express the real implications of functional recovery than neuroregeneration.
3) Believing that randomizing double-blind control studies are the only assessment method for a top clinical study and that self-comparison cannot be used as an assessment method for such studies. Recently, Rama's clinical study paper with a self-comparison design was published in the *New England Journal of Medicine* (Rama P et al., 2010). Self-comparison is sometimes a better option for some special clinical conditions. Its value is fully recognized and accepted for clinical studies of some incurable diseases, such as heart, kidney, liver, and cornea transplant, and lesions that require surgical intervention (Huang H, 2010). Inclusion of a sham operation may be ethically questionable, as it inflicts unnecessary harm on the controls (Huang H et al., 2012).

# 9. The Principle of Cell-Based Comprehensive Neurorestorative Strategies

Over 30 different types of cells have been studied in neurorestoratology, among them olfactory ensheathing cells, umbilical cord stromal cells, umbilical cord blood mononuclear cells, Schwann cells, neural stem/progenitor cells, and bone marrow mononuclear cells or stromal cells, encompassing some thousands of patients. Despite their diversity in number, clinical status of subjects, route of cell administration (cells can be transplanted into the parenchyma of the brain or spinal cord, the ventricle or subarachnoid space, or blood vessels), and criteria to evaluate efficacy, from the cellular biology viewpoint several unanswered questions for cell transplantation remain: what kind of cells would be the best source, what is the best therapeutic time window, what is the most suitable selection for patient and disease, and what are the optimal route and dose. Importantly, the main conclusion drawn from these clinical studies is that such therapies are safe, feasible, and have some neurological functional improvement or restoration along with an improvement in the quality of life to a varying extent for human CNS lesions (single-cell therapy including varying cells or single strategy was proposed as the first generation of the neurorestoratology regime) (Huang H et al., 2012).

The second generation of the neurorestoratology regime (ABFMMC) should be recommended now and in the future as the principle of cell-based comprehensive neurorestoration, which includes appropriate time for intervention, best cellular combination, full cellular dosage, multiple route cell implantation, multiple process and the optimizing combination with the most appropriate nerve stimulation, neurorehabilitation (for example, Active movement-target enhancement- neurorehabilitation therapy (AMTENT)) and drugs, according to the personal medical status of each patient. Development of the second generation neurorestoratology regime relies on the exploration of vast basic and clinical translation studies and its more evidence-based medicine should be obtained by multicenter collaborating studies around the world.

# 10. Developing Phases and Directions of Neurorestoratology

*Hongyun Huang and Lin Chen*

The future progression of neurorestoratology may embrace six different phases.

Phase 1: the concept changing period has concluded, the aim of which was to explore if neurorestoration was achievable or CNS neurorestorable theory was correct and feasible.

Phase 2: the therapeutic exploring period is in progress, in which the goal is to explore the therapeutic effect of various methods though clinical trials or experimental treatments.

Phase 3: the comparing and integrating period is ready to begin, in which the objective is to explore the more effective comprehensive therapeutic methods with evidence-based medicine.

Phase 4: it is to be hoped that the standardizing treatment period will not be too far into the future, with the goal of establishing and improving clinical therapeutic guidelines.

Phase 5: the popularizing period is likely to be a very long future process, with the objective of extensively popularizing neurorestoratology as a routine clinical treatment, continually studying the mechanisms, constantly increasing restorative methods and continuously raising the effective degree of neurorestoration.

Phase 6: the clinical cure period may possibly come true in the far future, in which physicians will totally understand the nature of diseases and can manage them, make personal treatments and effect clinical cure.

According to the above developing phases, directions or tasks for neurorestoratology should be the following now and in the near future.

1) Compare and integrate available neurorestorative methods to look for the optimizational regimes by multicenter collaborating studies throughout the world, and edit and publish clinical therapeutic standards or guidelines of neurorestoratology.
2) Combine neurorestoratology with active movement-target enhancement neurorehabilitation to optimize functional recovery.
3) Push for more physicians, medicinal centers, and countries globally to raise neurorestorative effects.
4) Rapidly translate the potential methods that have been demonstrated in basic research into clinical trials and application under appropriate guidelines.
5) Actively explore new advanced methods and their mechanism of action.

At this very early stage of neurorestoratology, its development and maturation will rely on wisdom, patience and strenuous efforts of scientists and clinical physicians in neurorestoratology, who dedicate themselves to its success (Huang H et al., 2012).

# 11. Hypothesis in Discipline of Neurorestoratology

In the process of changing traditional thinking, the development of the discipline of neurorestoratology is undergoing a continuous distillation from practice to theory and from theory to further practice and more progress. The formation of new terms and phrases is a theoretical qualitative leap, which will greatly promote advancing the discipline.

In recent years, a large amount of basic research, especially clinical translation practice has rapidly and greatly enriched and updated our understanding of neurorestoratology, and constantly promoted the in-depth development of these disciplines. Based on our own research, and extensive references and relevant literature, we put forward some new theories and principles of the new terminology, and new hypothesis inference, which require further testing and verification.

*The clinical classification of neurorestoratology:* general neurorestoratology, pediatric neurorestoratology, gerontoneurorestoratology/geriatric neurorestoratology, traumatic neurorestoratology, pain neurorestoratology, psycho-neurorestoratology, epilepsy neuro-restoratology, stroke neurorestoratology, etc.

*Epilepsy Neurorestoratology:* A new regime for some types of intractable epilepsy, i.e., temporal lobe epilepsy and immune-mediated epilepsies. The candidates for clinical therapeutic agents include neural stem / progenitor cells, mononuclear bone marrow cells, interneuronal precursors, etc. The known mechanisms of anti-seizure effect following cell transplantation include immune-modulating, neural repair for structures and circuits, and neuroprotection.

*Pain Neurorestoratology (PN):* A crucial branch of neurorestoratology is how to intervene in pain, especially refractory neuropathic pain, under the new theories and methods of neurorestorative therapy.

The fundamental principles of PN are to promote nerve repair, immune regulation, improve microcirculation, and modulate neurotransmission. PN treatment is not completely identical to etiological treatment. PN is more active on the treatment of ideas, which is not equal to the straightforward anatomical structure repair, but emphasizes neural painless remodeling and benign neural net plasticity. PN treatment is etiological treatment plus benign neural network plasticity.

*Psycho-Neurorestoratology:* also known as psychorestoratology, this is an emerging branch of neurorestoratology to study neural repair intervention in a variety of mental illnesses including organic mental disorders (Alzheimer's disease, mental disorders attributed to cerebral vascular disease, and mental disorders due to other brain disorders) and mental retardation, autism, schizophrenia, and obsessive-compulsive disorder. Current research evidence strongly suggests that mental illnesses have a pathological and/or pathophysiological basis, e.g., abnormalities of neuronal circuits, internal environment neurotransmitters, and neuroimmune function.

The main potential intervention strategies of psycho-neurorestoratology include cytotherapy (olfactory ensheathing cells, umbilical cord stromal cells, bone marrow stromal cells, peripheral blood stromal cells, and neural stem/progenitor cells), nerve stimulation, or nerve modulation. The latest clinical data show the positive effect of neurorestoration in selected organic mental disorders, autism, and obsessive-compulsive disorder, which comprehensively upgrades the thinking of traditional mental illness treatment.

## 12. Hypothesis in Strategies of Neurorestoratology

***Hongyun Huang and Lin Chen***

*Key point for neural network restoration:* Diseases of the CNS, such as cerebral palsy, amyotrophic lateral sclerosis, ataxia, multiple sclerosis, dementia, and epilepsy, although varied in etiology and pathologic findings, ultimately effect similar elements in the brain such as neurons and nerve fibers of the cerebral cortex, spinal cord, cerebellum, pons, brain stem nuclei, red nucleus, substantia nigra, and basal ganglia.

An anatomic structure, located at anterior 1/4–1/3 of ateral ventricle and 23–27 mm away from the midline, is where the frontal corona radiata pyramidal tract passes through, and represents a point at which numerous projection fibers, association fibers, and commissural fibers converge, which is presumed be a key point among these elements where cell grafts should be delivered for cell-based therapy. Clinical practice has shown that, after being transplanted into this important "point" in the brain, the cells will initiate an extensive bidirectional remodeling in the entire neural network, including cerebrum, cerebellum, and spinal cord. Therefore, the key point of cell transplantation should be of great importance in approaching functional neurorestoration.

*Theory of qualitative critical point for neurorestoration:* the neurorestorative process is to follow the law of quantitative to qualitative changes and the neurorestorative curve or trajectory to its critical point. From lying down, sitting, standing and finally moving, many critical points are involved in the neurorestorative process. That means long, arduous and unremitting accumulation of exercise every day, never giving up faith. Every uninterrupted quantitative change, from the meager to the many, once accumulated to a critical point, will complete a qualitative leap.

Like eating, to the one hundredth meal, the previous ninety-nine represent a cumulative process. The hundredth mouth is a qualitative change, and therefore we cannot ignore the value of each, as we should cherish every small progress.

*Theory of river dredging:* neurorestoration is like river repair. The river will not recover until both the main obstruction point and sediment deposition and aquatic plants upstream and downstream are dredged together with adding water. Only in this way, can the entire river eventually recover some or all of its current.

In accordance with the "river theory," the longer the river, the more difficult the repair. A human is much longer than a mouse, so it is probably more difficult to repair their nerves, even without the species' differences.

*Principle of mutual foundation between neurorestoration and conventional therapy:* To greatly enhance neurological rehabilitation and symptomatic treatment, neurorestoration is the only way to bring about a curative effect. As with peripheral muscle and joint movement, which in turn also affect nerve remodeling, neurorestoration must be closely integrated with the highest level of neurorehabilitation and symptomatic treatment (e.g., anticonvulsant drug injection).

This will reduce long-term abnormal joint movement in these patients to achieve the best functional improvement. This is particularly important for cerebral palsy. Because these patients' brains, from an early age, do not have a normal neurological control loop, rehabilitation training for normal movement should be done under the neurorestorative premise.

*Principle of the same goal or conclusion from different approaches in treatment of nervous system illness*: many neurological diseases have a varied onset, but in the end undermine the same thing (all rivers run into the sea). So many treatments are the same or similar; their mechanism of action also includes protection, regeneration, repair, replacement, activation, changes in the microenvironment, immune regulation, and other aspects.

*Principle of cells used as medicine:* One of the main mechanisms of cell transplantation is the release of factors to change the microenvironment. Due to the number of cells implanted, these will gradually decrease after a certain time and the neurorestorative effect will also gradually weaken. As with using a drug, cell transplantation may be required to be repeated at regular intervals.

*Theory of stream of vehicles obstruction:* a small blocking node is likely to seriously affect all traffic, while the dredge is a huge time-consumer.

*Principle of golden two hours to use cells from lab to clinic:* cell products from collection to implantation in the patient's body should not exceed two hours. After this time cell survival and functional status decline rapidly. Significant work should continue on extending this time period through cryopreservation and other methods.

*The goal of treatment of spinal cord injury patients with neurorestoration three steps (three-step ladder) program:* let the people lying down, sit up; let the people sitting, stand up; let the people standing up, walk. Besides neurorestoration, guidance for the treatment of patients, with clear direction, will improve clinical outcomes.

*Active movement-target enhancement-neurorehabilitation therapy (AMTENT):* a neurorehabilitative therapy to improve paralyzed limb dysfunction through intensive training therapy following preset goals based on neurorestoration. For example, for patients with spinal cord injury, the treatment goal of a three-step ladder is set, which enables the patient to first sit up, then stand up, then re-walk. For patients with involvement of lower cervical, thoracic, and lumbar areas, injury-intensive standing up training is required to recover standing and walking functions, with a support and/or brace that is as short as possible. For stroke patients, enforcement of intensive training and use of impaired limbs are required, frequently by limiting movement of the contralateral limb, to improve motor function for activities of daily living.

Repeated short-term training can be focused to strengthen limbs, routinely 120-240 minutes per day, 5-7 days per week, for 8-12 consecutive weeks. Subsequently, the load of training is adjusted according to first-stage efficacy. AMTENT develops individual training programs by selecting different plastic tasks which highlight daily living actions. Behavioral training methods of shaping technique with preset action or behavior objectives can be achieved through efforts of the patient.

*Painless active movement-target enhancement-neurorehabilitation therapy (PAMTENT):* a more advanced concept of rehabilitation medicine that adds the new idea of “pain-free rehabilitation treatment” into the strategy of AMTENT. PAMTENT emphasizes close monitoring during the procedure of AMTENT for management of pain stress response. The regime requires the control of the pain within the limitation of pain-free during active rehabilitation training, which includes comprehensive treatments for prevention of pain, real-time pain control, and early pain relief.

Its fundamental goal is to maximize improvement of patient utility function, but without possible joint and muscle injury caused by AMTENT.

# 13. Hypothesis in Mechanisms of Neurorestoratology

*Hongyun Huang and Lin Chen*

*Hypothesis of the sensation promoting movement:* the nervous system through sensory afferent perceives existence and the central issue of a movement signal continues to strengthen, correcting and curing. Therefore, exercise without effective sensory stimulation will limit incoming motor nerve remodeling which does not conform to the natural process of learning in the nerve.

Because sense determines the direction of nerve regeneration, we should strengthen sensory stimulation after cell implantation. It should be emphasized that patients have a sufficient amount of sensory stimulation in order to facilitate correct motor nerve regeneration. Thus, exercise alone is not enough.

*Hypothesis of local neural network node activation:* the cells after parenchymal transplantation activate a local neural network node, reverse the direction of polarization, and inhibit the epileptic discharge process.

*Principle of remodeling following activation:* after adequate or multiple cellular transplantations, drugs, and electromagnetic stimulation, correct and fully functional training must be continued to achieve neural remodeling, otherwise “good” cells around the “bad” environment are likely to be assimilated.

*Nerve hibernation:* for nervous tissue suffering from trauma or other pathological damage, some of its neurons or nerve fiber pathways are in a quiescent or dormant state of low metabolism, functionality, conductivity and vigor state, which is similar to an animal’s hibernation.

Nerve hibernation is not death and disappearance, as cells and nerve fibers are morphologically integral; due to lack of energy or harmful factors acting in an inhibitory state in the acute phase, they cannot exercise their original normal function. If there is a suitable environment, such as an activation factor, directly or indirectly, to stimulate them, they can restore a functional condition.

This is one of the physiological bases of neural plasticity, neural modulation and nerve repair. Compare this with the so-called ischemic penumbra, i.e., the concept of "sleep" or "semi-sleep" in the super-acute or acute phase of stroke: nerve hibernation is a state of nerve disease in a chronic or sub-acute period. This state of normal neural structure backup belongs to the generalized neural hibernate category, that is, the process of neural development in the hibernating nerve.

*Principle of both inside and outside neural repair:* this important part refers to brain and spinal cord cellular repair treatment that should be done based on the comprehensive implementation of the disposal principle, i.e., both parenchymal and extraparenchymal transplantation. Emphasize the direct local implantation of cells in brain and spinal cord with the peripheral blood and cerebrospinal fluid, thereby combining the overall mobilization of systemic factors and focus on activation of local factors to reach the best therapeutic effect.

In summary, under the efforts of several generations of pioneers, Neurorestoratology has been set up and become one of the most important disciplines in medicine, and the neurorestorative door has been opened. Now we clearly know our final target and its direction; what we should do now is to explore the road reaching our destination, that is, to find the best strategies which help patients get the optimal benefits in each step.

## Note

This chapter was primarily written by Huang and Chen.

## References

Aldini, J. Essai théoriqueet expérimental sur le galvanisme, avec une série d'expériences faites devant des commissaires del'Institut nationale de France, et en divers amphithéâtres anatomiques de Londres. *Paris:Fournier Fils*;1804.

Altman, J; Das, GD. Autoradiographic and histological evidence of postnatal hippocampal neurogenesis in rats. *J. Comp. Neurol.* 1965;124:319-335.

Anderberg, L; Aldskogius, H; Holtz, A. Spinal cord injury–scientific challenges for the unknown future. *Ups. J. Med. Sci.* 2007;112(3):259-288.

Andres, RH; Meyer, M; Ducray, AD; Widmer, HR. Restorative neuroscience: Concepts and perspectives. *Swiss Med. Wkly.* 2008;138(11–12):155-172.

Bechtereva, NP; Bondartchuk, AN; Smirnov, VM; Meliutcheva, LA; Shandurina, A. N. Method of electrostimulation of the deep brain structures in treatment of some chronic diseases. *Confin. Neurol.* 1975;37(1-3):136-40.

Bechtereva, NP; Zontov, VV. The relationship between certain forms of potentials and the variations in brain excitability (based on EEG, recorded during photic stimuli triggered by rhythmic brain potentials). *Electroencephalogr. Clin. Neurophysiol.* 1962;14:320-30.

Bendel, O; Bueters, T; von Euler, M; Ove Ogren, S; Sandin, J; von Euler, G. Reappearance of hippocampal CA1 neurons after ischemia is associated with recovery of learning and memory. *J. Cereb. Blood Flow Metab.* 2005; 25(12):1586-95.

Björklund, A. Neural transplantation–an experimental tool with clinical possibilities. *Trends Neurosci.* 1991;14(8):319-22.

Blomer, U; Naldini, L; Verma, IM; Trono, D; Gage, FH. Applications of gene therapy to the CNS. *Hum. Mol. Genet.* 1996;5:1397-1404.

Borlongan, CV; McWhirter, C; Fultz-Carver, C; FitzGerald, KT; Sanberg, PR. The Case for an Ethics Research Consortium for Emerging Technologies: Public Perception of Stem Cell Research and Development. *Techno. and Innov*. 2010;12:21-28.

Bornstein, MB; Raine, CS. Experimental allergic encephalomyelitis: demyelination, remyelination and sclerosis in cultured mammalian CNS tissue. *Trans. Am. Neurol. Assoc.* 1969; 94:46-7.

Cajal, SRY. *Degeneration and regeneration of the nervous system* (RM May, Trans.). London: Oxford University Press; 1928.

Chen L., Huang H. Neurorestoratology: new concept and bridge from bench to bedside. Chin. *J. Repar. Reconstr. Surg.,* 2009;23(3):366-370.

Croll, RP; Baker, MW. Axonal regeneration and sprouting following injury to the cerebral-buccal connective in the snail Achatina fulica. *J. Comp. Neurol.* 1990; 300(2): 273-86.

D'Angelo, E. The human *Funct. Neurol.* 2012; 27(4):205.

David, S; Aguayo, AJ. Axonal elongation into peripheral nervous system "bridges" after central nervous system injury in adult rats. *Science.* 1981;214(4523):931-3.

Dimitrijevic, MR. *Recent achievements of restorative neurology*. Switzerland: Karger; 1985.

Fernández, CI; Soto, J; González, O; González, ME; Quijano, Z. Neurorestorative techniques as experimental approach to Alzheimer disease treatment. *Mol. Chem. Neuropathol.* 1995; 24(2-3):241-4.

Honmou, O; Felts, PA; Waxman, SG; Kocsis, JD. Restoration of normal conduction properties in demyelinated spinal cord axons in the adult rat by transplantation of exogenous Schwann cells. *J. Neurosci.* 1996; 16(10):3199-208.

WMA General Assembly. WMA Declaration of Helsinki–Ethical Principles for Medical Research Involving Human Subjects. 2014 June 23. Available from: http://www.wma.net/en/30publications/10policies/b3/index.html

Huang, H; Chen, L; Sanberg, P. Cell therapy from bench to bedside translation in CNS Neurorestoratology era. *Cell Med.* 2010;1:15-46.

Huang, H; Chen, L; Sanberg, P. Clinical achievements, Obstacles, falsehoods, and future directions of cell–based neurorestoratology. *Cell Transplant.* 2012;21(S1):S3-S11.

Huang, H; Chen, L; Wang, H; Xiu, B; Li, B, Wang, R; Zhang, J; Zhang, F; Gu, Z; Li, Y; Song, Y; Hao, W; Pang, S; Sun, J. Influence of patients' age on functional recovery after transplantation of olfactory ensheathing cells into injured spinal cord injury. *Chin. Med. J. (Engl.).* 2003;116:1488-91.

Huang, H. Chen, L. Neurorestoratology–new subject, new principle, new field in 21st century. *Chinese Journal of Reparative and Reconstructive Surgery.* 2008; 22:439-445.

Huang, H; Sharma, HS. Neurorestoratology: one of the most promising new disciplines at the forefront of neuroscience and medicine. *Journal of Neurorestoratology*. 2013; 1:37-41.

Huang, H. Neurorestoratology, a distinct discipline and a new era: A brief introduction to the first IANR section. *Cell Transplant.* 2010; 19:129-131.

IANR (International Association of Neurorestoratology). Beijing declaration of international association of neurorestoratology (IANR). *Cell Transplant.* 2009; 18:487.

Jiménez-Jiménez, FJ. Molina, JA. Neuroprotective and neurorestorative therapy in Parkinson's disease. *Rev. Neurol.* 1997; 25 Suppl. 2:S185-93.

Katayama, Y. Deep brain stimulation therapy: Control of human brain function by chronically implanted electrodes. *No To Shinkei*. 2000; 52(4):297-305.

Langmoen, IA; Ohlsson, M; Westerlund, U; Svensson, M. A new tool in restorative neurosurgry: creating niches for neuronal stem cells. *Neurosurgery*. 2003; 52(5):1150-1153.

Levi-Montalcini, R; Hamburger, V. Selective growth stimulating effects of mouse sarcoma on the sensory and sympathetic nervous system of the chick embryo. *J. Exp. Zool.* 1951; 116: 321-361.

Liberson, WT. More on restorative neurosurgery. *Electromyogr. Clin. Neurophysiol.* 1987; 27(6-7): 323-325.

Liepert, J. Pharmacotherapy in restorative neurology. *Curr. Opin. Neurol.* 2008;21(6):639-643.

Liu, CN; Chambers, WW. Intraspinal sprouting of dorsal root axons; development of new collaterals and preterminals following partial denervation of the spinal cord in the cat. *AMA Arch. Neurol. Psychiatry*. 1958; 79(1):46-61.

Luque, JM; Gime´nezy Ribotta, M. Neural stem cells and the quest for restorative neurology. *Histol. Histopathol.* 2004; 19(1):271-280.

Marquez, YD; Wang, MY; Liu, CY. Cellular signaling in neural stem cells: Implications for restorative neurosurgery. *Neurosurg. Focus*. 2005; 19(3):E2.

Muller-Putz, GR; Scherer, R; Pfurtscheller, G; Neuper, C; Rupp, R. Non-invasive control of neuroprostheses for the upper extremity: temporal coding of brain patterns. *Conf. Proc. IEEE Eng. Med. Biol. Soc.* 2009;2009:3353-6.

Naftchi, NE. Functional restoration of the traumatically injured spinal cord in cats by clonidine. *Science*. 1982;217(4564):1042-4.

Nicholls, JG. Neural repair. Based on a discussion meeting. Kolimbari, Crete, March 1987. *J. Exp. Biol.* 1987; 132:1-289.

Palladini, G; Caronti, B; Pozzessere, G; Teichner, A; Buttarelli, FR; Morselli, E; Valle, E; Venturini, G; Fortuna, A; Pontieri, FE. Treatment with cyclosporine A promotes axonal regeneration in rats submitted to transverse section of the spinal cord–II–Recovery of function. *J. Hirnforsch*. 1996; 3147(1):5-53.

Raisman, G. Neuronal plasticity in the septal nuclei of the adult rat. *Brain Res.* 1969; 14(1):25-48.

Rama, P; Matuska, S; Paganoni, G; Spinelli, A; De Luca, M; Pellegrini, G. Limbal stem-cell therapy and long-term corneal regeneration. *N. Engl. J. Med.* 2010;363:47-55.

Reswick, JB. Functional electrical stimulation–neural prosthesis for the disabled. *Bull. Prosthet. Res.* 1976; (10-25):1-4.

Richardson, RM; Varenika, V; Forsayeth, JR; Bankiewicz, KS. Future applications: Gene therapy. *Neurosurg. Clin. N. Am.* 2009; 20(2):205-210.

Sanberg, PR. Stem cell research reversal of fortune. *The Scientist*. 2005; 19:12-15.

Sanberg, PR. Students' views on fetal neural tissue transplantation. *The Lancet*. 1990; 1:1594.

Sironi, VA. Origin and evolution of deep brain stimulation. *Front. Integr. Neurosci.* 2011;5:42.

Taira, T; Hori, T. Clinical application of drug pump for spasticity, pain, and restorative neurosurgery: Other clinical applications of intrathecal baclofen. *Acta Neurochir. Suppl.* 2003; 87:37-38.

Taylor, SM. Electroconvulsive therapy, brain-derived neurotrophic factor, and possible neurorestorative benefit of the clinical application of electroconvulsive therapy. *J. ECT.* 2008; 24(2):160-165.

The BRAIN Initiative. The BRAIN Initiative: BAM or BUST? June 30, 2014, Available from: http://blogs.

Thompson, TP; Lunsford, LD; Kondziolka, D. Restorative neurosurgery: Opportunities for restoration of function in acquired, degenerative, and idiopathic neurological diseases. *Neurosurgery.* 1999; 45(4):741-752.

Yamamoto, M; Raisman, G; Li, D; Li, Y. Transplanted olfactory mucosal cells restore paw reaching function without regeneration of severed corticospinal tract fibres across the lesion. *Brain Res.* 2009; 1303:26-31.

Young, W; Flamm, ES. Effect of high-dose corticosteroid therapy on blood flow, evoked potentials, and extracellular calcium in experimental spinal injury. *J. Neurosurg.* 1982 ; 57(5):667-73.

Zhang, ZG; Chopp, M. Neurorestorative therapies for stroke: Underlying mechanisms and translation to the clinic. *Lancet Neurol.* 2009; 8(5):491-500.

In: Neurorestoratology, volume 1
Editors: H. Huang, G. Raisman, P. R. Sanberg et al.
ISBN: 978-1-63463-599-8


*Chapter 2*

# Initiation and Development of CNS Neurorestorative Strategies

***Lin Chen*[1,2] *and Hongyun Huang*[3,4*]**
[1]Tsinghua University Yuquan Hospital, Beijing, China
[2]Medical Center, Tsinghua University, Beijing, China
[3]Beijing Rehabilitation Hospital of Capital Medical University, Beijing, China
[4]Beijing Hongtianji Neuroscience Academy, Beijing, China

## Introduction

During the past 100 years, in particular the last 30 years, numerous neurorestorative strategies have emerged demonstrating their positive potential in the central nervous system (CNS) (Table 1] through various possible mechanisms. In this chapter, we briefly describe their history and pioneers who brought them forward to the clinic.

**Table 1. Classification of neurorestorative strategies**

| |
|---|
| cell or tissue transplantation |
| neuromodulation therapy (electric /magnetic stimulation) and neuroprosthesis |
| factors and neurorestorative pharmacotherapy |
| tissue engineering therapy |
| bio-engineering therapy |
| neurorestorative surgery |
| neurorehabilitation |

* Corresponding author: Hongyun Huang. E-mail: hongyunh@gmail.com.

# 1. Cell or Tissue Transplantation

Since Gilman Thompson published his article on successful intracerebral transplantation in mammals in 1890 (Björklund A, 1991), Ramon Y Cajal (1928) later first described the axonal regeneration-promoting effects of peripheral nerve implants in spinal cord. Presently, over 30 types of cells and tissues have been successfully used in preclinical experiments and/or clinical trials/treatment (Table 2]. The first clinical trial of neural tissue transplantation was done by Olson's team (Olson L et al., 1984; Backlund EO et al., 1985). The earliest clinical trials or studies of neural cell (olfactory ensheathing cell) transplantation into spinal cord or brain parenchyma were started for spinal cord injury (SCI) by Huang and Rabinovich (Huang H et al., 2003; Rabinovich SS et al., 2003); olfactory mucosa tissue transplantation was done by Lima in 2001 (Lima C et al., 2006). Cell-based neurorestorative therapy is now the core strategy and has become a new trend and the most promising direction in this field.

Increasing data worldwide strongly prove that it has a pivotal therapeutic value in CNS diseases (Huang H et al., 2010). The principle kinds of cells or tissues for neurorestoration are described below.

**Table 2. Current neurorestorative cells/tissues**

| |
|---|
| fetal/embryonic cells or tissue |
| induced pluripotent stem cells |
| neural stem cells |
| neural progenitor/precursor cells |
| adipose-derived precursor cells |
| hair follicle stem cells |
| skin-derived precursor/stem cells |
| dental stem cells |
| myoblast or muscle-derived stem cells |
| Sertoli cells |
| T cell vaccination |
| macrophages |
| bone marrow mononuclear or stromal cells |
| umbilical cord mesenchymal stromal cells |
| placenta-derived mesenchymal stromal cells |
| umbilical cord blood cells |
| menstrual blood cells |
| amniotic epithelial cells |
| hematopoietic stem cells |
| peripheral blood mononuclear cells |
| olfactory ensheathing cells |
| oligodendrocytes |
| tanycytes |
| microglia |
| astrocytes |
| Schwann cells |
| neurons or neuron-like cells |
| dopamine cells |
| Purkinje cells |
| endothelial progenitor cells |
| retinal pigment epithelial cells |
| fibroblasts |
| embryonic brain or fetal brain cells |
| embryonic spinal cord cells |
| chimeric stem cells |

## 1.1. Fetal/Embryonic Brain Tissue

The first evidence was presented by Nygren LG, et al. (1977) that grafts of fetal brain tissue to the adult CNS could counteract a neurological deficit. More studies have convincingly shown that grafting of fetal/embryonic brain cells/tissue into the brain and/or spinal cord is a useful alternative therapy for neural degenerative and traumatic disorders (Michejda M, 1987; López-Lozano JJ, et al., 1995; Madrazo I, et al., 1995).

## 1.2. Fetal/Embryonic Spinal Cord Tissue

The first successful transplantation of fetal spinal cord into adult spinal cord was reported by Patel U et al. in 1983. The grafted tissue stimulated partial regression of an established glial scar (Houlé JD et al., 1988), replaced missing motoneurons (Sieradzan K et al., 1989), formed myelin (Rosenbluth J, et al., 1990), restores some degree of anatomical continuity (Reier PJ et al., 1986), and rescued axotomized host neurons that otherwise would have died (Tessler A, 1991). Falci S et al. (1997) reported the first use of solid human embryonic cord grafts in a patient with a posttraumatic cyst.

## 1.3. Olfactory Ensheathing Cells

Olfactory ensheathing cells (OECs) are novel cells that display Schwann cell and astrocyte-like properties. The initial OEC transplantation with histological and functional analysis in animals started in the 1990s. Ramón-Cueto reported that regeneration of injured dorsal root axons into the adult spinal cord was possible after OEC transplantation (Ramón-Cueto A and Nieto-Sampedro M 1994). OEC transplants successfully led to functional and structural recovery after complete spinal cord transection in adult rats (Ramón-Cueto A et al., 2000). Franklin et al. (1996) first provided in vivo evidence that olfactory bulb-ensheathing cells are able to produce peripheral-type myelin sheaths around demyelinated spinal cord axons of the appropriate diameter. The team of Raisman subsequently reported that damaged corticospinal axons grew through the transplant and continued to regenerate into the denervated caudal host tract. Rats with transplanted cells exhibited directed forepaw reaching on the lesioned side (Li Y et al., 1997, 1998). OECs are the pioneer cell for neurological disease and damage in animal models and clinical studies.

## 1.4. Schwann Cells

Aguayo proved that peripheral nerves with Schwann cells (SCs) could help axons of damaged spinal cord regenerate (Aguayo AJ et al., 1981). These cells also could form myelin in a demyelinated CNS animal model (Imaizumi T et al., 2000).

But astrocytes inhibite transplanted SCs migration into CNS white matter, so more efforts have focused on enhancing their migration and functional integration into the lesioned CNS (Luo J et al., 2011).

SC ability attracts more studies for repair of CNS damage; At the clinical level, Zhang WC et al. (1994) reported that co-grafting of SCs and human fetal adrenal medullary tissue could significantly improve symptoms of Parkinson's disease. Saberi H et al. (2008) reported autologous SC transplantation for patients with stable chronic SCI.

## 1.5. Oligodendrocyte/Precursor Cells

Oligodendrocytes or precursor cells can migrate from the implantation site to the lesion over a distance of several millimeters (Crang AJ et al., 1991; Duncan ID, 1996) to remyelinate the CNS (Franklin RJ et al., 1995; Sasaki M et al., 2010; Miron VE et al., 2011; Banisadr G et al., 2011). Thus these cells have potential for myelin repair in demyelinating diseases.

## 1.6. Astrocytes

Cultured astrocytes can alter the microenvironment (Bradbury EJ et al., 1995), survive and migrate following transplantation (Davies SJ et al., 2011; Ridet JL et al., 2003).

## 1.7. Macrophages

Activated macrophages/microglial cells can provide a beneficial environment at a SCI site to promote sensory axon regeneration (Gensel JC et al., 2009; Prewitt CM et al., 1997). A phase I, open-label non-randomized clinical trial of incubated autologous macrophage cell therapy for patients with acute complete SCI has been reported. Some adverse events were noted, such as pulmonary embolism and osteomyelitis (Knoller N et al., 2005).

## 1.8. Tanycytes

Tanycytes are specialized ependymal glia in the CNS and mostly located in the ventral wall of the 3rd ventricle and median eminence (Changaris DG et al., 1978; Gross DS, 1976). Tanycytes transplanted into the adult rat spinal cord can support lesioned axons to regenerate (Prieto M et al., 2000) and significantly improve motor functions (Xu XX et al., 2010).

## 1.9. Dopaminergic Neurons

Björklund first transplanted monoaminergic neurons into the adult rodent hippocampus (Björklund A et al., 1976; Stenevi U et al., 1976).

Dopaminergic neurons/cells nowadays perform as an alternative regime for Parkinson's disease in the clinic (Chou J et al., 2011; Nikkhah G et al., 2009; Strömberg I et al., 2010) and can be considered as an emerging choice for transplantation (Cai J et al., 2010; Hwang DY et al., 2010; Kubo A et al., 2009; Liste I et al., 2004; Rhee YH et al., 2011; Zhao J et al., 2011). Cell therapy focuses on counteracting symptoms of Parkinson's disease and slowing down disease progression by neuroprotection or neurorestoration (Ren Z et al., 2009).

## 1.10. GABAergic Neurons

Grafts of GABAergic neurons were first transplanted by Frotscher M and Zimmer J (1987), which induced recovery of sensorimotor function in brain injury (Becerra GD et al., 2007) and might be an effective method to block seizure generalization (Baraban SC et al., 2009; Löscher W et al., 1998).

## 1.11. Embryonic Stem Cells

Embryonic stem cells (ESCs) were transplanted for SCI by McDonald JW (1999). ESCs can differentiate into neural stem cells and further generate functional neurons, astrocytes, and oligodendrocytes (Fluckiger AC et al., 2003; Liu S et al., 2000; López-González R et al., 2009) and have the beneficial properties to secrete neurotrophic and neural growth factors (Newman MB et al., 2008).

ESCs may provide a potential restorative therapy for neurological conditions. However, ESC-based therapy still faces several problems; the major hurdle is tumor formation (Li JY et al., 2008).

## 1.12. Neural Stem/Progenitor Cells

Groves AK reported neural progenitor cell transplantation for SCI in 1993 (Groves, 1993). Neural stem/progenitor cells (NSPCs) in the adult CNS are capable of generating new neurons, astrocytes, and oligodendrocytes (Trujillo CA et al., 2009) and can be used for neurodegenerative diseases and trauma.

## 1.13. Bone Marrow Mononuclear or Stromal Cells

Bone marrow cells transplanted intravenously could enter the brain (Eglitis MA et al., 1997), and migrate from the injection site into the surrounding parenchyma (Azizi SA et al.,

1998). These cells could improve functional recovery for ischemic brain by intrastriatal transplantation (Li Y et al., 2000).

Bone marrow stromal cells or mononuclear cell transplantation showed beneficial outcome (Karussis D et al., 2008; Takizawa S, 2003; Torrente Y et al., 2008).

## 1.14. Umbilical Cord Mesenchymal Stromal Cells

Weiss ML (2003) transplanted porcine umbilical cord matrix cells into the normal rat brain; then Fu YS (2006) and Weiss ML (2006) tested human umbilical cord mesenchymal stromal cells for Parkinson's disease. A clinical study showed its safety and effects in patients with spinocerebellar ataxia and multiple system atrophy-cerebellar type (Dongmei H et al., 2011). Umbilical cord including arteries, veins, and Wharton's jelly is a convenient, efficient source of mesenchymal stromal cells (Girdlestone J et al., 2009; Ishige I et al., 2009) and can be a viable alternative therapy for CNS trauma and neurodegenerative diseases (Low CB et al., 2008; Nekanti U et al., 2010; Peng J et al., 2011).

## 1.15. Umbilical Cord Blood Cells

Intravenous human umbilical cord blood cells improved functional recovery for stroke (Chen J et al., 2001), Alzheimer's disease and Huntington's disease in animal study (Ende N et al., 2001a; 2001b). Umbilical cord blood cells may promote neural repair (Sanberg PR et al., 2005; Peterson DA, 2004) for CNS injury and neurodegenerative diseases (Lee JH et al., 2011; Rosenkranz K et al., 2011; Sanberg PR et al., 2011). Nowadays, umbilical cord blood cells have been used for some neurological diseases (Kang KS et al., 2005; Papadopoulos KI et al., 2011; Yang, WZ et al., 2011).

## 1.16. Hematopoietic Stem Cells

Hematopoietic stem cells (HSCs) have been proposed to treat multiple sclerosis (Burt RK et al., 1999, 2005; Mandalfino P et al., 2000; Tyndall A et al., 2002), SCI and ischemic brain lesions (Koshizuka S et al., 2004) whose putative underlying mechanisms (Haas S et al., 2005) are interwoven with sites of motoneuron pathology (Appel SH et al., 2008). Clinical trials of autologous HSC transplantation for severe progressive multiple sclerosis patients have been shown to improve their quality of life (Saccardi R et al., 2005; Loh YS et al., 2007); however the effects were dependent on patient-selection, time of transplantation and conditioning regimens used (Rogojan C et al., 2009). Patients with chronic complete SCI and amytrophic lateral sclerosis received benefits from autologous bone marrow-derived HSC transplantation (Deda H et al., 2008, 2009).

## 1.17. Adipose-Derived Adult Stromal/Precursor Cells

Adipose-derived adult stromal cells (ADAs) show characteristics of multipotent adult stromal cells, similar to those of MSCs (de Villiers JA et al., 2009; Franco Lambert AP et al., 2009; Kokai LE et al., 2005; Locke M et al., 2009; Yu JM et al., 2011) and have been tested for various neurologic disorders (Kim WS et al., 2009; Mizuno H, 2009; Ogawa R, 2006; Safford KM, 2005). Clinical ADA therapy remains an emerging tool for neurology (Brown SA et al., 2010).

## 1.18. Skin-Derived Precursors

Skin-derived precursors (SKPs) can migrate to the lesion site and differentiate mainly into cells expressing glia and neuronal markers (Gorio A et al., 2004), which share characteristics with embryonic neural crest stem cells (Hunt DP et al., 2009; Zavan B et al., 2010). After transplantation, SKPs has been identified as a novel, accessible, and potentially autologous source for neurorestoration (Proulx S et al., 2011).

## 1.19. Amniotic Epithelial Cells

Kakishita K transplanted human amniotic epithelial cells (hAECs) in the brain of a rat Parkinson's disease model (Kakishita K et al., 2000). Nakama H (2006) transplanted encapsulized immortalized hAECs in the mice brain for lysosomal storage diseases. hAECs have low immunogenicity, anti-inflammatory function (Meng XT et al., 2007; Miki T et al., 2006; Toda A et al., 2007) and therapeutic potential for CNS disorders (Yang X et al., 2010; Yu SJ et al., 2009).

## 1.20. Sertoli Cells

Sertoli cells provide local immunoprotection for tissue grafts (Borlongan CV et al., 1996; Halberstadt C et al., 2004; Mital P et al., 2010; Sanberg PR et al., 1996, 1997; Willing AE et al., 1998) and act as a viable graft source for Parkinson's disease, Huntington's disease, and other neurodegenerative diseases.

## 1.21. Induced Pluripotent Stem Cells

Wernig M (2008) reported the use of induced pluripotent stem (iPS) cells in a rat model of Parkinson's disease. iPS cells appear to be able to indefinitely self-renew and to differentiate into all types of cells in the body, and are almost identical to ESCs (Czepiel M et al., 2011; Kiefer JC et al., 2011; Ogawa S et al., 2011; Wang A et al., 2011) and may be a new avenue as a highly effective and immune rejection-free cell therapy for Parkinson's disease, SCI, stroke, spinal muscular atrophy, and hearing impairment (Chen LW et al., 2011; El-Amraoui A et al., 2010; Hernándeza J et al., 2011; Hunt CJ, 2011; Sendtner M, 2010;

Tomaskovic-Crook E et al., 2011). As with ESCs, the intrinsic property of teratoma formation (Masip M et al., 2010) is currently an insurmountable obstacle for iPS clinical use.

## 1.22. Hair Follicle Stem Cells

Hair follicle stem cells were transplanted for peripheral nerve and SCI may be better than embryonic stem cells and induced pluripotent stem cells (Amoh Y et al., 2005, 2008, 2010, 2012; Liu F et al., 2011).

## 1.23. Menstrual Blood Cells

Stem cells from menstrual blood cells could significantly reduce behavioral and histological impairments in ischemic stroke in adult rats (Borlongan CV et al., 2010; Sanberg PR et al., 2011) with high replicative ability (Toyoda M et al., 2007).

## 1.24. Placenta-Derived Mesenchymal Stromal Cells

Human placenta-derived mesenchymal stromal cells were transplanted for into the ischemic rat brain and showed partial recovery (Yarygin KN et al., 2009).

## 1.25. Dental Stem Cells

Dental stem cells, including dental pulp stem cells and dental follicle cells could rescue motoneurons in SCI (Nosrat IV et al., 2001), protect primary neurons in Alzheimer's and Parkinson's disease models (Apel C et al., 2009) or cerebral ischemia (Yalvac ME et al., 2009) and help peripheral nerve regeneration (Sasaki R et al., 2008).

## 1.26. Retinal Pigment Epithelial Cells

Retinal pigment epithelial cells have been transplanted for Parkinson's disease in animal studies (Marchionini DM et al., 1999; Subramanian T et al., 1998, 2002; Subramanian T, 2001) and clinical trials (Stover NP et al., 2005).

# 2. Neuromodulation and Neuroprosthesis

## 2.1. Brain or Spinal Cord Electrical Stimulation

Aldini in 1804 first reported that cortical stimulation evoked horrible facial grimaces (Aldini J, 1804). The first case of brain stimulation in a patient was reported by Bartholow in 1874 (Bartholow R, 1874; Zimmermann M, 1982). Direct electrical stimulation or transcranial direct current stimulation to cerebral cortex or spinal cord could exert potassium release (Cicardo VH and Torino A, 1942), antiapoptotic, angiogenic, anti-inflammatory effects, and synaptic plasticity (Baba T et al., 2009; Rothwell JC, 2010) and induce or promote axon outgrowth (Borgens RB et al., 1986; Hamid S et al., 2008; Li Q et al., 2010) to restore motor function (Fehlings MG et al.,1988; Carmel JB et al., 2010; Polanía R et al., 2011). Brain stimulation (called electroshock) was the first therapeutic application for severe psychosis (Cerletti, 1940; Sironi VA, 2011) and then for pain in 1954 (Wallace BA et al., 2004). Epidural stimulation of spinal cord could induce stepping-like movements in patients with complete SCI (Minassian K et al., 2004; von Wild K et al., 2002). Transcranial direct current stimulation is a non-invasive technique and is increasingly being used in the treatment of some neurological/psychiatric conditions, e.g. chronic pain, epilepsy, depression, motor rehabilitation after stroke, SCI and Parkinson's disease (Knotkova H et al., 2010).

## 2.2. Deep Brain Stimulation

Deep brain stimulation was first used as a diagnostic method by Delgado (Delgado JM et al., 1952; Sironi VA, 2011) and as a treatment method for motor disorders (Bekhtereva NP et al., 1963; Sironi VA, 2011).

Recent studies have demonstrated its potential for treating epilepsy, depression and obsessive-compulsive disorder (Dowling J, 2008; Coffey RJ, 2009; Sironi VA, 2011).

## 2.3. Magnetic Stimulation

The magnetic stimulator was reported for stimulating neural elements in 1982 (Polson MJ et al., 1982). Transcranial magnetic stimulation was first used in the clinic by Barker et al. (Barker AT et al., 1985). In recent years, repetitive Transcranial magnetic stimulation has been used as a therapeutic tool for a variety of psychiatric and neurological disorders, such as Parkinson's disease (Strafella AP et al., 2006), amyotrophic lateral sclerosis (Di Lazzaro V et al., 2006), traumatic brain injury (Pape TL et al., 2006), stroke (Lefaucheur JP, 2006; Zhang X et al., 2007), pain (Lefaucheur JP, 2006), dystonia (Tyvaert L et al., 2006), and epilepsy (Fregni F et al., 2006).

## 2.4. Neuroprosthesis

Nashold BS reported electromicturition by a spinal neuroprosthesis implantation for paraplegia in 1971 (Nashold et al., 1971). Recently it was shown that brain-machine interfaces with neuroprosthetic limbs could help patients with long-term paralysis to recover the natural and intuitive command signals for hand placement, orientation, and reaching, allowing them to perform activities of partial daily living (Collinger JL et al., 2013; Hochberg LR et al.,2006; Onose G et al., 2012; Simeral JD et al., 2011).

# 3. Factors and Pharmacological Agents

## 3.1. Neurotrophic Factors

Sixty years ago the discovery of nerve growth factor (NGF) led to the formulation of the "Neurotrophic Factor Hypothesis". Neurotrophic factors (NTFs) include: first, NGF and the other members of the neurotrophin family, i.e., brain derived neurotrophic factor (BDNF), neurotrophin-3 (NT-3), neurotrophin-4/5; second, the neurokines ciliary neurotrophic factor (CNTF) and leukemia inhibitory factor; and third, the transforming growth factors-beta and their distant relative, glial cell line-derived neurotrophic factor (GDNF).

Understanding NTF regulation and actions on neurons has led to their use in clinical trials of human neurological diseases. NTFs may emerge as important therapies to prevent neuronal cell dysfunction and death (Frostick SP et al., 1998; Yuen EC et al.,1996).

*NGF*

Levi-Montalcini R and Hamburger V discovered that NGF could promote the survival and differentiation of sensory and sympathetic neurons (Cohen S et al., 1954,1957; Levi-Montalcini R et al., 1951) and was first used in clinical trials by Olson L. et al. in 1991.

*BDNF*

Lindsay RM, et al. (1985) found that primary sensory neurons were responsive to BDNF. Later its physico-chemical characteristics were shown to be close to those of the monomer of NGF (Thoenen H et al., 1987) BDNF appears to play a role in rescuing dopaminergic neurons following damage (Fusco M et al., 1993), in Alzheimer's disease and in small fiber sensory neuropathy (Lindsay RM, 1994).

*CNTF*

CNTF was purified and cloned by Watters and Lin (Lin LF et al., 1989; Watters DJ et al., 1987). It is a 22-kDa protein with neurotrophic activities distinct from NGF and BDNF. CNTF can prevent degeneration of motoneurons (Sendtner M et al., 1991) and slow symptoms of motor neuron dysfunction in genetic models, such as Parkinson's disease, amyotrophic lateral sclerosis, Alzheimer's disease, and Huntington's disease (Kuzis K et al., 1996; Lindsay RM, 1994; Sariola H et al., 1994).

*NT-3*

Maisonpierre PC et al. (1990) reported that NT-3 is neurotrophic factor distinct from NGF and BDNF.

*GDNF*

Lin LF, et al. (1993) purified and cloned GDNF. GDNF promotes the survival and morphological differentiation of dopaminergic neurons and increases their high-affinity dopamine uptake, which may be of utility in the treatment of neurodegenerative diseases such as Parkinson's disease, amyotrophic lateral sclerosis, and cholinergic deficit-related dementia (Lapchak PA, 1996; Grondin R et al., 1998).

*Insulin-Like Growth Factor-I*

Rinderknecht E and Humbel RE (1978) determined the complete amino acid sequence of human insulin-like growth factor-I, which demonstrated efficacy in amyotrophic lateral sclerosis (Yuen EC et al., 1995; Di Giulio AM et al., 2000) and focal brain ischemia (Kooijman R et al., 2009).

*Fibroblast Growth Factor*

Gospodarowicz D (1974, 1975) discovered and purified fibroblast growth factor, which could prevent apoptosis and promote neurogenesis after injury (Alzheimer C et al., 2002).

*Vascular Endothelial Growth Factor*

Chen described the presence of vascular endothelial growth factor in the retina in 1987, which prevented neuron death under critical conditions such as hypoxia and glucose deprivation (Góra-Kupilas K et al., 2005), and stimulated the proliferation and survival of neural stem cells (Zachary I, 2005). Vascular endothelial growth factor might be a promising treatment method for neurodegenerative disorders and stroke (Namiecińska M et al., 2005).

### 3.2. Neurorestorative Drugs

*Methylprednisolone*

High-dose methylprednisolone therapy showed neuroprotection for SCI in an animal study in 1982 and progressed to a clinical trial in 1988 by Young W. et al. (Young W et al., 1982; 1988). Then more neurorestorative drugs, such as ganglioside GM1, granulocyte-colony stimulating factor, and erythropoietin have been used for neurodegenerative disease or damage.

## 4. Tissue Engineering and Bioengineering Therapy

Rosenberg MB et al. (1988) reported that implanting fibroblasts genetically modified with NGF into rat brain could prevent cholinergic neuron degeneration. Emerich DF et al. found (1997) that transplanting polymer-encapsulated fibroblasts genetically modified with human CNTF into striatum had a protective effect in a Huntington's disease animal model.

Later, Bloch J et al. (2004) carried out a clinical trial for Huntington's disease by transplanting this kind of polymer-encapsulated cells engineered with CNTF. Tuszynski MH et al. (2005) reported a I phase clinical trial by gene therapy with NGF for Alzheimer's disease.

# 5. Neurorestorative Surgery

## 5.1. Cordotomy or Myelotomy

The first report about cordotomy or myelotomy in an animal study was by Freeman LW et al. (1953), which showed a protective effect for injured spinal cord. Tachibana S et al. (1984) did posterior longitudinal myelotomy for patients with cervical acute complete spinal cord.

## 5.2. Neurotisation or Nerve Bridging

Carlsson CA and Sundin T (1967) reported reconstructing nerve bridging to the urinary bladder in a paraplegic child and reconstructed nerve bridging to the urinary bladder for another two paraplegic patients in 1980 (Carlsson and Sundin, 1980). Then Zhang S, Brunelli and others followed or improved neurotisation or nerve bridging for patients with SCI.

# 6. Neurorehabilitation

Brackett EG (1918) first mentioned rehabilitation for soldiers injured in war. Ueda S (1963) summarized rehabilitation in neural diseases. Luzhetskaia TA et al. (1974) first introduced neurorehabilitation as a therapeutic method for neural diseases and damage.

# 7. Cell-Based Comprehensive Neurorestorative Strategies

Single cell therapy or single neurorestorative strategy has shown some effects for patients with neurodegenerative diseases or sequel of CNS damage as listed above, but the extent of improvement cannot satisfy the high expectations. Cell-based comprehensive neurorestorative strategies or combined neurorestorative therapies should be recommended for clinical study, in order that patients may obtain more benefits or neurological functions (Huang H, 2013).

In summary, the pioneers have unyieldingly explored many neurorstorative strategies. Even some of them look very rough in current view, but they initiate or guide the direction for the younger generation. Exploring the best combined strategies have been the targets of Neurorestoratology now and in near future.

# References

Aguayo, AJ; David, S; Bray, G M. Influences of the glial environment on the elongation of axons after injury: transplantation studies in adult rodents. *J. Exp. Biol.* 1981; 95:231-40.

Aldini, J. Essai théoriqueet expérimental sur le galvanisme, avec une série d'expériences faites devant des commissaires del'Institut nationale de France, et en divers amphithéâtres anatomiques de Londres. *Paris: Fournier Fils*; 1804.

Alzheimer, C; Werner, S. Fibroblast growth factors and neuroprotection. *Adv. Exp. Med. Biol.* 2002;513:335-51.

Amoh, Y; Aki, R; Hamada, Y; Niiyama, S; Eshima, K; Kawahara, K; Sato, Y; Tani, Y; Hoffman, R M; Katsuoka, K. Nestin-positive hair follicle pluripotent stem cells can promote regeneration of impinged peripheral nerve injury. *J. Dermatol.* 2012;39 (1): 33-8.

Amoh, Y; Katsuoka, K; Hoffman, R M. The advantages of hair follicle pluripotent stem cells over embryonic stem cells and induced pluripotent stem cells for regenerative medicine. *J Dermatol Sci.* 2010; 60(3):131-7.

Amoh, Y; Li, L; Campillo, R; Kawahara, K et al. Implanted hair follicle stem cells form Schwann cells that support repair of severed peripheral nerves. *Proc. Natl. Acad. Sci. US.* 2005;102(49):17734-8.

Amoh, Y; Li, L; Katsuoka, K; Hoffman, R M. Multipotent hair follicle stem cells promote repair of spinal cord injury and recovery of walking function. *Cell Cycle.* 2008;7(12): 1865-9.

Apel, C; Forlenza, OV; de Paula, V J et al. The neuroprotective effect of dental pulp cells in models of Alzheimer's and Parkinson's disease. *J. Neural. Transm.* 2009;116(1):71-8.

Appel, SH; Engelhardt, J I; Henkel, J S et al. Hematopoietic stem cell transplantation in patients with sporadic amyotrophic lateral sclerosis. *Neurology.* 2008;71(17):1326-34.

Azizi, SA; Stokes, D; Augelli, BJ; DiGirolamo, C; Prockop, DJ. Engraftment and migration of human bone marrow stromal cells implanted in the brains of albino rats--similarities to astrocyte grafts. *Proc. Natl. Acad. Sci. US.* 1998;95(7):3908-13.

Baba, T; Kameda, M; Yasuhara, T et al. Electrical stimulation of the cerebral cortex exerts antiapoptotic, angiogenic, and anti-inflammatory effects in ischemic stroke rats through phosphoinositide 3-kinase/Akt signaling pathway. *Stroke.* 2009;40(11):e598-605.

Backlund, EO; Granberg, PO; Hamberger, B; Knutsson, E; Mårtensson, A; Sedvall, G; Seiger, A; Olson, L. Transplantation of adrenal medullary tissue to striatum in parkinsonism. First clinical trials. *J. Neurosurg.* 1985;62(2):169-73.

Banisadr, G; Frederick, TJ; Freitag, C et al. The role of CXCR4 signaling in the migration of transplanted oligodendrocyte progenitors into the cerebral white matter. *Neurobiol. Dis.* 2011;44(1):19-27.

Baraban, SC; Southwell, DG; Estrada, RC et al. Reduction of seizures by transplantation of cortical GABAergic interneuron precursors into Kv1.1 mutant mice. *Proc. Natl. Acad. Sci. US.* 2009;106(36):15472-7.

Barker, AT; Jalinous, R; Freeston, IL. Non-invasive magnetic stimulation of the human motor cortex. *Lancet.* 1985; i: 1106-7.

Bartholow, R. Experimental investigations into the functions of the human brain. *Am. J. Med. Sci.* 1874; 134: 305-313.

Becerra, GD; Tatko, LM; Pak, ES et al. Transplantation of GABAergic neurons but not astrocytes induces recovery of sensorimotor function in the traumatically injured brain. *Behav. Brain Res.* 2007;179(1):118-25.

Bekhtereva, NP; Grachev, KV; Orlova, AN; Iatsuksl. Utilization of multiple electrodes implanted in the subcortical structure of the human brain for the treatment of hyperkinesis. *Zh. Nevropatol. Psikhiatr. Im. S. S. Korsakova*. 1963;63:3-8.

Björklund, A; Stenevi, U; Svendgaard, N. Growth of transplanted monoaminergic neurones into the adult hippocampus along the perforant path. *Nature*. 1976;262 (5571): 787-90.

Björklund, A. Neural transplantation--an experimental tool with clinical possibilities. *Trends Neurosci.* 1991;14(8):319-22.

Bloch, J; Bachoud-Lévi, AC; Déglon, N; Lefaucheur, JP; Winkel, L; Palfi, S; Nguyen, JP; Bourdet, C; Gaura, V; Remy, P; Brugières, P; Boisse, MF; Baudic, S; Cesaro, P; Hantraye, P; Aebischer, P; Peschanski, M. Neuroprotective gene therapy for Huntington's disease, using polymer-encapsulated cells engineered to secrete human ciliary neurotrophic factor: results of a phase I study. *Hum. Gene. Ther.* 2004;15(10):968-75.

Borgens, RB; Blight, AR; Murphy, DJ; Stewart, L. Transected dorsal column axons within the guinea pig spinal cord regenerate in the presence of an applied electric field. *J. Comp. Neurol.* 1986; 250(2):168-80.

Borlongan, CV; Kaneko, Y; Maki, M et al. Menstrual blood cells display stem cell-like phenotypic markers and exert neuroprotection following transplantation in experimental stroke. *Stem Cells Dev.* 2010;19(4):439-52.

Borlongan, CV; Stahl, CE; Cameron, DF et al. CNS immunological modulation of neural graft rejection and survival. *Neurol. Res.* 1996;18(4):297-304.

Brackett, EG. Rehabilitation of diseased and injured soldiers to the war. *Am. J. Public Health* (NY). 1918;8(1):11-3.

Bradbury, EJ; Kershaw, TR; Marchbanks, RM;Sinden, JD. Astrocyte transplants alleviate lesion induced memory deficits independently of cholinergic recovery. *Neuroscience*. 1995;65(4):955-72.

Brown, SA; Levi, B; Lequeux, C et al. Basic science review on adipose tissue for clinicians. *Plast. Reconstr. Surg.* 2010;126(6):1936-46.

Burt, RK; Cohen, B; Rose, J et al. Hematopoietic stem cell transplantation for multiple sclerosis. *Arch. Neurol.* 2005;62(6):860-4.

Burt, R. K., Traynor, A. E. Hematopoietic stem cell transplantation: a new therapy for autoimmune disease. *Stem Cells*. 1999;17(6):366-72.

Cai, J; Yang, M; Poremsky, E; Kidd, S;Schneider, J S; Iacovitti, L. Dopaminergic neurons derived from human induced pluripotent stem cells survive and integrate into 6-OHDA lesioned rats. *Stem Cells Dev.* 2010;19(7):1017-23.

Carlsson, CA; Sundin, T. Reconstruction of afferent and efferent nervous pathways to the urinary bladder in two paraplegic patients. *Spine* (Phila. Pa 1976). 1980;5(1):37-41.

Carlsson, CA; Sundin, T. Reconstruction of efferent pathways to the urinary bladder in a paraplegic child. *Rev. Surg.* 1967;24(1):73-6.

Carmel, J B; Berrol, LJ; Brus-Ramer, M; Martin, J H. Chronic electrical stimulation of the intact corticospinal system after unilateral injury restores skilled locomotor control and promotes spinal axon outgrowth. *J. Neurosci.* 2010;30(32):10918-26.

Cerletti, U. L'elettroshock. *Riv. Sper. Freniatr. Med. Leg. Alien. Ment.* 1940; I: 209-310.

Changaris, DG; Keil, LC; Severs, WB. Angiotensin II immunohistochemistry of the rat brain. *Neuroendocrinology*. 1978;25(5):257-74.

Chen, J; Sanberg, P R; Li, Y et al. Intravenous administration of human umbilical cord blood reduces behavioral deficits after stroke in rats. *Stroke*. 2001;32(11):2682-8.

Chen, LW; Kuang, F; Wei, LC et al. Potential application of induced pluripotent stem cells in cell replacement therapy for Parkinson's disease. *CNS Neurol. Disord. Drug Targets*. 2011;10(4):449-58.

Chou, J; Greig, NH; Reiner, D et al. Enhanced survival of dopaminergic neuronal transplants in hemi-Parkinsonian rats by the p53 inactivator PFT-α. *Cell Transplant*. 2011; 20(9):1351-9.

Cicardo, VH; Torino, A. Release of potassium by the brain of the dog during electrical stimulation. *Science*. 1942;95(2477):625.

Coffey, RJ. Deep brain stimulation devices: a brief technical history and review. *Artif. Organs*. 2009;33(3):208-20.

Cohen, S; Levi-Montalcini, R; Hamburger, V. A nerve growth-stimulating factor isolated from sarcom as 37 and 180. *Proc. Natl. Acad. Sci. US*. 1954;40(10):1014-8.

Cohen, S;Levi-Montalcini, R. Purification and properties of a nerve growth-promoting factor isolated from mouse sarcoma 180. *Cancer Res.* 1957;17(1):15-20.

Collinger, JL; Wodlinger, B; Downey, JE; Wang, W; Tyler-Kabara, EC; Weber, DJ;McMorland, AJ;Velliste, M; Boninger, ML; Schwartz, AB. High-performance neuroprosthetic control by an individual with tetraplegia. *Lancet*. 2013;381:557-64.

Crang, AJ; Blakemore, WF. Remyelination of demyelinated rat axons by transplanted mouse oligodendrocytes. *Glia*. 1991;4(3):305-13.

Czepiel, M; Balasubramaniyan, V; Schaafsma, W et al. Differentiation of induced pluripotent stem cells into functional oligodendrocytes. *Glia*. 2011;59(6):882-92.

Davies, SJ; Shih, CH; Noble, M et al. Transplantation of specific human astrocytes promotes functional recovery after spinal cord injury. *PLoS One*. 2011;6(3):e17328.

De Villiers, JA; Houreld, N; Abrahamse, H. Adipose derived stem cells and smooth muscle cells: implications for regenerative medicine. *Stem Cell Rev*. 2009;5(3):256-65.

Deda, H; Inci, MC; Kürekçi, AE et al. Treatment of amyotrophic lateral sclerosis patients by autologous bone marrow-derived hematopoietic stem cell transplantation: a 1-year follow-up. *Cytotherapy*. 2009;11(1):18-25.

Deda, H; Inci, MC; Kürekçi, AE et al. Treatment of chronic spinal cord injured patients with autologous bone marrow-derived hematopoietic stem cell transplantation: 1-year follow-up. *Cytotherapy*. 2008;10(6):565-74.

Delgado, JM; Hamlin, H; Chapman, WP. Technique of intracranial electrode implacement for recording and stimulation and its possible therapeutic value in psychotic patients. *Confin. Neurol*. 1952;12(5-6):315-9.

Di Giulio, AM; Germani, E; Lesma, E et al. Glycosaminoglycans co-administration enhance insulin-like growth factor-I neuroprotective and neuroregenerative activity in traumatic and genetic models of motor neuron disease: a review. *Int. J. Dev. Neurosci*. 2000; 18(4-5):339-46.

Di Lazzaro, V; Dileone, M; Pilato, F et al. Repetitive transcranial magnetic stimulation for ALS. A preliminary controlled study. *Neurosci. Lett*. 2006;408(2):135-40.

Dongmei, H; Jing, L; Mei, X et al. Clinical analysis of the treatment of spinocerebellar ataxia and multiple system atrophy-cerebellar type with umbilical cord mesenchymal stromal cells. *Cytotherapy*. 2011;13(8):913-7.

Dowling, J. Deep brain stimulation: current and emerging indications. *Mo. Med.* 2008;105 (5):424-8.

Duncan, ID. Glial cell transplantation and remyelination of the central nervous system. *Neuropathol. Appl. Neurobiol.* 1996;22(2):87-100.

Eglitis, MA., Mezey, E. Hematopoietic cells differentiate into both microglia and macroglia in the brains of adult mice. *Proc. Natl. Acad. Sci. US*. 1997;94(8):4080-5.

El-Amraoui, A; Petit, C. Stem cell therapy in the inner ear: recent achievements and prospects. *Med. Sci.* (Paris). 2010;26(11):981-5.

Emerich, DF; Winn, SR; Hantraye, PM; Peschanski, M; Chen, EY; Chu, Y; McDermott, P; Baetge, EE; Kordower, JH. Protective effect of encapsulated cells producing neurotrophic factor CNTF in a monkey model of Huntington's disease. *Nature*. 1997;386(6623):395-9.

Ende, N; Chen, R; Ende-Harris, D. Human umbilical cord blood cells ameliorate Alzheimer's disease in transgenic mice. *J. Med.* 2001a;32(3-4):241-7.

Ende, N; Chen, R. Human umbilical cord blood cells ameliorate Huntington's disease in transgenic mice. *J. Med.* 2001b;32(3-4):231-40.

Falci, S; Holtz, A; Akesson, E; Akesson, E; Azizi, M; Ertzgaard, P; Hultling, C; Kjaeldgaard, A; Levi, R; Ringden, O; Westgren, M; Lammertse, D; Seiger, A. Obliteration of a posttraumatic spinal cord cyst with solid human embryonic spinal cord grafts: first clinical attempt. *J. Neurotrauma*. 1997;14(11):875-84.

Fehlings, MG; Tator, CH., Linden, RD. The effect of direct-current field on recovery from experimental spinal cord injury. *J. Neurosurg*. 1988;68(5):781-92.

Fluckiger, AC; Dehay, C; Savatier, P. Embryonic stem cells and cell replacement therapies in the nervous system. *Med. Sci.* (Paris). 2003;19(6-7):699-708.

Franco Lambert, AP; Fraga Zandonai, A; Bonatto, D et al. Differentiation of human adipose-derived adult stem cells into neuronal tissue: does it work? *Differentiation*. 2009; 77(3):221-8.

Franklin, RJ; Bayley, SA; Milner, R et al. Differentiation of the O-2A progenitor cell line CG-4 into oligodendrocytes and astrocytes following transplantation into glia-deficient areas of CNS white matter. *Glia*. 1995;13(1):39-44.

Franklin, RJ; Gilson, JM; Franceschini, IA; Barnett, SC. Schwann cell-like myelination following transplantation of an olfactory bulb-ensheathing cell line into areas of demyelination in the adult CNS. *Glia*. 1996; 17(3): 217-24.

Freeman, LW; Wright, TW. Experimental observations of concussion and contusion of the spinal cord. *Ann. Surg*. 1953;137(4):433-43.

Fregni, F; Otachi, PT; Do Valle, A et al. A randomized clinical trial of repetitive transcranial magnetic stimulation in patients with refractory epilepsy. *Ann. Neurol.* 2006; 60(4):447-55.

Frostick, SP; Yin, Q; Kemp, GJ. Schwann cells, neurotrophic factors, and peripheral nerve regeneration. *Microsurgery*. 1998;18(7):397-405.

Frotscher, M; Zimmer, J. GABAergic nonpyramidal neurons in intracerebral transplants of the rat hippocampus and fascia dentata: a combined light and electron microscopic immunocytochemical study. *J. Comp. Neurol.* 1987;259(2):266-76.

Fu, YS; Cheng, YC; Lin, M Y C et al. Conversion of human umbilical cord mesenchymal stem cells in Wharton's jelly to dopaminergic neurons in vitro: potential therapeutic application for Parkinsonism. *Stem Cells*. 2006;24(1):115-24.

Fusco, M; Vantini, G; Schiavo, N; Zanotti, A; Zanoni, R; Facci, L; Skaper, S D. Gangliosides and neurotrophic factors in neurodegenerative diseases: from experimental findings to clinical perspectives. *Ann. N Y Acad. Sci*. 1993. 24;695:314-7.

Gensel, JC; Nakamura, S; Guan, Z et al. Macrophages promote axon regeneration with concurrent neurotoxicity. *J. Neurosci*. 2009;29(12):3956-68.

Girdlestone, J; Limbani, VA; Cutler, AJ; Navarrete, CV. Efficient expansion of mesenchymal stromal cells from umbilical cord under low serum conditions. *Cytotherapy*. 2009;11(6):738-48.

Góra-Kupilas, K; Jośko, J. The neuroprotective function of vascular endothelial growth factor (VEGF). *Folia Neuropathol*. 2005;43(1):31-9.

Gorio, A; Torrente, Y; Madaschi, L et al. Fate of autologous dermal stem cells transplanted into the spinal cord after traumatic injury (TSCI). *Neuroscience*. 2004;125(1):179-89.

Gospodarowicz, D. Localisation of a fibroblast growth factor and its effect alone and with hydrocortisone on 3T3 cell growth. *Nature*. 1974;249(453):123-7.

Gospodarowicz, D. Purification of a fibroblast growth factor from bovine pituitary. *J. Biol. Chem*. 1975;250(7):2515-20.

Grondin, R; Gash, DM. Glial cell line-derived neurotrophic factor (GDNF): a drug candidate for the treatment of Parkinson's disease. *J. Neurol*. 1998;245(11 Suppl. 3):P35-42.

Gross, DS. Distribution of gonadotropin-releasing hormone in the mouse brain as revealed by immunohistochemistry. *Endocrinology*. 1976;98(6):1408-17.

Groves, AK; Barnett, SC; Franklin, RJ; Crang, AJ; Mayer, M; Blakemore, WF; Noble, M. Repair of demyelinated lesions by transplantation of purified O-2A progenitor cells. *Nature*. 1993;362(6419):453-5.

Haas, S; Weidner, N; Winkler, J. Adult stem cell therapy in stroke. *Curr. Opin. Neurol*. 2005;18(1):59-64.

Halberstadt, C; Emerich, DF; Gores, P. Use of Sertoli cell transplants to provide local immunoprotection for tissue grafts. *Expert Opin. Biol. Ther*. 2004;4(6):813-25.

Hamid, S;Hayek, R. Role of electrical stimulation for rehabilitation and regeneration after spinal cord injury: an overview. *Eur. Spine J*. 2008;17(9):1256-69.

Hernándeza, J; Torres-Espína, A; Navarro, X. Adult Stem Cell Transplants for Spinal Cord Injury Repair: Current State in Preclinical Research. *Curr. Stem Cell Res. Ther*. 2011;6(3):273-87.

Hochberg, LR; Serruya, MD; Friehs, GM; Mukand, JA; Saleh, M; Caplan, AH; Branner, A; Chen, D; Penn, RD; Donoghue, J P. Neuronal ensemble control of prosthetic devices by a human with tetraplegia. *Nature*. 2006;442:164-71.

Houlé, JD, Reier, PJ. Transplantation of fetal spinal cord tissue into the chronically injured adult rat spinal cord. *J. Comp. Neurol*. 1988;269(4):535-47.

Huang, H; Chen, L; Sanberg, P. Cell Therapy From Bench to Bedside Translation in CNS Neurorestoratology Era. *Cell Medicine, Part B of Cell Transplantation*. 2010; 1(1): 15–46.

Huang, H; Chen, L; Wang, H et al. Influence of patients' age on functional recovery after transplantation of olfactory ensheathing cells into injured spinal cord injury. *Chin. Med. J. (Engl.)*. 2003;116(10):1488-91.

Huang, H. Progress in Cellular Neurorestoratology: A Brief Introduction to the IANR Supplement Issue. *Cell Transplantation*, 2013; 22:S1-S3.

Hunt, CJ. Cryopreservation of Human Stem Cells for Clinical Application: A Review. *Transfus. Med. Hemother.* 2011;38(2):107-123.

Hunt, DP; Jahoda, C; Chandran, S. Multipotent skin-derived precursors: from biology to clinical translation. *Curr. Opin. Biotechnol.* 2009;20(5):522-30.

Hwang, DY; Kim, DS;, Kim, DW. Human ES and iPS cells as cell sources for the treatment of Parkinson's disease: current state and problems. *J. Cell. Biochem.* 2010; 109 (2):292-301.

Imaizumi, T; Lankford, KL; Kocsis, JD et al. Comparison of myelin-forming cells as candidates for therapeutic transplantation in demyelinated CNS axons. *No To Shinkei.* 2000;52(7):609-15.

Ishige, I; Nagamura-Inoue, T; Honda, M J et al. Comparison of mesenchymal stem cells derived from arterial, venous, and Wharton's jelly explants of human umbilical cord. *Int. J. Hematol.* 2009;90(2):261-9.

Kakishita, K; Elwan, M A; Nakao, N et al. Human amniotic epithelial cells produce dopamine and survive after implantation into the striatum of a rat model of Parkinson's disease: a potential source of donor for transplantation therapy. *Exp. Neurol.* 2000;165 (1):27-34.

Kang, KS; Kim, SW; Oh, YH et al. A 37-year-old spinal cord-injured female patient, transplanted of multipotent stem cells from human UC blood, with improved sensory perception and mobility, both functionally and morphologically: a case study. *Cytotherapy.* 2005;7(4):368-73.

Karussis, D; Kassis, I; Kurkalli, BG; Slavin, S. Immunomodulation and neuroprotection with mesenchymal bone marrow stem cells (MSCs): a proposed treatment for multiple sclerosis and other neuroimmunological/neurodegenerative diseases. *J. Neurol. Sci.* 2008; 265 (1-2):131-5.

Kiefer, JC. Primer and interviews: Promises and realities of induced pluripotent stem cells. *Dev. Dyn.* 2011;240(8):2034-41.

Kim, WS; Park, BS; Sung, JH. The wound-healing and antioxidant effects of adipose-derived stem cells. *Expert Opin. Biol. Ther.* 2009;9(7):879-87.

Knoller, N; Auerbach, G; Fulga, V et al. Clinical experience using incubated autologous macrophages as a treatment for complete spinal cord injury: phase I study results. *J. Neurosurg. Spine.* 2005;3(3):173-81.

Knotkova, H; Cruciani, RA. Non-invasive transcranial direct current stimulation for the study and treatment of neuropathic pain. *Methods Mol. Biol.* 2010;617:505-15.

Kokai, LE; Rubin, JP; Marra, KG. The potential of adipose-derived adult stem cells as a source of neuronal progenitor cells. *Plast. Reconstr. Surg.* 2005;116(5):1453-60.

Kooijman, R; Sarre, S; Michotte, Y; De Keyser, J. Insulin-like growth factor I: a potential neuroprotective compound for the treatment of acute ischemic stroke? *Stroke.* 2009; 40 (4):e83-8.

Koshizuka, S; Okada, S; Okawa, A et al. Transplanted hematopoietic stem cells from bone marrow differentiate into neural lineage cells and promote functional recovery after spinal cord injury in mice. *J. Neuropathol. Exp. Neurol.* 2004;63(1):64-72.

Kubo, A; Yoshida, T; Kobayashi, N et al. Efficient generation of dopamine neuron-like cells from skin-derived precursors with a synthetic peptide derived from von Hippel-Lindau protein. *Stem Cells Dev.* 2009;18(10):1523-32.

Kuzis, K; Eckenstein, FP. Ciliary neurotrophic factor as a motor neuron trophic factor. *Perspect. Dev. Neurobiol.* 1996;4(1):65-74.

Lapchak, PA. Therapeutic potentials for glial cell line-derived neurotrophic factor (GDNF) based upon pharmacological activities in the CNS. *Rev. Neurosci.* 1996;7(3):165-76.

Lee, JH; Chung, WH; Kang, EH; C et al. Schwann cell-like remyelination following transplantation of human umbilical cord blood (hUCB)-derived mesenchymal stem cells in dogs with acute spinal cord injury. *J. Neurol. Sci.* 2011;300(1-2):86-96.

Lefaucheur, JP. Stroke recovery can be enhanced by using repetitive transcranial magnetic stimulation (rTMS). *Neurophysiol. Clin.* 2006;36(3):105-15.

Lefaucheur, JP. The use of repetitive transcranial magnetic stimulation (rTMS) in chronic neuropathic pain. *Neurophysiol. Clin.* 2006;36(3):117-24.

Levi-Montalcini, R; Hamburger, V. Selective growth stimulating effects of mouse sarcoma on the sensory and sympathetic nervous system of the chick embryo. *J. Exp. Zool.* 1951; 116(2):321-61.

Li, JY; Christophersen, NS; Hall, V; Soulet, D; Brundin, P. Critical issues of clinical human embryonic stem cell therapy for brain repair. *Trends Neurosci.* 2008;31(3):146-53.

Li, Q; Brus-Ramer, M; Martin, JH; McDonald, JW. Electrical stimulation of the medullary pyramid promotes proliferation and differentiation of oligodendrocyte progenitor cells in the corticospinal tract of the adult rat. *Neurosci. Lett.* 2010;479(2): 128-33.

Li, Y; Chopp, M; Chen, J; Wang, L; Gautam, SC; Xu, YX; Zhang, Z. Intrastriatal transplantation of bone marrow nonhematopoietic cells improves functional recovery after stroke in adult mice. *J. Cereb. Blood Flow Metab.* 2000;20(9):1311-9.

Li, Y;Field, PM; Raisman, G. Regeneration of adult rat corticospinal axons induced by transplanted olfactory ensheathing cells. *J. Neurosci.* 1998;18(24):10514-24.

Li, Y; Field, PM; Raisman, G. Repair of adult rat corticospinal tract by transplants of olfactory ensheathing cells. *Science.* 1997;277(5334):2000-2.

Lima, C; Pratas-Vital, J; Escada, P; Hasse-Ferreira, A; Capucho, C; Peduzzi, JD. Olfactory mucosa autografts in human spinal cord injury: a pilot clinical study. *J. Spinal Cord Med.* 2006;29:191-203.

Lin, LF; Doherty, DH; Lile, JD, et al. GDNF: a glial cell line-derived neurotrophic factor for midbrain dopaminergic neurons. *Science.* 1993; 260(5111):1130-2.

Lin, LF; Mismer, D; Lile, JD; Armes, LG; Butler, ET. 3rd, Vannice, J. L; Collins, F. Purification, cloning, and expression of ciliary neurotrophic factor (CNTF). *Science.* 1989;246(4933):1023-5.

Lindsay, RM; Thoenen, H; Barde, Y A. Placode and neural crest-derived sensory neurons are responsive at early developmental stages to brain-derived neurotrophic factor. *Dev. Biol.* 1985;112(2):319-28.

Lindsay, RM. Neurotrophic growth factors and neurodegenerative diseases: therapeutic potential of the neurotrophins and ciliary neurotrophic factor. *Neurobiol. Aging.* 1994; 15 (2):249-51.

Liste, I; García-García, E; Martínez-Serrano, A. The generation of dopaminergic neurons by human neural stem cells is enhanced by Bcl-XL, both in vitro and in vivo. *J. Neurosci.* 2004;24(48):10786-95.

Liu, F; Uchugonova, A; Kimura, H; Zhang, C; Zhao, M; Zhang, L; Koenig, K; Duong, J; Aki, R; Saito, N; Mii, S; Amoh, Y; Katsuoka, K; Hoffman, R M. The bulge area is the major hair follicle source of nestin-expressing pluripotent stem cells which can repair the spinal cord compared to the dermal papilla. *Cell Cycle*. 2011;10(5):830-9.

Liu, S; Qu, Y; Stewart, TJ; Howard, MJ; Chakrabortty, S; Holekamp, TF; McDonald, JW. Embryonic stem cells differentiate into oligodendrocytes and myelinate in culture and after spinal cord transplantation. *Proc. Natl. Acad. Sci. US*. 2000;97(11):6126-31.

Locke, M; Windsor, J; Dunbar, PR. Human adipose-derived stem cells: isolation, characterization and applications in surgery. *ANZ J. Surg*. 2009;79(4):235-44.

Loh, YS; Hwang, W Y; Ratnagopal, P. Autologous haematopoietic stem cell transplantation for the treatment of multiple sclerosis. *Ann. Acad. Med. Singapore*. 2007; 36(6):421-6.

López-González, R;Kunckles, P; Velasco, I. Transient recovery in a rat model of familial amyotrophic lateral sclerosis after transplantation of motor neurons derived from mouse embryonic stem cells. *Cell Transplant*. 2009;18(10):1171-81.

López-Lozano, JJ; Bravo, G; Brera, B et al. Long-term follow-up in 10 Parkinson's disease patients subjected to fetal brain grafting into a cavity in the caudate nucleus: the Clinica Puerta de Hierro experience. CPH Neural Transplantation Group. *Transplant. Proc*. 1995;27(1):1395-400.

Löscher, W; Ebert, U; Lehmann, H et al. Seizure suppression in kindling epilepsy by grafts of fetal GABAergic neurons in rat substantia nigra. *J. Neurosci. Res*. 1998;51(2):196-209.

Low, CB; Liou, YC; Tang, BL. Neural differentiation and potential use of stem cells from the human umbilical cord for central nervous system transplantation therapy. *J. Neurosci. Res*. 2008;86(8):1670-9.

Luo, J; Bo, X; Wu, D; Yeh, J; Richardson, P M; Zhang, Y. Promoting survival, migration, and integration of transplanted Schwann cells by over-expressing polysialic acid. *Glia*. 2011;59(3):424-34.

Luzhetskaia, TA; Gorbunov, FE; Knyshenko, V I. Neurorehabilitation. *Med. Sestra*. 1974; 33(10):15-20.

Madrazo, I; Franco-Bourland, RE; Castrejon, H et al. Fetal striatal homotransplantation for Huntington's disease: first two case reports. *Neurol. Res*. 1995;17(4):312-5.

Maisonpierre, PC; Belluscio, L; Squinto, S; Ip, NY; Furth, ME; Lindsay, RM; Yancopoulos, GD. Neurotrophin-3: a neurotrophic factor related to NGF and BDNF. *Science*. 1990;247(4949 Pt 1):1446-51.

Mandalfino, P; Rice, G; Smith, A et al. Bone marrow transplantation in multiple sclerosis. *J. Neurol*. 2000;247(9):691-5.

Marchionini, DM; Subramanian, T; Bumette, B et al. Dopaminergic properties of retinal pigmented epithelial cells attached to microcarriers (RPE-M) transplanted into parkinsonian animals. *Exp. Neurol*. 1999; 3: 559-608.

Masip, M; Veiga, A; Izpisúa Belmonte, JC; Simón, C. Reprogramming with defined factors: from induced pluripotency to induced transdifferentiation. *Mol. Hum. Reprod*. 2010;16(11):856-68.

McDonald, JW; Liu, XZ; Qu, Y; Liu, S; Mickey, SK; Turetsky, D; Gottlieb, DI; Choi, DW. Transplanted embryonic stem cells survive, differentiate and promote recovery in injured rat spinal cord. *Nat. Med*. 1999; 5:1410-2.

Meng, XT; Chen, D; Dong, ZY; Liu, JM. Enhanced neural differentiation of neural stem cells and neurite growth by amniotic epithelial cell co-culture. *Cell Biol. Int*. 2007;31(7): 691-8.

Michejda, M. Treatment of Parkinson's disease in adult patients by transplantation of human fetal brain tissue obtained from elective abortions. *Fetal Ther.* 1987;2(3):129-34.

Miki, T; Strom, SC. Amnion-derived pluripotent/multipotent stem cells. *Stem Cell Rev.* 2006;2(2):133-42.

Minassian, K; Jilge, B; Rattay, F; Pinter, MM; Binder, H; Gerstenbrand, F; Dimitrijevic, MR. Stepping-like movements in humans with complete spinal cord injury induced by epidural stimulation of the lumbar cord: electromyographic study of compound muscle action potentials. *Spinal Cord.* 2004; 42:401-16.

Miron, VE; Kuhlmann, T; Antel, JP. Cells of the oligodendroglial lineage, myelination, and remyelination. *Biochim. Biophys. Acta.* 2011;1812(2):184-93.

Mital, P; Kaur, G; Dufour, JM. Immunoprotective sertoli cells: making allogeneic and xenogeneic transplantation feasible. *Reproduction.* 2010;139(3):495-504.

Mizuno, H. Adipose-derived stem cells for tissue repair and regeneration: ten years of research and a literature review. *J. Nippon Med. Sch.* 2009;76(2):56-66.

Nakama, H; Ohsugi, K; Otsuki, T; Date, I; Kosuga, M; Okuyama, T; Sakuragawa, N. Encapsulation cell therapy for mucopolysaccharidosis type VII using genetically engineered immortalized human amniotic epithelial cells. *Tohoku J. Exp. Med.* 2006; 209 (1):23-32.

Namiecińska, M; Marciniak, K; Nowak, JZ. VEGF as an angiogenic, neurotrophic, and neuroprotective factor. *Postepy Hig. Med. Dosw.* (Online). 2005;59:573-83.

Nashold, BS; Friedman, H; Glenn, JF; Grimes, JH; Barry, WF; Avery, R. Electromicturition in paraplegia: implantation of a spinal neuroprosthesis. *Proc. Veterans Adm. Spinal Cord Inj. Conf.* 1971;18:161-5.

Nekanti, U; Mohanty, L; Venugopal, P et al. Optimization and scale-up of Wharton's jelly-derived mesenchymal stem cells for clinical applications. *Stem Cell Res.* 2010; 5(3):244-54.

Newman, MB; Bakay, RA. Therapeutic potentials of human embryonic stem cells in Parkinson's disease. *Neurotherapeutics.* 2008;5(2):237-51.

Nikkhah, G; Rosenthal, C;Falkenstein, G et al. Microtransplantation of dopaminergic cell suspensions: further characterization and optimization of grafting parameters. *Cell Transplant.* 2009;18(2):119-33.

Nosrat, IV; Widenfalk, J; Olson, L; Nosrat, CA. Dental pulp cells produce neurotrophic factors, interact with trigeminal neurons in vitro, and rescue motoneurons after spinal cord injury. *Dev. Biol.* 2001;238(1):120-32.

Nygren, LG; Olson, L; Seiger, A. Mnoaminergic reinnervation of the transected spinal cord by homologous fetal brain grafts. *Brain Res.* 1977;129(2):227-35.

Ogawa, R. The importance of adipose-derived stem cells and vascularized tissue regeneration in the field of tissue transplantation. *Curr. Stem Cell Res. Ther.* 2006;1(1):13-20.

Ogawa, S; Tokumoto, Y; Miyake, J; Nagamune, T. Induction of oligodendrocyte differentiation from adult human fibroblast-derived induced pluripotent stem cells. *In Vitro Cell Dev. Biol. Anim.* 2011;47(7):464-9.

Olson, L; Backlund, EO; Ebendal, T; Freedman, R; Hamberger, B; Hansson, P; Hoffer, B; Lindblom, U; Meyerson, B; Strömberg, I et al. Intraputaminal infusion of nerve growth factor to support adrenal medullary autografts in Parkinson's disease. One-year follow-up of first clinical trial. *Arch. Neurol.* 1991;48(4):373-81.

Olson, L; Backlund, EO; Sedvall, G; Herrera-Marschitz, M; Ungerstedt, U; Strömberg, I; Hoffer, B; Seiger, Å. Intrastriatal chromaffin grafts in experimental and clinical Parkinsonism: first impressions. In: E. Usdin, A. Carlsson, A. Dahlström, J. Engel, eds. *Alan. Catecholamines. Part C. Neuropharmacology and Central Nervous System-Therapeutic Aspects.* New York: Alan R Liss. Inc.: 1984; pp. 195-201.

Onose, G; Grozea, C; Anghelescu, A; Daia, C; Sinescu, CJ; Ciurea, AV; Spircu, T; Mirea, A; Andone, I; Spânu, A; Popescu, C; Mihăescu, AS; Fazli, S; Danóczy, M; Popescu, F. On the feasibility of using motor imagery EEG-based brain-computer interface in chronic tetraplegics for assistive robotic arm control: a clinical test and long-term post-trial follow-up. *Spinal Cord.* 2012;50:599-608.

Papadopoulos, KI; Low, SS; Aw, TC; Chantarojanasiri, T. Safety and feasibility of autologous umbilical cord blood transfusion in 2 toddlers with cerebral palsy and the role of low dose granulocyte-colony stimulating factor injections. *Restor. Neurol. Neurosci.* 2011;29(1):17-22.

Pape, TL; Rosenow, J; Lewis, G. Transcranial magnetic stimulation: a possible treatment for TBI. *J. Head Trauma Rehabil.* 2006;21(5):437-51.

Peng, J; Wang, Y; Zhang, L et al. Human umbilical cord Wharton's jelly-derived mesenchymal stem cells differentiate into a Schwann-cell phenotype and promote neurite outgrowth in vitro. *Brain Res. Bull.* 2011;84(3):235-43.

Peterson, DA. Umbilical cord blood cells and brain stroke injury: bringing in fresh blood to address an old problem. *J. Clin. Invest.* 2004;114(3):312-4.

Polanía, R; Paulus, W; Nitsche, MA. Modulating cortico-striatal and thalamo-cortical functional connectivity with transcranial direct current stimulation. *Hum. Brain Mapp.* 2011.

Polson, MJ; Barker, AT; Freeston, IL. Stimulation of nerve trunks with time-varying magnetic fields. *Med. Biol. Eng. Comput.* 1982;20(2):243-4.

Prewitt, CM; Niesman, IR; Kane, CJ; Houlé, JD. Activated macrophage/microglial cells can promote the regeneration of sensory axons into the injured spinal cord. *Exp. Neurol.* 1997;148(2):433-43.

Prieto, M; Chauvet, N; Alonso, G. Tanycytes transplanted into the adult rat spinal cord support the regeneration of lesioned axons. *Exp. Neurol.* 2000;161(1):27-37.

Proulx, S; Fradette, J; Gauvin, R et al. Stem cells of the skin and cornea: their clinical applications in regenerative medicine. *Curr. Opin. Organ Transplant.* 2011; 16(1): 83-9.

Rabinovich, SS; Seledtsov, VI; Poveschenko, O V et al. Transplantation treatment of spinal cord injury patients. *Biomed. Pharmacother.* 2003;57(9):428-33.

Ramon y Cajal, S. *Degeneration and regeneration of the nervous system.* Volume 2. New York, US: Haffner Publishing Co.; 1928.

Ramón-Cueto, A; Cordero, MI; Santos-Benito, FF; Avila, J. Functional recovery of paraplegic rats and motor axon regeneration in their spinal cords by olfactory ensheathing glia. *Neuron.* 2000;25(2):425-35.

Ramón-Cueto, A; Nieto-Sampedro, M. Regeneration into the spinal cord of transected dorsal root axons is promoted by ensheathing glia transplants. *Exp. Neurol.* 1994;127(2):232-44.

Reier, PJ; Bregman, BS; Wujek, JR. Intraspinal transplantation of embryonic spinal cord tissue in neonatal and adult rats. *J. Comp. Neurol.* 1986;247(3):275-96.

Ren, Z; Zhang, Y. Cells therapy for Parkinson's disease--so close and so far away. *Sci. China C Life Sci.* 2009;52(7):610-4.

Rhee, Y H; Ko, J Y; Chang, M Y et al. Protein-based human iPS cells efficiently generate functional dopamine neurons and can treat a rat model of Parkinson disease. *J. Clin. Invest.* 2011;121(6):2326-35.

Ridet, JL; Sarkis, C; Serguera, C et al. Transplantation of human adult astrocytes: efficiency and safety requirements for an autologous gene therapy. *J. Neurosci. Res.* 2003;72(6):704-8.

Rinderknecht, E; Humbel, RE. The amino acid sequence of human insulin-like growth factor I and its structural homology with proinsulin. *J. Biol. Chem.* 1978; 253 (8): 2769-76.

Rogojan, C; Frederiksen, JL. Hematopoietic stem cell transplantation in multiple sclerosis. *Acta Neurol. Scand.* 2009;120(6):371-82.

Rosenberg, MB; Friedmann, T; Robertson, R C; Tuszynski, M; Wolff, J A; Breakefield, X O; Gage, FH. Grafting genetically modified cells to the damaged brain: restorative effects of NGF expression. *Science.* 1988;242(4885):1575-8.

Rosenbluth, J; Hasegawa, M; Shirasaki, N et al. Myelin formation following transplantation of normal fetal glia into myelin-deficient rat spinal cord. *J. Neurocytol.* 1990;19(5):718-30.

Rosenkranz, K; Meier, C. Umbilical cord blood cell transplantation after brain ischemia-From recovery of function to cellular mechanisms. *Ann. Anat.* 2011;193(4):371-9.

Rothwell, JC. Plasticity in the human motor system. *Folia Phoniatr. Logop.* 2010;62(4): 153-7.

Saberi, H; Moshayedi, P; Aghayan, HR et al. Treatment of chronic thoracic spinal cord injury patients with autologous Schwann cell transplantation: an interim report on safety considerations and possible outcomes. *Neurosci. Lett.* 2008;443(1):46-50.

Saccardi, R; Mancardi, GL; Solari, A et al. Autologous HSCT for severe progressive multiple sclerosis in a multicenter trial: impact on disease activity and quality of life. *Blood.* 2005;105(6):2601-7.

Safford, KM; Rice, HE. Stem cell therapy for neurologic disorders: therapeutic potential of adipose-derived stem cells. *Curr. Drug Targets.* 2005;6(1):57-62.

Sanberg, PR; Borlongan, CV; Othberg, A I et al. Testis-derived Sertoli cells have a trophic effect on dopamine neurons and alleviate hemiparkinsonism in rats. *Nat. Med.* 1997; 3(10):1129-32.

Sanberg, PR; Borlongan, CV; Saporta, S; Cameron, DF. Testis-derived Sertoli cells survive and provide localized immunoprotection for xenografts in rat brain. *Nat. Biotechnol.* 1996;14(13):1692-5.

Sanberg, PR; Eve, D J;Willing, AE et al. The treatment of neurodegenerative disorders using umbilical cord blood and menstrual blood-derived stem cells. *Cell Transplant.* 2011; 20(1):85-94.

Sanberg, PR; Willing, AE; Garbuzova-Davis, SS et al. Umbilical cord blood-derived stem cells and brain repair. *Ann. NY Acad. Sci.* 2005;1049:67-83.

Sariola, H;Sainio, K; Arumäe, U; Saarma, M. Neurotrophins and ciliary neurotrophic factor: their biology and pathology. *Ann. Med.* 1994;26(5):355-63.

Sasaki, M; Lankford, K L; Brown, R J et al. Focal experimental autoimmune encephalomyelitis in the Lewis rat induced by immunization with myelin oligodendrocyte glycoprotein and intraspinal injection of vascular endothelial growth factor. *Glia.* 2010;58(13):1523-31.

Sasaki, R; Aoki, S; Yamato, M et al. Tubulation with dental pulp cells promotes facial nerve regeneration in rats. *Tissue Eng. Part A*. 2008;14(7):1141-7.

Sendtner, M; Arakawa, Y; Stöckli, KA; Kreutzberg, GW; Thoenen, H. Effect of ciliary neurotrophic factor (CNTF) on motoneuron survival. *J. Cell Sci. Suppl*. 1991;15:103-9.

Sendtner, M. Therapy development in spinal muscular atrophy. *Nat. Neurosci*. 2010;13(7): 795-9.

Sieradzan, K; Vrbová, G. Replacement of missing motoneurons by embryonic grafts in the rat spinal cord. *Neuroscience*. 1989;31(1):115-30.

Simeral, JD; Kim, SP; Black, MJ; Donoghue, JP; Hochberg, LR. Neural control of cursor trajectory and click by a human with tetraplegia 1000 days after implant of an intracortical microelectrode array. *J. Neural Eng*. 2011;8:025027.

Sironi, VA. Origin and evolution of deep brain stimulation. *Front. Integr. Neurosci*. 2011;5: 42.

Stenevi, U; Björklund, A; Svendgaard, NA. Transplantation of central and peripheral monoamine neurons to the adult rat brain: techniques and conditions for survival. *Brain Res*. 1976;114(1):1-20.

Stover, NP; Bakay, R A; Subramanian, T; Raiser, CD; Cornfeldt, ML; Schweikert, AW; Allen, RC; Watts, RL. Intrastriatal implantation of human retinal pigment epithelial cells attached to microcarriers in advanced Parkinson disease. *Arch. Neurol*. 2005;62(12):1833-7.

Strafella, AP; Ko, JH; Monchi, O. Therapeutic application of transcranial magnetic stimulation in Parkinson's disease: the contribution of expectation. *Neuroimage*. 2006; 31 (4):1666-72.

Strömberg, I; Bickford, P; Gerhardt, GA. Grafted dopamine neurons: Morphology, neurochemistry, and electrophysiology. *Prog. Neurobiol*. 2010;90(2):190-7.

Subramanian, T; Bumette, B; Miller, GW et al. Characterization of the dopaminergic properties of human retinal pigmented epithelial(hRPE)cells and the efect of intrastriatal transplantation of hRPE cells in hemiparkinsonian (HP)monkeys. *Mov. Disord*. 1998; 13 (2): 268.

Subramanian, T; Marchionini, D; Potter, EM; Cornfeldt, M L. Striatal xenotransplantation of human retinal pigment epithelial cells attached to microcarriers in hemiparkinsonian rats ameliorates behavioral deficits without provoking a host immune response. *Cell Transplant*. 2002;11(3):207-14.

Subramanian, T. Cell transplantation for the treatment of Parkinson's disease. *Semin. Neurol*. 2001;21(1):103-15.

Tachibana, S; Okada, K; Ohwada, T; Yada, K. Posterior longitudinal myelotomy as a surgical treatment of acute cervical spinal cord injury. *No Shinkei Geka*. 1984;12(2):183-8.

Takizawa, S. Differentiation of adult bone marrow cells into neurons and endothelial cells in rat brain after stroke in the presence of cytokines. *Rinsho Shinkeigaku*. 2003;43(11):830-1.

Tessler, A. Intraspinal transplants. *Ann. Neurol*. 1991;29(2):115-23.

Thoenen, H; Barde, YA; Davies, AM; Johnson, JE. Neurotrophic factors and neuronal death. *Ciba Found. Symp*. 1987;126:82-95.

Toda, A; Okabe, M; Yoshida, T; Nikaido, T. The potential of amniotic membrane/amnion-derived cells for regeneration of various tissues. *J. Pharmacol. Sci*. 2007;105(3):215-28.

Tomaskovic-Crook, E; Crook, JM. Human embryonic stem cell therapies for neurodegenerative diseases. *CNS Neurol. Disord. Drug Targets*. 2011;10(4):440-8.

Torrente, Y; Polli, E. Mesenchymal stem cell transplantation for neurodegenerative diseases. *Cell Transplant*. 2008;17(10-11):1103-13.

Toyoda, M; Cui, Ch; Umezawa, A. Myogenic transdifferentiation of menstrual blood-derived cells. *Acta Myol*. 2007;26(3):176-8.

Trujillo, CA; Schwindt, TT; Martins, AH et al. Novel perspectives of neural stem cell differentiation: from neurotransmitters to therapeutics. *Cytometry A*. 2009;75(1):38-53.

Tuszynski, MH; Thal, L; Pay, M; Salmon, D P; U. H. S; Bakay, R; Patel, P; Blesch, A; Vahlsing, HL; Ho, G; Tong, G; Potkin, SG; Fallon, J; Hansen, L; Mufson, EJ; Kordower, JH; Gall, C; Conner, J. A phase 1 clinical trial of nerve growth factor gene therapy for Alzheimer disease. *Nat. Med*. 2005;11(5):551-5.

Tyndall, A; Koike, T. High-dose immunoablative therapy with hematopoietic stem cell support in the treatment of severe autoimmune disease: current status and future direction. *Intern. Med*. 2002;41(8):608-12.

Tyvaert, L; Houdayer, E; Devanne, H et al. The effect of repetitive transcranial magnetic stimulation on dystonia: a clinical and pathophysiological approach. *Neurophysiol. Clin*. 2006; 36(3):135-43.

Ueda, S. Rehabilitation in neural diseases, with emphasis on apoplexy. *Sogo Igaku*. 1963;20: 107-20.

Von Wild, K; Rabischong, P; Brunelli, G; Benichou, M; Krishnan, K. Computer added locomotion by implanted electrical stimulation in paraplegic patients (SUAW). *Acta Neurochir. Suppl*. 2002; 79:99-104.

Wallace, BA; Ashkan, K; Benabid, AL. Deep brain stimulation for the treatment of chronic, intractable pain. *Neurosurg. Clin. N. Am*. 2004;15(3):343-57, vii.

Wang, A; Tang, Z; Park, IH et al. Induced pluripotent stem cells for neural tissue engineering. *Biomaterials*. 2011;32(22):5023-32.

Watters, DJ; Hendry, IA. Purification of a ciliary neurotrophic factor from bovine heart. *J. Neurochem*. 1987;49(3):705-13.

Weiss, ML; Medicetty, S; Bledsoe, AR; Rachakatla, RS; Choi, M; Merchav, S; Luo, Y; Rao, MS; Velagaleti, G; Troyer, D. Human umbilical cord matrix stem cells: preliminary characterization and effect of transplantation in a rodent model of Parkinson's disease. *Stem Cells*. 2006;24(3):781-92.

Weiss, ML; Mitchell, KE; Hix, JE; Medicetty, S; El-Zarkouny, SZ; Grieger, D; Troyer, DL. Transplantation of porcine umbilical cord matrix cells into the rat brain. *Exp. Neurol*. 2003;182(2):288-99.

Wernig, M; Zhao, JP; Pruszak, J; Hedlund, E; Fu, D; Soldner, F; Broccoli, V; Constantine-Paton, M; Isacson, O; Jaenisch, R. Neurons derived from reprogrammed fibroblasts functionally integrate into the fetal brain and improve symptoms of rats with Parkinson's disease. *Proc. Natl. Acad. Sci. US*. 2008 ;105(15):5856-61.

Willing, AE; Cameron, DF; Sanberg, PR. Sertoli cell transplants: their use in the treatment of neurodegenerative disease. *Mol. Med. Today*. 1998;4(11):471-7.

Xu, XX; Shao, XM; Yu, F et al. Effects of tanycytes transplantation on the motor function score and rubrospinal motor evoked potentials of adult rats after spinal cord completely transected. *Zhongguo Ying Yong Sheng Li Xue Za Zhi*. 2010;26(4):433-5.

Yalvac, ME; Rizvanov, A A; Kilic, E et al. Potential role of dental stem cells in the cellular therapy of cerebral ischemia. *Curr. Pharm. Des*. 2009;15(33):3908-16.

Yang, WZ; Zhang, Y; Wu, F et al. Human umbilical cord blood-derived mononuclear cell transplantation: case series of 30 subjects with hereditary ataxia. *J. Transl. Med.* 2011; 9: 65.

Yang, X; Song, L; Wu, N et al. An experimental study on intracerebroventricular transplantation of human amniotic epithelial cells in a rat model of Parkinson's disease. *Neurol. Res*. 2010;32(10):1054-9.

Yarygin, KN; Kholodenko, IV; Konieva, AA et al. Mechanisms of positive effects of transplantation of human placental mesenchymal stem cells on recovery of rats after experimental ischemic stroke. *Bull. Exp. Biol. Med*. 2009;148(6):862-8.

Young, W; DeCrescito, V; Flamm, ES; Blight, AR; Gruner, JA. Pharmacological therapy of acute spinal cord injury: studies of high dose methylprednisolone and naloxone. *Clin. Neurosurg*. 1988;34:675-97.

Young, W; Flamm, ES. Effect of high-dose corticosteroid therapy on blood flow, evoked potentials, and extracellular calcium in experimental spinal injury. *J. Neurosurg*. 1982; 57 (5):667-73.

Yu, JM; Bunnell, BA; Kang, SK. Neural differentiation of human adipose tissue-derived stem cells. *Methods Mol. Biol*. 2011;702:219-31.

Yu, S J; Soncini, M; Kaneko, Y et al. Amnion: a potent graft source for cell therapy in stroke. *Cell Transplant*. 2009;18(2):111-8.

Yuen, EC; Howe, CL; Li, Y et al. Nerve growth factor and the neurotrophic factor hypothesis. *Brain Dev*. 1996;18(5):362-8.

Yuen, EC; Mobley, WC. Therapeutic applications of neurotrophic factors in disorders of motor neurons and peripheral nerves. *Mol. Med. Today*. 1995;1(6):278-86.

Zachary, I. Neuroprotective role of vascular endothelial growth factor: signalling mechanisms, biological function, and therapeutic potential. *Neurosignals*. 2005;14(5): 207-21.

Zavan, B; Michelotto, L; Lancerotto, L et al. Neural potential of a stem cell population in the adipose and cutaneous tissues. *Neurol. Res*. 2010;32(1):47-54.

Zhang, WC; Ding, YJ;Cao, JK et al. Intracerebral co-grafting of Schwann's cells and fetal adrenal medulla in the treatment of Parkinson's disease. *Chin. Med. J*. (Engl.). 1994; 107(8):583-8.

Zhang, X; Mei, Y; Liu, C; Yu, S. Effect of transcranial magnetic stimulation on the expression of c-Fos and brain-derived neurotrophic factor of the cerebral cortex in rats with cerebral infarct. *J. Huazhong Univ. Sci. Technolog. Med. Sci*. 2007;27(4):415-8.

Zhao, J; Xu, Q. Emerging restorative treatments for Parkinson's disease: manipulation and inducement of dopaminergic neurons from adult stem cells. *CNS Neurol. Disord. Drug Targets*. 2011;10(4):509-16.

Zimmermann, M. Electrical stimulation of the human brain. *Hum. Neurobiol*. 1982;1 (4):227-9.

In: Neurorestoratology, Volume 1
Editors: H. Huang, G. Raisman, P. R. Sanberg et al.
ISBN: 978-1-63463-599-8


*Chapter 3*

# Neurorestorative Process, Law and Mechanisms

***Hongyun Huang*[1,2*] *and Lin Chen*[3,4]**
[1]Beijing Rehabilitation Hospital of Capital Medical University, Beijing, China
[2]Beijing Hongtianji Neuroscience Academy, Beijing, China
[3]Tsinghua University Yuquan Hospital, Beijing, China
[4]Medical Center,Tsinghua University, Beijing, China

The concept of neurorestoration was merely taken as a strategy at the beginning, which means that cellular and structural elements that have been lost are replaced, and their function is restored after treatment in degenerative diseases (e.g. Parkinson's disease) (Liu CY, et al. 2003). Because there was a loss of the dopamine phenotype in patients with PD initially, the neurorestoration therapy restored the dopamine phenotype through changing the pathophysiological environment or through cell transplantation or endogenously repopulating dopamine neurons (Airavaara M et al., 2012).

Today the term "Neurorestoration" means partly or completely restoring or maintaining the integrity of neurological functions and/or structures, with the emphasis on functional integrity by neurorestorative strategies, which include physical (i.e, electronic or magnetic), chemical (for instance medicine and factors), biological (such as cell therapy, molecule, bioengineering and tissue engineering), surgical and other kinds of interventions (International Association of Neurorestoratology, 2009). Currently known neurorestorative mechanisms as the basis of *CNS Neurorestorable theory* include neuroprotection, neuroplasticity (neurosynapsis, neural circuit or network reconstruction), neuromodulation, immunomodulation, axonal regeneration, sprouting, remyelination or neurorepair, neuroregeneration or neurogenesis, neuroreplacement, angiogenesis and so on (Huang H et al., 2010; Karussis D et al., 2010; Lima C et al., 2006).

* Corresponding author: Hongyun Huang hongyunh@gmail.com.

Herein, we introduce the Neurorestorative Process and Law, and describe briefly several important neurorestorative mechanisms, including neuromodulation, neuroprotection, neuroplasticity, and neurogenesis/ neuroregeneration.

# 1. The Term of Neurorestorative Process and Law

No matter what reasons cause the neural insults, they most likely make neurons (its soma and fiber) and glia or environment to present at the physiological stage or different stages of pathophysiological change. That is, neurons in part or all may be in unhealthy, excitotoxicity, abnormal autophagy or death (necrosis and apoptosis). At the same time, restoring by nature or intervention occurs through a wide variety of neurorestorative mechanisms. Unfortunately, those mechanisms in response to different insults have been studied and viewed in isolation. All those related factors are not independents and have close relation with one another, so the entire attacking or insults and restoring mechanisms should be put and generalized as a whole in this *Neurorestorative Process.* The concept "*Neurorestorative Process"* refers to the entire changing process of the dynamic interaction between neural insults and restorative mechanisms, which are divided into a physiological state and three types of – early, middle, and final – pathophysiological states in Figure 1-1.

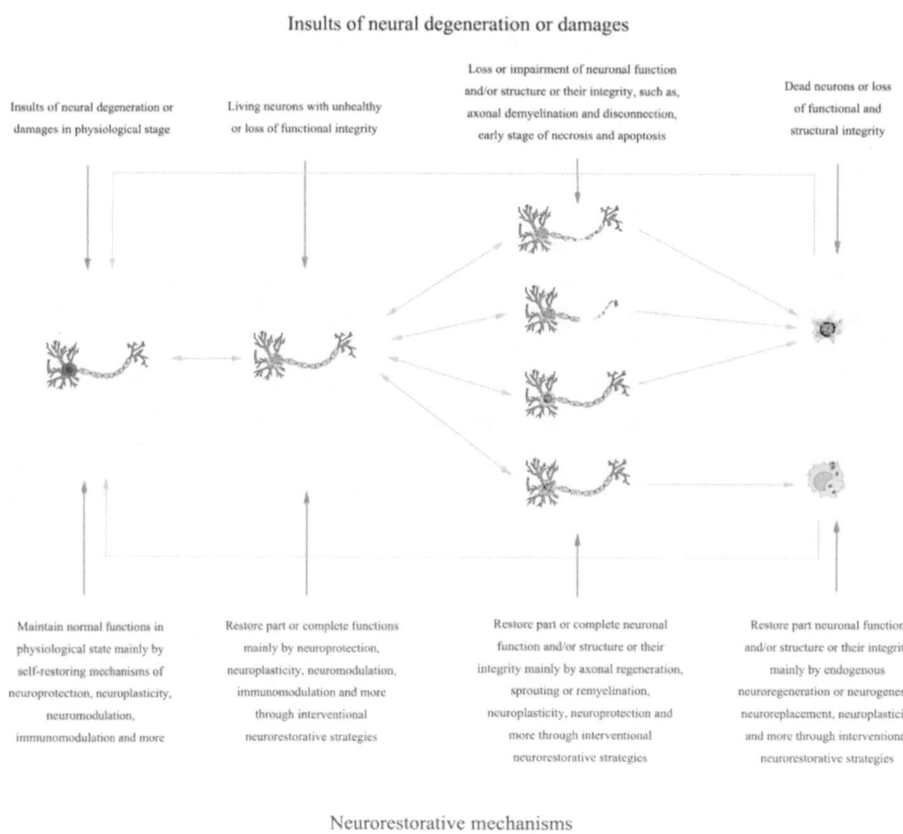


Figure 1.1. Neurorestorative process.

*Neurorestorative Process* illustrates the full dynamic neural changing course for all animal lives, including humans' and all neural activity in the physiological and pathophysiological states. More importantly, from the *Neurorestorative Process*, it is clearly to find that insults and restoration are two aspects of a contradiction unity. As long as insults occur, they must be accompanied by restoration. Self-restoration may not be enough in serious situation, so appropriate intervention should be taken to enhance functional restoration. Excitingly we have revealed the *Neurorestorative Law* from the *Neurorestorative Process, that is, more or less self-restoring always occurs by nature while facing insults, further active (appropriate) medical intervention better restores functions (this law may be simplified as: facing insults, self-restore by nature; appropriate intervention better restore functions).* The *Neurorestorative Law* fits the past, the present, and the future in all physiological, psychological, spiritual neural activities. The exploration by this law is endless, which includes time, neurorestorative extent, mechanisms, and strategies.

## Physiological State

To maintain normal functions in physiological state mainly by neuroprotection, neuroplasticity neuromodulation, and/or immunomodulation through self-restoring mechanisms while facing insults of physiological neural degeneration or damages.

## Pathophysiological States

When neurons, via self-restoring mechanism, cannot keep their physiological functions from attacking insults, they will be worsening at the pathophysiological states.

1) **The early stage:** the past or ongoing insults which resulted in unhealthy but living neurons or neurons losing function but maintaining structural integrity, can be limited to further deterioration, or be able to restored partial or complete functions by neuroprotection, neuroplasticity, neuromodulation, immunomodulation and etc.
2) **The middle stage:** the past insults which caused the loss or impairment of neuronal function and/or structure or their integrity, can be completely or partly restored through axonal regeneration, sprouting, remyelination, neurorepair, neuroplasticity and etc.
3) **The final stage:** the past insults which have ceased and have no prospect of recurring but led to dead neurons or loss of functional and structural integrity can be restored through endogenous neuroregeneration or neurogenesis, neuroplasticity, neuroreplacement and etc.

In view of the entire process of neuron lifespan from the normal state to the final death in Figure 1-1, which is probably an example of the entire nervous system, restoring mechanisms are throughout the whole process.

It is only neurorestoration that can accurately elucidate and expresses the real implications of the whole neurorestorative process. Each important neurorestorative mechanism plays certain role in the physiological or different pathophysiological stages, but only limited to certain parts, not as a whole.

Unfortunately, this process of dynamic changing interactions between neural insults and restorative mechanisms has been ignored over a century. Why? There are four main reasons. Firstly, conventional viewpoint has denied the possibility of CNS neurorestoration. Secondly, no overview has been presented in this field, attentions on shredded tactical or local details. Thirdly, all those mechanisms in response to different insults were studied and viewed in isolation. Fourthly, in the past and even now, the majority in the neuroscience have paid more attention on or overemphasized neuroregeneration, and taken it as the main direction for neuroscience.

As showed in Figure 1-1 that no one kind of neurorestorative mechanism, such as, neuroprotection, neuroplasticity, neuromodulation or neuroregeneration, can reflect or exert all roles in the neurorestorative process. For example, neuroregeneration or neurogenesis may only serve at the final stage of neuron death. Yet, we do not know whether or how much neuroregeneration or neurogenesis can occur?

Even if it really happens; it is not equal to having a functional restoration. So, overemphasizing neuroregeneration has possibly become a centurial directional mistake. It should no longer direct the development of neuroscience in the future.

In addition, Figure 1-1 shows some more important information.

(1) In view of the process of disease development, the insults for each or several cells can be clearly seen at some states, but insults for the entire nervous system must be seen in the mixtural states whose clinical presentation are shown as main attacks and impairments.
(2) In view of the action mode of different neurorestorative mechanisms, theoretically, they can be clearly separated, but in reality, they often play joint roles and should not be separated from one another in clinical practices.
(3) In view of the preferences at different insult stages, different neurorestorative mechanisms often prefer to play roles at different stages. For example, neuroprotection prefers at the physiological stage or at the early stage of function loss, which still maintain structure integrity. Importantly, it is neuroprotection, neuroplasticity, neuromodulation, and immunomodulation, but not neuroregeneration or neurogenesis that exerts main roles in the entire neurorestorative process.
(4) In view of the time and degree of difficulty of neurorestoration, we believe that the earlier, the better; and the earlier, the easier. In the early or middle pathophysiological stages, the damaged cells have a better chance to recover through appropriate interventional strategies. This implies that early interventional neurorestorative strategies should be recommended, and even more, preventative interventional neurorestorative strategies or those stimulate endogenous neurorestorative mechanisms should be recommended for anti-ageing treatment.
(5) In view of balance of disease changing process, if neurorestorative mechanisms with appropriate interventional strategies are stronger than insults, the balance of whole neurorestorative process will return as shown in Figure 1-2; otherwise, the insults will become worse as shown in Figure 1-3.

(6) In view of getting optimal neurorestoration result, one strategy may function through several mechanisms, but joint comprehensive strategies are likely to restore more functions. So combination should be paid more attention.

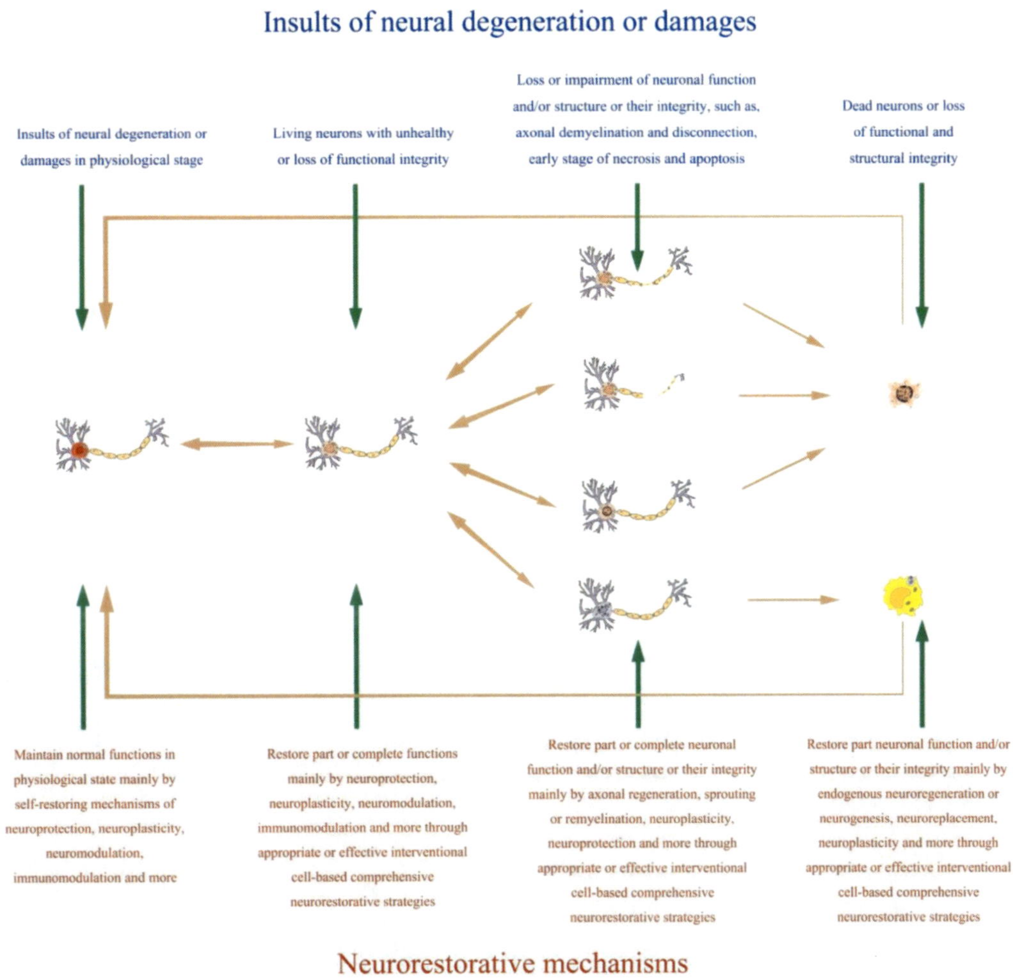


Figure 1.2. Neurorestorative process with effective interventional strategies.

For decades, people have been expecting quick success in structural repair of damaged CNS, particularly the spinal cord. So far, though the dream of such high expectation has not been realized, some neural functional restorations have occurred in chronic spinal cord injured patients who received the cell therapy after their natural neurological recoveries had plateaued (Huang et al., 2003; Huang et al., 2006; Lima et al., 2006; Guest et al., 2006). For those complete chronic SCI patients, their early functional recovery mainly are from signalling repair, neuromodulation or unmasking by neurotrophins and local microenvironment change from the cell therapy, but not from neuroregeneration or neurogenesis, because patients started to recover their functions in a few days after cell transplantation (Huang et al., 2003; Huang et al., 2006; Guest et al., 2006).

Under general condition in CNS, the mechanisms of patient clinical neurorestoration are very complex and comprehensive as showed in Figure 1-1 and Figure 5 in chapter 1 of section one. One strategy may restore neurological functions through several neurorestorative mechanisms; also different strategies may share the same mechanism.

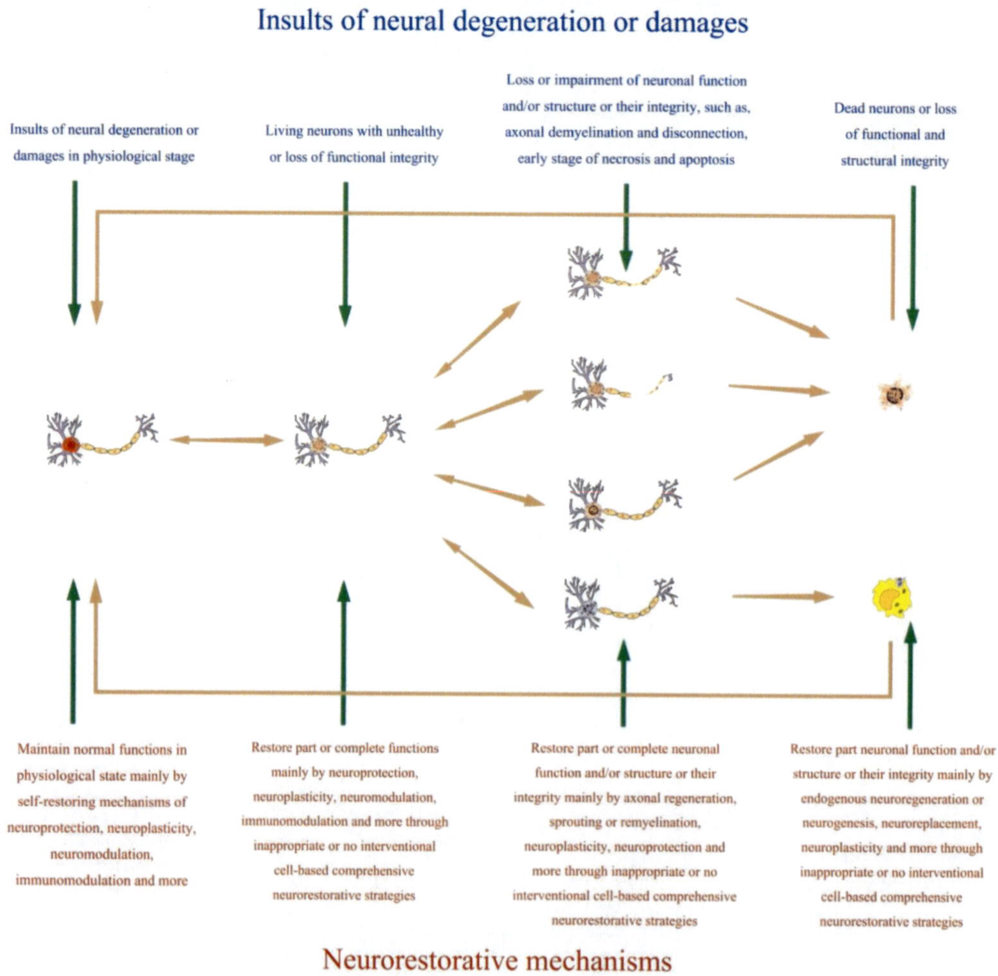


Figure 1.3. Neurorestorative process with inappropriate or no interventional strategies.

Any kind of neurorestoration may originate from one or all of the mechanisms as listed above. But current patients' functional recovery is mostly gained from neuromodulation, neuroprotection, and immunomodulation, and secondarily from neuroplasticity, axonal regeneration, sprouting, remyelination or neurorepair, while only a few cases are resulted from neurogenesis or neuroregeneration and angiogenesis (Toft A et al., 2007; Yamamoto M et al., 2009). Neuroreplacement can be an important tool or mechanism for PD, but probably not a major mechanism for neurorestoration in other CNS diseases or damages.

# 2. Neuromodulation

Neuromodulation was considered as the physiological process for regulating neural activities through neuromodulators or neurotransmitters thirty years ago (Zimmerman EA et al., 1978). Neuromodulators or neurotransmitters include acetylcholine (ACh), norepinephrine (NE), histamine, serotonin (5-HT), dopamine (DA), and a variety of neuropeptides (Linster C and Fontanini A. 2014; Santos-Carvalho A et al., 2014; Schmidt SL et al., 2013), glutamate, D-serine (Bardawee SK, et al., 2014), GABA (Dacks AM et al., 2013), glycine (Turpin F, et al., 2012), and others. Drugs targeting the neurotransmitters can affect the related neurological systems.

At that time it was also considered as a therapeutic method for restoring neurological functions by neurostimulators (Schröttner O 1978). Neurostimulators include auditory brainstem implant (ABI), brain computer interface (BCI), deep brain stimulation (DBS), functional electrical stimulation (FES), repetitive transcranial magnetic stimulation (rTMS), peripheral nerve stimulation (PNS), spinal cord stimulation (SCS), transcranial direct current stimulation (tDCS) and intrathecal drug delivery systems (ITDS) (http://www.neuromodulation.com/treatment).

Until the last decade, neuromodulation was still considered as a method that carries out interactions based on principles of neruo cell physiology and achieved by neuromodulation techniques which include implantable devices-neurostimulation and chronic drug delivery (Rise MT. 2000), and as a mechanism for neurological functional recovery gained by controlled electrical stimulation (Andrews RJ. 2003).

Neuromodulation defined by the International Neuromodulation Society is a therapeutic alteration of activities through stimulation or medication introduced by implanted devices, to modulate neural function (http://www.neuromodulation.com/about-neuromodulation). More accurately speaking, neuromodulation should also include physically or interventionaly regulating neural functions through neuromodulators, neurotransmitters or cell therapy (Huang, et al., 2003). The implanted devices are not always required.

So neuromodulation should be defined as the mechanisms and strategies that are used to activate neural functions by implanted devices, neurotransmitters, neuromodulators and cell therapy. As a neurorrestorative mechanism, neuromodulation modulates functions by adjusting stimulation on-off switch or volume, using implantable-devices-induced neurostimulation and medication, or by modulating ongoing neuronal spiking through acting on local postsynaptic receptors by neurotransmitters or neuromodulators. Further, the implantable-devices-induced neurostimulation and medication also may play roles by the mechanism of causing neuronal spiking and/or modulating ongoing neuronal spiking.

# 3. Neuroprotection

Neuroprotection means both the mechanisms and strategies protecting against neuronal injury or degeneration in the neurological system, including all acute neural disorders and chronic neurodegenerative diseases.

As one of the neurorestorative mechanisms, it restricts excitotoxicity and oxidative stress, moderates inflammatory changes, iron accumulation, and protein aggregation, and adjusts mitochondrial dysfunction (Andersen JK 2004; Dunnett SB and Björklund A 1999; Hall R et al., 1990; Zádori D et al., 2012).

The goal of neuroprotection is to limit neuronal dysfunction/death, when damage or degeneration occurs, to preserve the most possible integrity of neural function.

As one of the neurorestorative therapeutic strategies, neuroprotection include free radical trappers/scavengers, anti-excitotoxic agents, apoptosis inhibitors, anti-inflammatory agents, neurotrophic factors, metal ion chelators, ion channel modulators, gene therapy, cell therapy and others (Lange KW, et al., 1992; Li Y et al., 2013, Ma Y et al., 2011).

# 4. Neuroplasticity

Neuroplasticity encompasses both synaptic and non-synaptic plasticity, which changes in neural pathways and synapses, due to changes in behaviour, environment and neural activating, as well as changes resulted from physical injuries. Neuroplasticity keeps, but declines throughout the age-span (Pascual-Leone A. et al., 2005; 2011). Neuroplasticity occurs at the cellular level, due to learning or large-scale cortical level in response to injuries in health development, learning, memory, and recovery from neural damage.

In 1890, William James proposed the idea that the brain and its functions were not fixed throughout one's adulthood (James W. 1890); but Ramón Y Cajal concluded in the early 20th century that the neuron of the CNS could not be regenerated (Cajal, 1928). However, Hebb and Konorski introduced the idea of neural plasticity at the functional level; Liu and Chambers observed sprouting; and Raisman showed details of sprouting based on experimental quantitative electron microscopic techniques (Raisman, 1969; Liu and Chamber, 1958; Hebb and Penfield, 1940: Konorski, 1948).

It was believed in the 20th century that brain structure was relatively immutable, after a critical period in early childhood. Now many findings have revealed that many aspects of the brain remain plastic even in one's adulthood, and keep the ability to change throughout the whole lifespan (Rakic P 2002). The neuroplasticity can be classified into two kinds. The first are the physiological processes which are obligational responses to neural development, learning, memory, sensory input, motor act, thinking, cognition association, awareness, and other neural activity. The second are the pathogenesis processes which are obligational responses to neural damage or degeneration insults. When an animal suffers from a disease or injury, the nature intervenes and offers an automatic mechanism to repair the damage in its structure and restore its function for survival.

There are two types of sprouting: terminal and collateral. Terminal sprouting is part of a normal growth of an axon in embryos during fetal development or axonal regeneration after injury. When injured and the terminal sprouting of the original axon fails to reach the targeted neuron, collateral sprouting of neighboring axons may step in, which the basis of neuroplasticity.

# 5. Neurogenesis and Neuroregeneration

Neurogenesis means that neurons are generated from neural stem cells and progenitor cells. The first evidence of adult mammalian neurogenesis in the cerebral cortex was presented by J Altman in 1962 (Altman J., 1962); then he found that adult neurogenesis occurred in the dentate gyrus of the hippocampus (Altman J., 1963)

Many factors have the ability to affect the rate of hippocampal neurogenesis. Cerebral ischemia (Jin K, et al., 2006), epileptic seizures (Parent JM et al., 2006) and bacterial meningitis (Gerber J et al., 2009) may induce neurogenesis. On the other hand, chronic stress and ageing can result in a decreased neuronal proliferation (Jiang, W et al., 2005; Lee AL, et al., 2002; Sheline YI et al., 2003). Exercise and an enriched environment can help the survival of the neurons, and promote newborn cells to be integrated into the existing hippocampus (Bjørnebekk A, 2005; Lazarov O, 2005; Van Praag, H, 1999; 2005).

The term of neuroregeneration is similar with the concept of neurogenesis, but broader: it includes generating new neurons, glia, axons, myelin, or synapses. Neurogeneration is generally considered as axonal regeneration (Aldskogius H, 2001). Neuroregeneration in the peripheral nervous system (PNS) occurs in a significant degree (Bradbury EJ and Mcmahon SB, 2006). Unlike the peripheral nervous system injuries, injuries to the CNS are not followed by extensive and robust regeneration. It is limited by the inhibitory influences of the glial and extracellular environment.

In summary, it is viable to promote functional neurorestorations through various strategies either in isolation or in combination, based on the *CNS neurorestorable theory*. The concepts of the *CNS Neurorestorable theory, the Neurorestorative Process and the Neurorestorative Law* help researchers to easily understand the real value of what they are doing, and where they stand. Moreover, the new perspectives offered by the *CNS Neurorestorable theory, the Neurorestorative Process* and the *Neurorestorative Law* can help researchers to capture great changes in many viewpoints of neurosciences and related clinical disciplines. The mechanisms of functional recovery vary at different pathophysiological stages as shown in Figure 1-1, 1-2 and 1-3.

Currently, their work cannot be well controlled or adjusted, because we are still on the way to understand those mechanisms. The definitions of mechanisms often overlap with each other, without clear circumscription. For example, in neuroregeneration, neuronal regeneration holds similar meaning to neurogenesis, and axonal regeneration to neuroplasticity. Given that the neurological patterns and routes likely vary individually, the neurorestoration can take any easiest route to reach the target, similar to the rule that, in hydrodynamics, fluid follows the path with the least resistance. Excitingly, researchers have paid more attention on comprehending neurorestorative mechanisms at a higher level, and are ready to explore how those mechanisms work in the near future.

# References

Airavaara M, Voutilainen MH, Wang Y, Hoffer B. Neurorestoration. *Parkinsonism Relat Disord.* 2012;18 Suppl 1:S143-6.

Aldskogius H. Microglia in neuroregeneration. *Microsc. Res. Tech.* 2001;54(1):40-6.

Altman J. Are new neurons formed in the brains of adult mammals? *Science.* 1962;135(3509):1127-8.

Altman J. Autoradiographic investigation of cell proliferation in the brains of rats and cats. *Anat Rec.* 1963;145:573-91.

Andersen JK. Oxidative stress in neurodegeneration: cause or consequence? *Nat. Med.* 2004;10 Suppl:S18-25.

Andrews RJ. Neuroprotection trek--the next generation: neuromodulation I. Techniques--deep brain stimulation, vagus nerve stimulation, and transcranial magnetic stimulation. *Ann. N Y Acad. Sci.* 2003; 993:1-13.

Bardawee SK, Alzweiri M, Ishaqat AA. D-serine in neurobiology: CNS neurotransmission and neuromodulation. *Can. J. Neurol. Sci.* 2014;41(2):164-76.

Bjørnebekk A, Mathé AA, Brené S. The antidepressant effect of running is associated with increased hippocampal cell proliferation. *Int. J. Neuropsychopharmacol.* 2005;8 (3): 357–68.

Bradbury EJ, MCMAHON, SB. Spinal cord repair strategies: why do they work? *Nature Reviews Neuroscience.* 2006;7: 644-653.

Cajal S.R. *Degeneration & regeneration of the nervous system* (transl. R. M. May). Oxford: Oxford University Press; 1928.

Dacks AM, Reale V, Pi Y, Zhang W, Dacks JB, Nighorn AJ, Evans PD. A characterization of the Manduca sexta serotonin receptors in the context of olfactory neuromodulation. *PLoS One.* 2013;8(7):e69422.

Dunnett SB, Björklund A. Prospects for new restorative and neuroprotective treatments in Parkinson's disease. *Nature.* 1999;399(6738 Suppl):A32-9.

Gerber J, Tauber SC, Armbrecht I, Schmidt H, Brück W, Nau R. Increased neuronal proliferation in human bacterial meningitis. *Neurology.* 2009; 73 (13): 1026–32.

Guest J, Herrera LP, Qian T. Rapid recovery of segmental neurological function in a tetraplegic patient following transplantation of fetal olfactory bulb-derived cells. *Spinal Cord.* 2006;44:135-42.

Hall R, Murdoch J. Brain protection: physiological and pharmacological considerations. Part II: The pharmacology of brain protection. *Can. J. Anaesth.* 1990;37(7):762-77.

Hebb DO, Penfield W. Human behaviour after extensive bilateral removal from the frontal lobes. *Archives of Neurology and Psychiatry.*1940; 44: 421–436.

Huang H, Chen L, Sanberg P. Cell therapy from bench to bedside translation in CNS neurorestoratology era. *Cell Med* 2010;1:15-46.

Huang H, Chen L, Wang H, Xiu B, Li B, Wang R, Zhang J, Zhang F, Gu Z, Li Y, Song Y, Hao W, Pang S, Sun J. Influence of patients' age on functional recovery after transplantation of olfactory ensheathing cells into injured spinal cord. *Chinese Medical Journal.* 2003, 116: 1488-1491.

Huang H, Wang H, Chen L, Gu Z, Zhang J, Zhang F, Song Y, Li Y, Tan K, Liu Y, Xi H. Influence factors for functional improvement after recovery after olfactory ensheathing cell for chronic spinal cord injury. *Chinese J Restorative and Reconstructive Surgery.*2006; 20: 434-438.

International Association of Neurorestoratology. Beijing Declaration of International Association of Neurorestoratology (IANR). *Cell Transplant.* 2009;18(4):487.

International Neuromodulation Society. About neuromodulation. July 30, 2014. Available from: http://www.neuromodulation.com/about-neuromodulation

International Neuromodulation Society. Neuromodulation: An Emerging Field. July 30, 2014. Available from: http://www.neuromodulation.com/treatment

James W. *The Principles of Psychology*. New York: Henry Holt; 1890.

Jiang, W., et al. Cannabinoids promote embryonic and adult hippocampus neurogenesis and produce anxiolytic- and antidepressant-like effects. *The Journal of Clinical Investigation.* 2005;115 (11): 3104–3116.

Jin K, Wang X, Xie L, et al. Evidence for stroke-induced neurogenesis in the human brain. *Proc. Natl. Acad. Sci. U.S.A.* 2006;103 (35): 13198–202.

Karussis, D.; Karageorgiou, C.; Vaknin–Dembinsky, A.; Gowda–Kurkalli, B.; Gomori, J. M.; Kassis, I.; Bulte, J. W.; Petrou, P.; Ben–Hur, T.; Abramsky, O.; Slavin, S. Safety and immunological effects of mesenchymal stem cell transplantation in patients with multiple sclerosis and amyotrophic lateral sclerosis. *Arch. Neurol.* 2010;67(10):1187–1194.

Konorski J. *Conditioned reflexes and neuron organization.* London: Cambridge University Press; 1948.

Lange KW, Youdim MB, Riederer P, Levi-Montalcini R, Booker B. Neurotoxicity and neuroprotection in Parkinson's disease. *Excessive J. Neural Transm Suppl.* 1992;38:27-44.

Lazarov O, Robinson J, Tang YP, Hairston IS, Korade-Mirnics Z, Lee VM, Hersh LB, Sapolsky RM, Mirnics K, Sisodia SS. "Environmental enrichment reduces Abeta levels and amyloid deposition in transgenic mice". *Cell.* 2005;120 (5): 701–13.

Lee AL, Ogle WO, Sapolsky RM. Stress and depression: possible links to neuron death in the hippocampus". *Bipolar Disord.* 2002;4 (2): 117–28.

Li Y, Chen L, Zhao Y, Bao J, Xiao J, Liu J, Jiang X, Zhou C, Wang H, Huang H. Intracranial transplant of olfactory ensheathing cells can protect both upper and lower motor neurons in amyotrophic lateral sclerosis. *Cell Transplant.* 2013;22 Suppl 1:S51-65.

Lima C, Pratas-Vital, Escada P, Hasse-Ferreira A, Capucho C, Peduzzi JD. Olfactory mucosa autografts in human spinal cord injury: a pilot clinical study. *J. Spinal Cord Medicine.*2006; 29: 191-203.

Linster C, Fontanini A. Functional neuromodulation of chemosensation in vertebrates. Curr Opin Neurobiol. 2014;29C:82-87.

Liu CN, Chambers WW. Intraspinal sprouting of dorsal root axons. *Arch. Neurol. Psychiat.*1958; 79: 46-61.

Liu CY, Apuzzo ML, Tirrell DA. Engineering of the extracellular matrix: working toward neural stem cell programming and neurorestoration--concept and progress report. *Neurosurgery.* 2003;52(5):1154-65.

Ma Y, Liu W, Wang Y, Chao X, Qu Y, Wang K, Fei Z. VEGF protects rat cortical neurons from mechanical trauma injury induced apoptosis via the MEK/ERK pathway. *Brain Res Bull.* 2011;86(5-6):441-6.

Parent JM; Elliott, RC; Pleasure, SJ; Barbaro, NM; Lowenstein, DH. Aberrant seizure-induced neurogenesis in experimental temporal lobe epilepsy. *Annals of Neurology.* 2006; 59 (1): 81–91.

Pascual-Leone A, Freitas C, Oberman L, Horvath JC, Halko M, Eldaief M, Bashir S, Vernet M, Shafi M, Westover B, Vahabzadeh-Hagh AM, Rotenberg A. Characterizing brain cortical plasticity and network dynamics across the age-span in health and disease with TMS-EEG and TMS-fMRI. *Brain Topogr.* 2011;24(3-4):302-15.

Pascual-Leone, A., Amedi, A., Fregni, F., & Merabet, L. B. The plastic human brain cortex. Annual *Review of Neuroscience.* 2005; 28,377-401.

Raisman, G. Neuronal plasticity in the septal nuclei of the adult rat. *Brain Res.* 1969; 14: 25-48.

Rakic, P. Neurogenesis in adult primate neocortex: an evaluation of the evidence. *Nature Reviews Neuroscience.* 2002; 3 (1): 65–71.

Rise MT. Instrumentation for neuromodulation. *Arch Med Res.* 2000;31(3):237-47.

Santos-Carvalho A, Álvaro AR, Martins J, Ambrósio AF, Cavadas C. Emerging novel roles of neuropeptide Y in the retina: from neuromodulation to neuroprotection. *Prog Neurobiol.* 2014;112:70-9.

Schmidt SL, Chew EY, Bennett DV, Hammad MA, Fröhlich F. Differential effects of cholinergic and noradrenergic neuromodulation on spontaneous cortical network dynamics. *Neuropharmacology.* 2013; 72:259-73.

Schröttner O. Electric neuromodulation - a new concept in the treatment of chronic pain. *Wien Med Wochenschr.* 1978;128(23):721-3.

Sheline YI, Gado MH, Kraemer HC. Untreated depression and hippocampal volume loss. *Am. J. Psychiatry.* 2003;160 (8): 1516–8.

Toft, A.; Scott, D. T.; Barnett, S. C.; Riddell, J. S. Electrophysiological evidence that olfactory cell transplants improve function after spinal cord injury. *Brain* 2007;130(Pt. 4):970–984.

Turpin F, Dallérac G, Mothet JP. Electrophysiological analysis of the modulation of NMDA-receptors function by D-serine and glycine in the central nervous system. *Methods Mol Biol.* 2012;794:299-312.

Van Praag, H.; Kempermann, G.; Gage, F. Running increases cell proliferation and neurogenesis in the adult mouse dentate gyrus. *Nature Neuroscience.* 1999; 2 (3): 266–270.

Van Praag, H.; Shubert, T.; Zhao, C.; Gage, F. Exercise enhances learning and hippocampal neurogenesis in aged mice. *Journal of Neuroscience.* 2005;25 (38): 8680–8685.

Yamamoto, M.; Raisman, G.; Li, D.; Li, Y. Transplanted olfactory mucosal cells restore paw reaching function without regeneration of severed corticospinal tract fibres across the lesion. *Brain Res.* 2009; 1303:26–31.

Zádori D, Klivényi P, Szalárdy L, Fülöp F, Toldi J, Vécsei L. Mitochondrial disturbances, excitotoxicity, neuroinflammation and kynurenines: novel therapeutic strategies for neurodegenerative disorders. *J. Neurol. Sci.* 2012;322(1-2):187-91.

Zimmerman EA, Liotta A, Krieger DT. beta-Lipotropin in brain: localization in hypothalamic neurons by immunoperoxidase technique. *Cell Tissue Res.* 1978;186(3):393-8.

# Section 2: Techniques and Effects of Neurorestorative Strategies

In: Neurorestoratology, volume 1
Editors: H. Huang, G. Raisman, P. R. Sanberg et al.
ISBN: 978-1-63463-599-8


Chapter 4

# Neurobiological Property of Cells

***Lin Chen[1,2], Hongyun Huang*[3,4], Rebecca Lamond[5], Susan C. Barnett[5], Julie G. Allickson[6], Natalie Yefimenko[6], Cesar V. Borlongan[6], Paul R. Sanberg[6], Elena R. Chernykh[7], Ekaterina Ya. Shevela[7], Lyudmila V. Sakhno[7], Marina A. Tikhonova[7], Yaroslav L. Petrovsky[7], Alexander A. Ostain[7], Vladimir A. Kozlov[7] and Lei Zhang[8]***

[1]Medical Center of Tsinghua University, Beijing, China
[2]Tsinghua University Yuquan Hospital, Beijing, China
[3]Beijing Rehabilitation Hospital of Capital Medical University, Beijing, China
[4]Beijing Hongtianji Neuroscience Academy, Beijing, China
[5]Institute of Infection, Immunity and Inflammation (III's), University of Glasgow,Scotland
[6]University of South Florida College of Medicine, US
[7]Research Institute of Clinical Iimmunology SB RAMS, Novosibirsk, Russia
[8]Tianjin Sinica Biotech Co., Ltd.,Tianjin, China

## Introduction

Cells as a tool for neurorestorative strategies can be divided into immature or mature functional cells, which include neural progenitor or precursor cells, olfactory ensheathing cells, Schwann cells, neurons, and etc.; mesenchymal or stromal cells, which include bone marrow, umbilical cord or peripheral blood mononuclear or stromal cells, umbilical cord stromal cells, adipose stromal cells and etc; and totipotent stem cells, which include embryonic stem cell and induced pluripotential cells. Immature or mature functional cells andmesenchymal or stromal cells have proven safe without many problems in plenty of experimental and clinical studies; however tumorigenicity of totipotent stem cellsremains

*Corresponding author: Hongyun Huang hongyunh@gmail.com.

a big safety problem. Thus they must be prohibited for use in clinical trials until the researchers find a definite method to prevent tumorigenicity occurrence, even though those cells have demonstrated some advantages for treating diseases and repair of damage in experimental studies(Chen LW et al., 2011; El-Amraoui A et al., 2010; Hernándeza J et al., 2011; Hunt CJ,2011; Sendtner M,2010;Tomaskovic-Crook E et al., 2011). Here we individually introduce their neurobiological properties in brief.

# 1. Immature or Mature Functional Cell

## 1.1. Neural Stem/Progenitor Cell

*Lin Chen, Hongyun Huang*

Neural stem/progenitor cells (NSPCs) are multipotential progenitor cells that proliferate and generate various kinds of cells within the central nervous system (CNS), including neurons, astrocytes, and oligodendrocytes (Trujillo CA et al., 2009). Because of these characteristics, there is increasing interest in NSPCs from the aspects of both basic developmental biology and therapeutic applications to the damaged brain (Okano H,2002). NSPCs are present not only in the developing nervous systems, but also in the adult central nervous system of mammals, including humans. So NSPCs can be isolated from both fetal and adult mammalian brain and cultured in chemically defined medium substituted with EGF and bFGF (Reynolds BA and Weiss S, 1996). NSPCs are mainly present in the subventricular zone and hippocampal dentate gyrus; and can be stimulated to proliferate in many CNS diseases. NSPCs in rodent brain migrate into damaged brain regions and possibly replace damaged or lost neurons; the source of them may come by activating endogenous NSPCs and/or transplanting vitro-expanded stem cells and/or their neuronal progeny (Jin K et al., 2007; Goh EL et al., 2003). Also transplanted adult NSCs can differentiate into vascular cells for vasculogenesis at sites of injury (Ii M,2009). Transplanting NSCs, their derivatives or stimulating endogenous stem cells are emerging treatments for neurodegenerative diseases and trauma, for example, acute and chronic experimental autoimmune encephalomyelitis (EAE), multiple sclerosis, spinal cord injury, hypoxic-ischemic brain injury (HIBI) or cerebral palsy, stroke and other nervous diseases (Pluchino Set al., 2003; Ader M et al., 2004; Okano H,2010; Kim BG et al., 2007; Daadi MM et al., 2010; Teng YD et al., 2002). The main mechanisms of neurorestoration may not be cell replacement as people expected before, but instead by neneuroprotective effect through immunomodulatory substances and neurotrophic growth factors(De Feo D,2012).

## 1.2. Olfactory Ensheathing Cell

*Rebecca Lamond, Susan C Barnett**

Olfactory ensheathing cells (OECs) were originally described as the Schwann cells (SCs) of the olfactory system due to their antigenic and morphological properties (Gasser, 1956; De

Lorenzo, 1957; Frisch, 1967), however it became clear from further research that they are in fact a distinct and specialized population of glial cell (Barnett S et al., 1993). OECs present in the nerve fiber layer of the olfactory bulb, as well as in the nasal olfactory mucosa, which show clearly in a simple schematic of the olfactory system of Figure 1. OECs are specialized glial cells that ensheath the axons of the first cranial nerve and guide the regeneration of non-myelinated olfactory axons from the peripheral nasal epithelium through the cribriform plate of the ethmoid bone and into the olfactory bulb (OB) (Doucette R,1990; 1991).

They are novel cells that display Schwann cell or astrocyte-like properties. While sharing many common properties, comparisons of the in vitro properties and in vivo fate between OECs and SCs suggest unique properties of OECs as compared to SCs. Immunohistochemically they display characteristics of astrocytes (GFAP expression), SCs (p75) and oligodendrocytes (O4) in Figure 2 (Franceschini F and Barnett S, 1996). Although normally these cells do not produce myelin when resident in the olfactory system,after transplantation, they are able to myelinate axons with the myelin morphologically similar to what is produced by SCs (Franklin RJ et al., 1996). A human OEC equivalent was identified to be able to myelinate spinal cord axons, producing clinical feasibility for translation to the clinic (Barnett S et al., 2000).

Recent studies have shown that SCs, but not OECs inhibit CNS myelination via the secreting of connective tissue growth factor. This suggests that, OECs, and not SCs, would be better for transplant-mediated CNS repair (Lamond R and Barnett SC, 2013). OECs also support the growth of axons and produce neurotrophic factors (Lipson AC et al., 2003). Depending on culture conditions or *in vivo* microenvironment, OEC can secrete varying amounts of NGF, BDNF, GDNF, CNTF, FGF and VEGF and adhesion molecules, which play a very important role as a neuronal support enhancing cellular survival.

Several studies have demonstrated the great potential of OECs to improve functional recovery and axonal regrowth after lesions of the CNS or PNS (Franssen EH et al., 2007; Radtke C et al., 2009; Radtke C et al., 2009). Evidence that OECs have distinct glial cell properties is provided with emphasis on their unique ability to interact with astrocytes and induce less of an astroglyotic response when compared to SCs (Lakatos A et al., 2003; Barnett SC,2004; Santos-Silva et al., 2007; Higginson JR et al., 2012). This is the most significant difference between the two cell types and is thought to be related to differences in the secretion of sulphated moieties (Higginson JR et al., 2012).

Transplanting these cells have been proven to have a neuroprotective effect, supporting axonal regeneration, remyelination of demyelinated axons, neuroplasticity, neuromodulation, neurogenesis, angiogenesis, anti-inflammatory response (e.g. moderating astrocyte activation), reducing scar/cavity formation, and strong phagocytic activity (Toft A et al., 2007; Franssen EH et al., 2008; Lankford KL et al., 2008; Leung JY et al., 2008; Pellitteri R et al., 2007, 2009; Ramer LM et al., 2004; Sasaki M et al., 2007; Vincent AJ et al., 2008; Wewetzer K et al., 2005, 2006; Yu XD, 2007; Chehrehasa F et al., 2010; Hale DM et al., 2011; Ziegler MD et al., 2011).

More important finding is that OEC can protect both upper and lower motor neurons in rat model of ALS through intracranial implantation (Li Y et al., 2013). OECs have been employed as a possible tool for inducing axonal regeneration in the injured adult CNS, resulting in significant functional recovery in some animal models and promising outcomes

* Susan.Barnett@glasgow.ac.uk.

from early clinical applications (Caracciolo PC et al., 2009; Basso DM et al., 1995; Barritt AW et al., 2006; Dasari VR et al., 2009; Boyd JG et al., 2003).

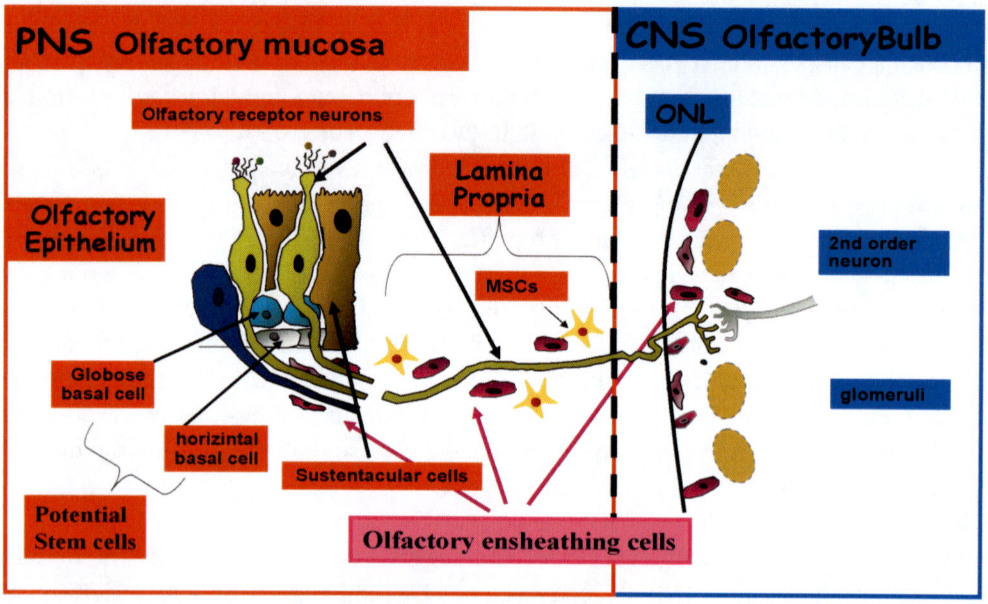


Figure 1. Schematic of the Peripheral Olfactory System (modified from Barnett et al., 2004). The olfactory mucosa consists of the epithelium layer (OE) and the lamina propria (LP). Sustentacular cells in the OE provide support for the olfactory receptor neurons (ORNs), whilst putative stem cells (globose basal cells (GBCs) and horizontal basal cells. HBCs) are thought to replace ORNs and olfactory glia, as well as the sustentacular cells. ORNs are able to extend their processes through the lamina propria, guided by OECs before crossing the cribriform plate (dashed line) to re-enter the CNS where they form functional connections with second order neurons in the olfactory bulb.

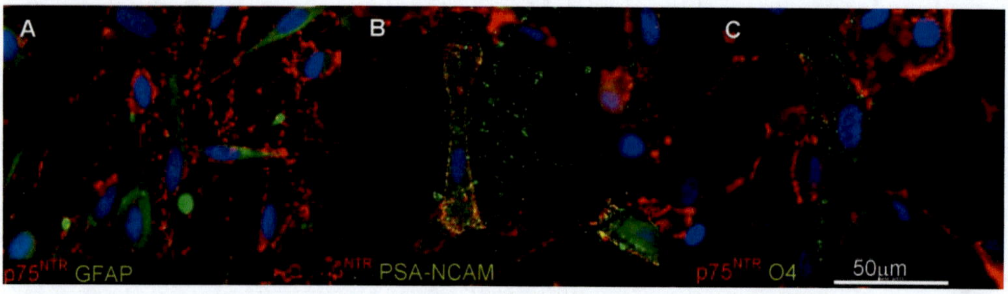


Figure 2. Antigenic profile of purified OECs taken from the olfactory bulb of neonatal rats. (A) Purified OECs express punctate $p75^{NTR}$ as well as diffuse glial fibrillary acidic protein (GFAP). Both PSA-N-CAM (B) and O4 (C) can be observed on the cell surface. Images were taken with an Olympus BX51 fluorescent microscope and Image Pro software using a x 60 objective.

However, there are other studies that suggest the transplantation of OECs alone would not be sufficient to promote CNS repair and a combined approach would be better. Thus, it would be an excellent candidate for transplantation together with other strategies.

It is a pioneer cell that has been used in animal models of neurological diseases and was first translated into the clinical study for patients with chronic spinal cord injury in 2001 (Huang H et al., 2003), which stimulated the enthusiasm of researchers. Later on, more clinical trials have been carried out in around the world with the main aim to test the practicability and safety of transplantation of autologous OECs into the human injured spinal cord (Mackay-Sim A et al., 2005;Féron F et al., 2005; Tabakow P et al., 2013). A more extensive clinical study was carried out in China to analyze if there was any therapeutic effect on damaged or diseased CNS or after fetal olfactory tissue (containing OECs) transplantation. Out of the 1255 participants from 71 countries or regions, 656 participants suffered from SCI and the rest with other diseases including amyotrophic lateral sclerosis, cerebral palsy, multiple sclerosis, sequelae of stroke, ataxia, and residual diseases (Huang H et al., 2009).

In summary, OECs are a highly specialised type of glial cell which are thought to aid the continual regeneration of the olfactory system by ensheathing the axons of unmyelinated olfactory receptor neurons, guiding them from the periphery back into the CNS to form secondary functional connections with the mitral cells in the olfactory bulb. In light of this, OECs are proposed to be a suitable candidate for transplant mediated repair of the CNS.

## 1.3. Schwann Cell

*Lin Chen and Hongyun Huang*

Schwann cells (SCs) play a pivotal role in the maintenance and regeneration of the axons in the peripheral nervous system (PNS) due to their ability to dedifferentiate, migrate, proliferate, express growth-promoting factors, and myelinate regenerating axons (Bryan DJ, et al., 1999). SCs are peripheral nervous elements, but they also exhibit good myelinating capacity in the CNS (Blakemore WF et al., 1985). SCs are key regulators of peripheral nerve development, being required for the survival of neurons, the distribution of ion channels along nerve fibers and formation of myelin sheath as well as stimulation of development of the connective tissue sheath (Bruska M and Woźniak W, 1999). They develop from the neural crest and differentiate into myelin- and non-myelin-forming cells. Myelinating and non-myelinating SCs of peripheral nerves are derived from the neural crest via an intermediate cell type, the SC precursor (Jessen KR et al., 1994). SC development in the PNS is dependent on contact-mediated signaling between SCs and the associated axons. SCs are involved in many important aspects of peripheral nerve biology - the conduction of nervous impulses along axons, nerve development and regeneration, trophic support for neurons, production of the nerve extracellular matrix, modulation of neuromuscular synaptic activity, and presentation of antigens to T-lymphocytes.

Ramon Y Cajal (1928) first described axonal regeneration-promoting effects of peripheral nerve implants in the spinal cord. SCs have been shown to form myelin after transplantation into the demyelinated CNS (Blakemore WF, 1977; 1984; 1985; Imaizumi T et al., 2000). Given SCs do not normally enter the CNS, and migration of SCs transplanted into the CNS white matter is inhibited by astrocytes, efforts are focused on enhancing their migration and functional integration into the lesion CNS (Blakemore WF and Crang AJ, 1989;Luo J et al., 2011). Ensheathment and myelination are specifically regulated by contact with axons, and SC is centrally involved in extracellular matrix production in the peripheral nerve trunk (Bunge RP, 1993). Additional Schwann cell functions include the promotion of both PNS and CNS regeneration, provision of a versatile source of trophic factors, the capacity to remyelinate CNS axons, and the restoration of electrophysiological conduction. SCs produce various growth factors or axonal growth-promoting factors such as nerve growth factor (Bandtlow CE et al., 1987), brain-derived neurotrophic factor (Acheson A et al., 1991; Meyer M et al., 1992), ciliary neurotrophic factor (Friedman M et al., 1992; Meyer M et al., 1992; Rende M et al., 1992), and glial cell line-derived neurotrophic factor (Widenfalk J et al., 2001), so they are widely used for CNS repair strategies (Bunge RP,1994; Oudega M and Xu XM, 2006). Therefore, efforts are focused on enhancing their migration and functional integration into the lesion CNS and leading in some cases to functional recovery in rodent and primate models (Lavdas AA et al., 2008). In addition, efforts are underway to use these cells as tissue engineer seeds and gene delivery vehicles for an array of molecules with repair potential (Bhatheja K et al., 2006; Deng LX et al., 2011).

In clinic, the initial data from Zhang WC et al. (1994) proved that intracerebral co-grafting of Schwann's cells and human fetal adrenal medullary tissue symptoms were improved significantly in Parkinson's disease patients within 1-6 months after grafting. Saberi H et al. (2008) reported 1-year follow-up outcome of four patients who had stable chronic spinal cord injury at mid-thoracic level and treated with autologous Schwann cell transplantation from sural nerve.

## 1.4. Oligodendrocyte /Precursor Cell

***Lin Chen and Hongyun Huang***

Both oligodendrocyte precursors and oligodendrocytes are able to remyelinate the CNS (Miron VE et al., 2011; Banisadr G et al., 2011; Franklin RJ et al., 1996). Oligodendrocytes or precursor cells have been shown to migrate from the implantation site to the lesion over a distance of several millimeters (Crang AJ et al., 1991; Duncan ID et al.,1988). In additional, many studies have demonstrated that transplanted oligodendrocytes survive in the host brain, migrate out of the graft and synthesize myelin (Franklin RJ et al., 1996). Thus these cells have potential for myelin repair in demyelinating diseases.

# 2. Mesenchymal or Stromal Cell

Mononuclear cells from bone marrow, cord blood and peripheral blood grossly include monocytes/macrophages, lymphocytes and a small amount stem cells. Unfortunately, many scientists or physicians often misname “mononuclear cell” as the term of “stem cell” in their published scientific papers. After expanding mononuclear cell in culture, even stem cells increase in number but most of them are a homogenous mix of cell types. Cells that are cultured and expanded from umbilical cord or adipose tissue are also a homogenous mix of cells. So we cannot identify or name both of them as purely “stem cells”. More commonly now, they are known as stromal cell (Salem H & Thiemermann C, 2010). Herein we use “mesenchymal, stromal or mononuclear cells” to describe those kinds of cells.

## 2.1. Bone Marrow Stromal (or Mononuclear) Cell

*Lin Chen and Hongyun Huang*

Bone marrow stromal cells (BMSCs) are a heterogeneous subpopulation of bone marrow cells including mesenchymal stromal or progenitor cells (Friedenstein AJ et al., 1976). BMSCs are a population of multipotential mesenchymal stromal and precursor cells (Kopen GC et al., 1999), which have shown to differentiate in vitro or in vivo into osteoblasts, chondrocytes, myocytes, adipocytes and beta-pancreatic islets cells and also transdifferentiate into glia, neuronal cells and SCs (Kassem M et al., 2008; Greco SJ et al., 2007). Although the concept of transdifferentiation is up for debate (Uccelli A et al., 2007) BMSCs spontaneously express certain neuronal phenotype markers in culture, in the absence of specialized induction reagents (Deng J et al., 2006).

When cultured in NSC culture conditions, 8% of BMSCs are able to generate neurospheres which express characteristic NSC antigens (nestin and musashi-1) and are capable of self-renewal and multi-lineage differentiation into neurons, astrocytes and oligodendrocytes. Differentiated neurons can form dendrites, axonal processes and synapses and fire action potentials or tetrodotoxin-sensitive action potentials (Shih CC et al., 2008; Wislet-Gendebien S et al., 2005).

BMSCs escape the immune system surveillance (Deans RJ et al., 2000; Li Y et al., 2002) and can be transplanted as an autograft, allograft and even xenograft (Azizi SA et al., 1998; Saito T et al., 2002).

BMSCs express an array of growth factors and cytokines to support sprouting axons and possess many advantages over other sources as minimal immunologic rejection and auto transplants with few ethical concerns (Ng TK et al., 2014). The possible mechanisms responsible for the beneficial outcome after BMSCs transplantation into neurodegenerating tissues include trophic factor delivery, immunomodulation and anti-inflammatory, neuroprotection, cell replacement, angiogenesis (Ng TK et al., 2014;Karussis D et al., 2008; Takizawa S,2003; Torrente Y et al., 2008), and remyelination (Sasaki M et al., 2001), however others suggest this is not possible (Hunt DP et al., 2008). BMSCs migrate to the area of CNS disease, close to the inflammatory infiltrate without significantly differentiating into neural cells. However they may foster survival of dying neurons, reduces neurodegeneration and be applied to neurodegenerative diseases (Dezawa M et al., 2005; Ng TK et al., 2014;Ramos AB et al., 2013).

## 2.2. Umbilical Cord Blood Mononuclear Cell

*Lin Chen and Hongyun Huang*

Umbilical cord blood mononuclear cells (UCBMCs) as well as the bone marrow and peripheral blood is a rich source of stem cells with great proliferative potential. There are at least three kinds of stem cells in the UCBMCs: hematopoietic, embryonic-like and mesenchymal stromal cell. UCBMCs are capable of differentiating across tissue lineage boundaries into neural, cardiac, epithelial, hepatocytic, and dermal tissue both in vitro and in vivo (Harris DT, 2008; Roszek K et al., 2008).

Its therapeutic potential for cell therapy extends regenerative medicine beyond the hematopoietic component (Bieback K et al., 2007). The expanding population of neural stem/progenitor cells can be selected from the human cord blood nonhematopoietic (CD34-negative) mononuclear fraction (Buzańska L et al., 2006).

UCBMCs or monocyte should be considered as a good candidate for incurable neural injuries and degenerative diseases owing to their easy of isolation, low immune rejection, and multiple characteristic advantages such as their anti-inflammatory properties by virtue of their unique immune and inflammatory immaturity, and their pro-angiogenic ability (Ali H et al., 2010).

Alternatively, UCBMCs or CD34(+) cells from UCBMC transplantation may promote neural repair by delivering neural protection, secreting neurotrophic factors, modulating immune function and inflammatory reaction, improving probability of neuromuscular transmission, remyelination, angiogenesis and neurogenesis (Lee JH et al., 2011; Peterson DA,2004; Rosenkranz K et al., 2011; Sanberg PR et al., 2005, 2011; Souayah N et al., 2011). Nowadays, several clinical centers have begun to transplant the UCBMCs and demonstrated some functional improvement in spinal cord injury (Kang KS et al., 2005), cerebral palsy (Papadopoulos KI et al., 2011), and hereditary ataxia (Yang WZ et al., 2011).

## 2.3. Hematopoietic Stem Cell

***Lin Chen and Hongyun Huang***

Hematopoietic stem cells (HSCs) are multipotent stem cells that give rise to all the blood cell types from myeloid (monocytes and macrophages, neutrophils, basophils, eosinophils, erythrocytes, megakaryocytes/platelets, dendritic cells), to lymphoid lineages (T-cells, B-cells, NK-cells) (Choi KD et al., 2011).

HSCs are present in the bone marrow, which includes femurs, hip, ribs, sternum, and other bones and can be obtained directly from bone marrow and blood following pre-treatment with cytokines, such as G-CSF (granulocyte colony-stimulating factors) (Zhang C et al., 2011) or ex-vivo expansion in 3D bioreactor (Damon LE et al., 2009). Various underlying mechanisms have been deciphered, such as transdifferentiation into neural lineages, neuroprotection through trophic support, cell fusion (Haas S et al., 2005) and entering into the sites of motoneuron pathology and doing immunomodulation (Appel SH et al., 2008). However trasndifferentation is still up for debate.

Engraftment of hematopoietic stem cells (HSCs) was proposed as a treatment for multiple sclerosis due to their neuroprotective effects in 1995 based on favorable results in animal models (Mandalfino P et al., 2000; Burt RK et al., 1999; Tyndall A et al., 2002; Burt RK et al., 2005).

Autologous HSC transplantation can induce a prolonged clinical stabilization in severe progressive MS patients (Saccardi R et al., 2005; Loh YS et al., 2007), however the effects of transplantation and transplantation-related morbidity are dependent on patient-selection, time of transplantation and conditioning regimens used (Rogojan C et al., 2009). Transplantation of HSCs from bone marrow is effective for spinal cord injury and ischemic brain lesions (Koshizuka S et al., 2004). Patients with chronic complete SCI and amyotrophic lateral sclerosis treated with autologous BM-derived hematopoietic progenitor cell transplantation showed neuorlogical improvement (Deda H et al., 2008, 2009).

## 2.4. Menstrual Blood Cell

### *Julie G. Allickson, Natalie Yefimenko, Cesar V. Borlongan and Paul R. Sanberg*

Adult stromalcells from menstrual blood were isolated, characterized and differentiated in 2008, which are able to differentiate into chondrogenic, adipogenic, osteogenic, neurogenic, and cardiogenic cell lineages and are positive for CD29, CD44, CD90, CD105, CD117, CD166, and MHC Class I and embryonic stem cell markers Oct-4 and SSEA-4 (Patel AN et al., 2008), Nanog and neuronal phenotypic markers (Nestin, MAP2) (Borlongan CV et al., 2010). Menstrual blood-derived stem cells can be transplanted either intracerebrally or intravenously without immunesuppression. Three neural growth factors from menstrual stem cell, that is, VEGF, BDNF, NT-3 may have contributed to reduce behavioral and histological impairments in adult ischemic stroke rats model after post intravenous (IV) and post intracerebral (IC) menstrual stem cell injection (Borlongan CV et al., 2010).

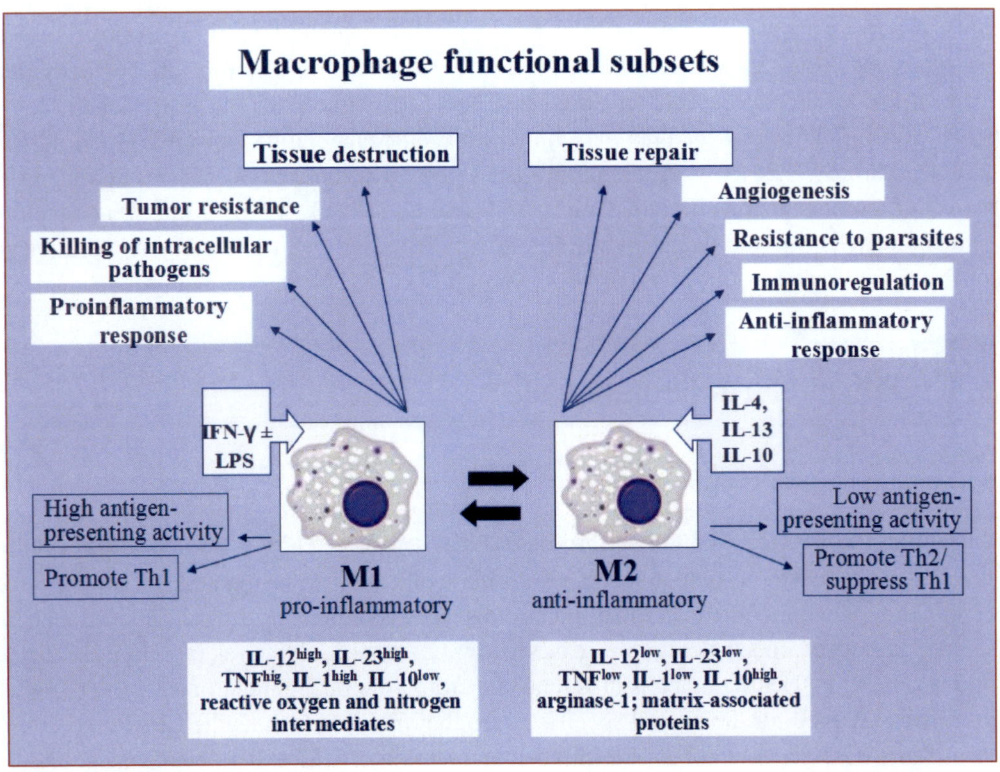


Figure 3. Macrophage functional subsets.

## 2.5. Macrophage

***Elena R. Chernykh, Ekaterina Ya. Shevela, Lyudmila V. Sakhno, Marina A. Tikhonova, Yaroslav L. Petrovsky, Alexander A. Ostain and Vladimir A. Kozlov***

Macrophage can be isolated in culture from peripheral blood mononuclear cells. There are at least two distinct functional macrophage subsets that are triggered in response to different stimuli, that is, classical pro-inflammatory (termed type 1 or M1) and nonclassical anti-inflammatory macrophages (termed type 2 or M2). Immune reactions may be beneficial and even essential for CNS repair (Yin Y et al., 2003; Bomstein Y et al., 2003; Vallières N et al., 2006; Barrette B et al., 2008) and more studies demonstrated that macrophages could enhance neuroprotection and promote long-distance axon growth, sprouting and remyelination (Kigerl KA et al., 2009; Shechter R et al., 2009). Mechanisms for functional neurorestoration include removing damaged cells, cell debris (Zupanc GK et al., 2003) and inhibitory molecules (Fan X et al., 2004), inactivating neurotoxic molecules (Griffiths MR et al., 2009), producing cytokines and growth/trophic factors with anti-inflammatory, neuroprotective and pro-regenerative activities (Fadok VA, et al., 1998; Freire-de-Lima CG et al., 2006; Golpon HA et al., 2004; Kerschensteiner M et al., 1999; Nakajima, 2004), recruiting stem cells and neural progenitor cells to the lesion site (Aarum J et al., 2003; Kotter MR et al., 2005; Ziv Y et al., 2006), and recruiting T cells to control innate immunity (Hohlfeld R et al., 2007; Kerschensteiner M et al., 1999; Moalem G et al., 2000). Diverse macrophage activities appear to be oppositional and have contradictory effects in nature (Figure3). Pro-inflammatory activity may cause the destructive potential in CNS pathology, whereas anti-inflammatory features may link with their regenerative capacity (Hohlfeld Ret al., 2007; Miron VE,2013). ‘‘Alternatively activated” macrophages could result in partial recovery of motor functions in paraplegic rats (Rapalino O et al., 1998). Moreover, injecting M2- macrophages into the damaged site for SCI patients was well tolerated and resulted in significant motor and sensory improvement (Knoller N et al., 2005).

## 2.6. Umbilical Cord Stromal Cell

***Lei Zhang***

Umbilical cord (UC) including arteries (UCA), veins (UCV), and Wharton's jelly (UCWJ) is a convenient, efficient source of stromal cells that can be expanded easily *in vitro* for clinical applications for non-hematopoietic diseases (Girdlestone J et al., 2009), such as CNS trauma and neurodegenerative diseases (Low CB et al., 2008; Nekanti U et al., 2010; Peng J et al., 2011). Neuroglial cells differentiated from umbilical cord stromal cells (UCSCs) are positively stained for the typical specific neuroglial markers such as the GFAP, the GAP-43 and NeuN (Gärtner A et al., 2012). Intrathecal injection of UCSC is safe and can delay the progression of neurologic deficits for SCA and MSA-C type patients (Dongmei H et al.,

2011). The mechanism of neurological function recovery may be from inhibiting inflammation and promoting angiogenesis.

## 2.7. Adipose Tissue-Derived Stromal/Precursor Cell

### *Lin Chen and Hongyun Huang*

Adipose tissue-derived stromal/precursor cells (ADSPCs) are isolated from the adipose tissue and can be greatly expanded in vitro, and induced to differentiate into multiple mesenchymal cell types, including osteogenic, chondrogenic, myogenic, adipogenic cells and neurogenic like cells (Gimble J et al., 2003; Safford KM et al., 2004; Yang LY et al., 2004; Yu JM et al., 2011). The cell surface phenotype of human ADSPCs is quite similar to MSCs (Zuk PA et al., 2002; De Ugarte DA et al., 2003). ADSPCs secrete a number of angiogenesis-related cytokines, such as VEGF and hepatocyte growth factor (HGF) (Nakagami H et al., 2006). ADSPCs may be to differentiate a particular lineage to replacing a damaged or ablated cell for their effect, but more acceptable mechanism is that paracrine release of growth factors from ADSPCs accelerates and directs tissue repair by endogenous cells (Gimble JM et al., 2012). ADSPCs have preclinical applications for the repair and regeneration of various neurologic disorders (Safford KM, 2005; Ogawa R,2006; Kim WS et al., 2009; Mizuno H,2009; Gimble JM et al., 2010;Yang YC et al., 2011). ADSPCs can reduce demyelination and axonal loss when given prior to disease onset (Constantin G et al., 2009) and intravenous injection for patients with multiple sclerosis is tolerated and may have some symptomatic benefit (Riordan NH et al., 2009). More clinical trials are going to do for neurologic diseases (Gimble JM et al., 2012).

## 2.8. Skin-Derived Precursor

### *Lin Chen and Hongyun Huang*

Skin-derived precursors (SKPs) share characteristics with fetal neural crest stem cells, including their ability to differentiate into neural crest derived cell types such as peripheral neurons, SCs, astrocytes, and endothelium (Fernandes KJ et al., 2008; Hunt DP et al., 2009; Zavan B et al., 2010). SKPs can be isolated and expanded from both neonatal and adult human skin (Joannides A et al., 2004; Toma JG et al., 2005). After transplantation, SKPs healthy cells migrate to the lesion site, and differentiate mainly into cells expressing glia and neuronal markers (Gorio A et al., 2004), so they should be considered as a novel, accessible and potentially autologous source for future nervous system repair (Proulx S et al., 2011; McKenzie IA et al., 2006; Biernaskie J et al., 2007).

# 3. Totipotent Stem Cell

*Lin Chen and Hongyun Huang*

## 3.1. Embryonic Stem Cell

Embryonic stem cells (ESCs) are obtained from the inner cell mass from the early embryo at blastocyst stage with two essential properties, that is, pluripotency and self-renewal. Successful derivation of the first stable mouse embryonic stem cell lines in 1981, and derived in human ESC lines for the first time in 1998, they can be maintained in culture in an undifferentiated state indefinitely (Evans MJ et al., 1981; Martin GR, 1981; Thomson JA et al., 1998). ESCs can efficiently differentiate into neural precursors which can further generate functional neurons, astrocytes, and oligodendrocytes (Fluckiger AC, et al., 2003; Liu S et al., 2000; López-González R et al., 2009) and have the beneficial properties of secreting neurotrophic and neural growth factors (Newman MB et al., 2008). Geron Corporation got permission to conduct SCI phase I trial by embryonic stem cell derivatives, but at last halted this trial (Lukovic D et al., 2014). ESC-based nervous system repair faces several problems now, in which the major hurdle is tumor formation (Yanai J et al., 1995; Li JY et al., 2008).

## 3.2. Induced Pluripotent Stem Cell

Induced pluripotent stem cells(iPSCs) were first produced in 2006 from mouse cells (Takahashi K et al., 2006) and in 2007 from human cells (Yu J et al., 2007; Takahashi K et al., 2007), commonly abbreviated as iPS cells, which are a type of pluripotent stem cell artificially derived from a non-pluripotent cell by a few transcription factors (Boucherie C et al., 2011; Cantz T et al., 2010) and similar to natural pluripotent stem cells, such as ESCs, in many respects, such as the expression of certain stem cell genes and proteins, chromatin methylation patterns, doubling time, embryoid body formation, teratoma formation, viable chimera formation, potency and differentiability and specific markers (Aoki T et al., 2010), and differentiate into all types of cells in the body, and are almost identical to ESCs (Kiefer JC, 2011; Ogawa S et al., 2011; Wang A et al., 2011; Czepiel M et al., 2011), but without any immunogenic responses.

The full extent of their relation to natural pluripotent stem cells is still being assessed (Takahashi K et al., 2006). iPSCs, like hESCs, may be differentiable into dopaminergic neurons (Ma L et al., 2011; Marchetto MC et al., 2011). Even iPSC therapy may be highly effective, and immune rejection-free for PD, SCI, stroke, spinal muscular atrophy, and hearing impairment (Chen LW et al., 2011; El-Amraoui A et al., 2010; Hernándeza J et al., 2011; Hunt CJ,2011; Sendtner M,2010;Tomaskovic-Crook E et al., 2011), the major hurdle for clinical application is its propensity to form tumors (Knoepfler PS,2009). A recent study indicated that iPS cells were far more tumorigenic than ESC with serious concern of safety (Gutierrez-Aranda I et al., 2010).

# References


Aarum, J;Sandberg, K;Haeberlein, SL;Persson, MA. Migration and differentiation of neural precursor cells can be directed by microglia. *Proc. Natl. Acad. Sci. USA*. 2003; 100:15983–15988.

Acheson, A;Barker, PA;Alderson, RF;Miller, FD;Murphy, RA. Detection of brain-derived neurotrophic factor-like activity in fibroblasts and Schwann cells: inhibition by antibodies to NGF. *Neuron*. 1991;7:265–275.

Ader, M;Schachner, M;Bartsch, U. Integration and differentiation of neural stem cells after transplantation into the dysmyelinated central nervous system of adult mice. *Eur. J. Neurosci*. 2004;20:1205–10.

Ali, H;Bahbahani, H. Umbilical cord blood stem cells - potential therapeutic tool for neural injuries and disorders. *Acta. Neurobiol. Exp.* (Wars). 2010;70(3):316-324.

Aoki, T;Ohnishi, H;Oda, Y;Tadokoro, M;Sasao, M;Kato, H;Hattori, K;Ohgushi, H. Generation of induced pluripotent stem cells from human adipose-derived stem cells without c-MYC. *Tissue Eng. Part A*. 2010;16(7):2197-2206.

Appel, SH;Engelhardt, JI;Henkel JS, et al. Hematopoietic stem cell transplantation in patients with sporadic amyotrophic lateral sclerosis. *Neurology*. 2008;71(17):1326-1334.

Azizi, SA;Stokes, D;Augelli, BJ;DiGirolamo, C;Prockop, DJ. Engraftment and migration of human bone marrow stromal cells implanted in the brains of albino rats--similarities to astrocyte grafts. *Proc. Natl. Acad. Sci. U S A*. 1998;95:3908–3913.

Bandtlow, CE;Heumann, R;Schwab, ME;Thoenen, H. Cellular localization of nerve growth factor synthesis by in situ hybridization. *EMBO J*. 1987;6:891–899.

Banisadr, G;Frederick, TJ;Freitag, C;Ren, D;Jung, H;Miller, SD;Miller, RJ. The role of CXCR4 signaling in the migration of transplanted oligodendrocyte progenitors into the cerebral white matter. *Neurobiol. Dis*. 2011;44(1):19-27.

Barette, B;Hébert, MA;Filali, M;Lafortune, K;Vallières, N;Gowing, G;Julien, JP;Lacroix, S. Requirement of myeloid cells for axon regeneration. *J Neurosci*. 2008; 28:9363–9376.

Barnett, SC;Hutchins, AM;Noble, M. Purification of olfactory nerve ensheathing cells from the olfactory bulb. *Dev. Biol*. 1993;155: 337-350.

Barnett, SC;Alexander, CL;Iwashita, Y;Gilson, JM;Crowther, J;Clark, L;Dunn, LT;Papanastassiou, V;Kennedy, PG;Franklin, RJ. Identification of a human olfactory ensheathing cell that can effect transplant-mediated remyelination of demyelinated CNS axons. *Brain*. 2000;123 ( Pt 8):1581-8.

Barnett, SC. Olfactory ensheathing cells: unique glial cell types? *J. Neurotrauma*. 2004;21(4):375-382.

Barritt, AW;Davies, M;Marchand, F;Hartley, R;Grist, J;Yip P, et al. Chondroitinase ABC promotes sprouting of intact and injured spinal systems after spinal cord injury. *J. Neurosci*. 2006;26(42):10856–10867.

Basso, DM;Beattie, MS;Bresnahan, JC. A sensitive and reliable locomotor rating scale for open field testing in rats. *J. Neurotrauma*. 1995;12((1)):1–21.

Bhatheja, K;Field, J. Schwann cells: origins and role in axonal maintenance and regeneration. *Int. J. Biochem. Cell. Biol*. 2006;38(12):1995-1999.

Bieback, K;Klüter, H. Mesenchymal stromal cells from umbilical cord blood. *Curr. Stem Cell. Res. Ther*. 2007;2(4):310-323.

Biernaskie, J;Sparling, JS;Liu, J;Shannon, CP;Plemel, JR;Xie, Y;Miller, FD;Tetzlaff, W. Skin-derived precursors generate myelinating Schwann cells that promote remyelination and functional recovery after contusion spinal cord injury.*J. Neurosci.* 2007;27(36):9545-9559.

Blakemore, WF;Crang, AJ. The relationship between type-1 astrocytes, Schwann cells and oligodendrocytes following transplantation of glial cell cultures into demyelinating lesions in the adult rat spinal cord. *J. Neurocytol.* 1989;18(4):519-28.

Blakemore, WF;Crang, AJ. The use of cultured autologous Schwann cells to remyelinate areas of persistent demyelination in the central nervous system. *J. Neurol. Sci.* 1985;70(2):207-223.

Blakemore, WF. Limited remyelination of CNS axons by Schwann cells transplanted into the sub-arachnoid space. *J. Neurol. Sci.* 1984; 64(3):265-76.

Blakemore, WF. Remyelination of CNS axons by Schwann cells transplanted from the sciatic nerve. *Nature.* 1977; 266(5597):68-9.

Bomstein, Y;Marder, JB;Vitner, K;Smirnov, I;Lisaey, G;Butovsky, O;Fulga, V;Yoles, E. Features of skin-coincubated macrophages that promote recovery from spinal cord injury. *J. Neuroimmunol.* 2003; 142:10–16.

Borlongan, CV;Kaneko, Y;Maki, M;Yu, SJ;Ali, M;Allickson, JG;Sanberg, CD;Kuzmin-Nichols, N;Sanberg, PR. Menstrual blood cells display stem cell-like phenotypic markers and exert neuroprotection following transplantation in experimental stroke. *Stem. CellsDev.* 2010; 19(4):439-52.

Boucherie, C;Sowden, JC;Ali, RR. Induced pluripotent stem cell technology for generating photoreceptors. *Regen. Med.* 2011;6(4):469-479.

Boyd, JG;Skihar, V;Kawaja, M;Doucette, R. Olfactory ensheathing cells: historical perspective and therapeutic potential. *Anat. Rec. B. New Anat.* 2003;271(1):49-60.

Bruska, M;Woźniak, W. Differentiation, maturation, and function of Schwann cells (lemmocytes). *Folia Morphol* (Warsz). 1999;58(3 Suppl 2):101-7.

Bryan, DJ;Wang, KK;Summerhayes, C. Migration of schwann cells in peripheral-nerve regeneration. *J. Reconstr. Microsurg.* 1999;15(8):591-596.

Bunge, RP. Expanding roles for the Schwann cell: ensheathment, myelination, trophism and regeneration. *Curr. Opin. Neurobiol.* 1993;3(5):805-9.

Bunge, RP. The role of the Schwann cell in trophic support and regeneration. *J. Neurol.* 1994;242(1 Suppl 1):S19-21.

Burt, RK;Cohen, B;Rose J, et al. Hematopoietic stem cell transplantation for multiple sclerosis. *Arch. Neurol.* 2005;62(6):860-864.

Burt, RK;Traynor, AE. Hematopoietic stem cell transplantation: a new therapy for autoimmune disease. *Stem. Cells.* 1999;17(6):366-372.

Buzańska, L;Jurga, M;Domańska-Janik, K. Neuronal differentiation of human umbilical cord blood neural stem-like cell line. *Neurodegener Dis.* 2006;3(1-2):19-26.

Cantz, T;Martin, U. Induced Pluripotent Stem Cells: Characteristics and Perspectives. *Adv Biochem Eng Biotechno*l. 2010;123:107-126.

Caracciolo, PC;Thomas, V;Vohra, YK;Buffa, F;Abraham, GA. Electrospinning of novel biodegradable poly(ester urethane)s and poly(ester urethane urea)s for soft tissue-engineering applications. *J. Mater Sci. Mater Med.* 2009;20(10):2129–2137.

Chehrehasa, F;Windus, LC;Ekberg JA, S et al. Olfactory glia enhance neonatal axon regeneration. *Mol. Cell. Neurosci.* 2010;45(3):277-288.

Chen, LW;Kuang, F;Wei, LC et al. Potential application of induced pluripotent stem cells in cell replacement therapy for Parkinson's disease. *CNS Neurol. Disord. Drug Targets.* 2011;10(4):449-458.

Choi, KD;Vodyanik, M;Slukvin, II. Hematopoietic differentiation and production of mature myeloid cells from human pluripotent stem cells. *Nat. Protoc.* 2011;6(3):296-313.

Constantin, G;Marconi, S;Rossi, B et al. Adipose-derived mesenchymal stem cells ameliorate chronic experimental autoimmune encephalomyelitis. *Stem Cells.* 2009;27:2624–2635.

Crang, AJ;Blakemore, WF. Remyelination of demyelinated rat axons by transplanted mouse oligodendrocytes. *Glia.* 1991;4(3):305-13.

Czepiel, M;Balasubramaniyan, V;Schaafsma, W et al. Differentiation of induced pluripotent stem cells into functional oligodendrocytes. *Glia.* 2011;59(6):882-892.

Daadi, MM;Davis, AS;Arac, A;Li, Z;Maag, AL;Bhatnagar, R;Jiang, K;Sun, G;Wu, JC;Steinberg, GK. Human neural stem cell grafts modify microglial response and enhance axonal sprouting in neonatal hypoxic-ischemic brain injury. *Stroke.* 2010;41(3):516-23.

Damon, LE;Damon, LE. Mobilization of hematopoietic stem cells into the peripheral blood. *Expert Rev Hematol.* 2009;2(6):717-733.

Dasari, VR;Veeravalli, KK;Tsung, AJ;Gondi, CS;Gujrati, M;Dinh, D et al. Neuronal apoptosis inhibited by cord blood stem cells after spinal cord injury. *J. Neurotrauma.* 2009 ;26(11):2057-2069.

De Feo, D;Merlini, A;Laterza, C;Martino, G. Neural stem cell transplantation in central nervous system disorders: from cell replacement to neuroprotection. *Curr. Opin. Neurol.* 2012;25(3):322-33.

De Lorenzo, AJ. Electron microscopic observations of the olfactory mucosa and olfactory nerve. *J. Biophys. Biochem. Cytol.* 1957; 3: 839-850.

De Ugarte, DA;Alfonso, Z;Zuk, PA;Elbarbary, A;Zhu, M;Ashjian, P;Benhaim, P;Hedrick, MH;Fraser, JK. Differential expression of stem cell mobilization-associated molecules on multi-lineage cells from adipose tissue and bone marrow. *Immunol Lett.* 2003; 89: 267–270.

Deans, RJ;Moseley, AB. Mesenchymal stem cells: Biology and potential clinical uses. *Exp. Hematol.* 2000;28:875–884.

Deda, H;Inci, MC;Kürekçi, AE et al. Treatment of amyotrophic lateral sclerosis patients by autologous bone marrow-derived hematopoietic stem cell transplantation: a 1-year follow-up. *Cytotherapy.* 2009;11(1):18-25.

Deda, H;Inci, MC;Kürekçi, AE et al. Treatment of chronic spinal cord injured patients with autologous bone marrow-derived hematopoietic stem cell transplantation: 1-year follow-up. *Cytotherapy.* 2008;10(6):565-574.

Deng, J;Petersen, BE;Steindler, DA;Jorgensen, ML;Laywell, ED. Mesenchymal stem cells spontaneously express neural proteins in culture and are neurogenic after transplantation. *Stem Cells.* 2006;24:1054–1064.

Deng, LX;Hu, J;Liu, N et al. GDNF modifies reactive astrogliosis allowing robust axonal regeneration through Schwann cell-seeded guidance channels after spinal cord injury. *Exp Neurol.* 2011;229(2):238-250.

Dezawa, M;Ishikawa, H;Hoshino, M;Itokazu, Y;Nabeshima, Y. Potential of bone marrow stromal cells in applications for neuro-degenerative, neuro-traumatic and muscle degenerative diseases. *Curr. Neuropharmacol.* 2005;3(4):257-266.

Dongmei, H;Jing, L;Mei, X;Ling, Z;Hongmin, Y;Zhidong, W;Li, D;Zikuan, G;Hengxiang, W. Clinical analysis of the treatment of spinocerebellar ataxia and multiple system atrophy-cerebellar type with umbilical cord mesenchymal stromal cells. *Cytotherapy.* 2011;13(8):913-7.

Doucette, R. Glial influences on axonal growth in the primary olfactory system. *Glia.* 1990;3:433–449.

Doucette, R. PNS-CNS transitional zone of the first cranial nerve. *J. Comp. Neurol.* 1991;312:451–466.

Duncan, ID;Hammang, JP;Jackson, KF;Wood, PM;Bunge, RP;Langford, L. Transplantation of oligodendrocytes and Schwann cells into the spinal cord of the myelin-deficient rat. *J. Neurocytol.* 1988;17(3):351-60.

El-Amraoui, A;Petit, C. Stem cell therapy in the inner ear: recent achievements and prospects. *Med. Sci.* (Paris). 2010;26(11):981-985.

Evans, MJ;Kaufman, M. Establishment in culture of pluripotential stem cells from mouse embryos. *Nature.* 1981;292(5819):151–156.

Fadok, VA;Bratton, DL;Konowal, A;Freed, PW;Westcott, JY;Henson, PM. Macrophages that have ingested apoptotic cells in vitro inhibit proinflammatory cytokine production through autocrine/paracrine mechanisms involving TGF-beta, PGE2, and PAF. *J. Clin. Invest.* 1998; 101:890–898.

Fan, X;Krahling, S;Smith, D;Williamson, P;Schlegel, RA. Macrophage surface expression of annexins I and II in the phagocytosis of apoptotic lymphocytes. *Mol. Biol. Cell.* 2004; 15(6):2863-72.

Fernandes, KJ;Toma, JG;Miller, FD. Multipotent skin-derived precursors: adult neural crest-related precursors with therapeutic potential. *Philos Trans R. Soc. Lond B. Biol. Sci.* 2008;363(1489):185-198.

Féron, F;Perry, C;Cochrane, J;Licina, P;Nowitzke, A;Urquhart, S;Geraghty, T;Mackay-Sim, A. Autologous olfactory ensheathing cell transplantation in human spinal cord injury. *Brain.* 2005; 128(Pt 12):2951-60.

Fluckiger, AC;Dehay, C;Savatier, P. Embryonic stem cells and cell replacement therapies in the nervous system. *Med. Sci.* (Paris). 2003;19(6-7):699-708.

Franceschini, IA;Barnett, SC. Low-affinity NGF-receptor and E-N-CAM expression define two types of olfactory nerve ensheathing cells that share a common lineage. *Dev. Biol.* 1996; 173(1):327-43.

Franklin, RJ;Gilson, JM;Franceschini, IA;Barnett, SC. Schwann cell-like myelination following transplantation of an olfactory bulb-ensheathing cell line into areas of demyelination in the adult CNS. *Glia.* 1996; 17(3): 217-224.

Franssen, EH;De Bree, FM;Essing, AH et al. Comparative gene expression profiling of olfactory ensheathing glia and Schwann cells indicates distinct tissue repair characteristics of olfactory ensheathing glia. *Glia.* 2008;56(12):1285-1298.

Franssen, EH;de Bree, FM;Verhaagen, J. Olfactory ensheathing glia: their contribution to primary olfactory nervous system regeneration and their regenerative potential following transplantation into the injured spinal cord. *Brain Res. Rev.* 2007;56:236–258.

Freire-de-Lima, CG;Xiao, YQ;Gardai, SJ;Bratton, DL;Schiemann, WP; Henson, PM. Apoptotic cells, through transforming growth factor-β, coordinately induce anti-inflammatory and suppress pro-inflammatory eicosanoid and NO synthesis in murine macrophages. *J. Biol. Chem.* 2006; 281:38376–38384.

Friedenstein, AJ;Gorskaja, JF;Kulagina, NN. Fibroblast precursors in normal and irradiated mouse hematopoietic organs. *Exp. Hematol*. 1976;4:267–274.

Friedman, B;Scherer, SS;Rudge, JS;Helgren, M;Morrisey, D;McClain, J;Wang DY;Wiegand, SJ;Furth, ME;Lindsay, RM. Regulation of ciliary neurotrophic factor expression in myelin-related Schwann cells in vivo. *Neuron*. 1992;9:295–305.

Frisch, D. Ultrastructure of mouse olfactory mucosa. *Am. J. Anat*. 1967;121: 87-120.

Gärtner, A;Pereira, T;Alves, MG;Armada-da-Silva, PA;Amorim, I;Gomes, R;Ribeiro, J;França, ML;Lopes, C;Carvalho, RA;Socorro, S;Oliveira, PF;Porto, B;Sousa, R;Bombaci, A;Ronchi, G;Fregnan, F;Varejão, AS;Luís, AL;Geuna, S;Maurício, AC. Use of poly(DL-lactide-ε-caprolactone) membranes and mesenchymal stem cells from the Wharton's jelly of the umbilical cord for promoting nerve regeneration in axonotmesis: in vitro and in vivo analysis. *Differentiation*. 2012;84(5):355-65.

Gasser, HS. Olfactory nerve fibers. *J. Gen. Physiol*. 1956; 39: 473-496.

Gimble, J;Guilak, F. Adipose-derived adult stem cells: isolation, characterization, and differentiation potential. *Cytotherapy*. 2003;5:362–369.

Gimble, JM;Bunnell, BA;Guilak, F. Human adipose-derived cells: an update on the transition to clinical translation. *Regen. Med*. 2012;7(2):225-35.

Gimble, JM;Guilak, F;Bunnell, BA. Clinical and preclinical translation of cell-based therapies using adipose tissue-derived cells. *Stem Cell. Res. Ther*. 2010;1(2):19

Girdlestone, J;Limbani, VA;Cutler, AJ;Navarrete, CV. Efficient expansion of mesenchymal stromal cells from umbilical cord under low serum conditions. *Cytotherapy*. 2009;11(6):738-48.

Goh, EL;Ma, D;Ming, GL;Song, H. Adult neural stem cells and repair of the adult central nervous system. *J. Hematother Stem. Cell Res*. 2003;12(6):671-679.

Golpon, HA;Fadok, VA;Taraseviciene-Stewart, L et al. Life after corpse engulfment: phagocytosis of apoptotic cells leads to VEGF secretion and cell growth. *The FASEB Journal*. 2004; 18:1716–1718.

Gorio, A;Torrente, Y;Madaschi, L et al. Fate of autologous dermal stem cells transplanted into the spinal cord after traumatic injury (TSCI). *Neuroscience*. 2004;125(1):179-189.

Greco, SJ;Rameshwar, P. Enhancing effect of IL-1alpha on neurogenesis from adult human mesenchymal stem cells: implication for inflammatory mediators in regenerative medicine. *J. Immunol*. 2007;179:3342–3350.

Griffiths, MR;Gasque, P;Neal, JW. The multiple roles of the innate immune system in the regulation of apoptosis and inflammation in the brain. *J. Neuropathol. Exp. Neurol*, 2009; 68: 217–226.

Gutierrez-Aranda, I;Ramos-Mejia, V;Bueno, C;Munoz-Lopez, M;Real, PJ;Mácia, A;Sanchez, L;Ligero, G;Garcia-Parez, JL;Menendez, P. Human induced pluripotent stem cells develop teratoma more efficiently and faster than human embryonic stem cells regardless the site of injection. *Stem Cells*. 2010;28(9):1568-1570.

Haas, S;Weidner, N;Winkler J. Adult stem cell therapy in stroke. *Curr. Opin. Neurol*. 2005;18(1):59-64.

Hale, DM;Ray, S;Leung, JY;Holloway, AF;Chung, RS;West, AK;Chuah, MI. Olfactory ensheathing cells moderate nuclear factor kappaB translocation in astrocytes. *Mol. CellNeurosci*. 2011;46(1):213-221.

Harris, DT. Cord blood stem cells: a review of potential neurological applications. *Stem CellRev*. 2008; 4(4):269-74.

Hernándeza, J;Torres-Espína, A;Navarro, X. Adult Stem Cell Transplants for Spinal Cord Injury Repair: Current State in Preclinical Research. *Curr. Stem. Cell Res. Ther.* 2011;6(3):273-287.

Higginson, JR;Thompson, SM;Santos-Silva, A;Guimond, SE;Turnbull, JE;Barnett, SC. Differential sulfation remodelling of heparan sulfate by extracellular 6-O-sulfatases regulates fibroblast growth factor-induced boundary formation by glial cells: implications for glial cell transplantation. *J. Neurosci.* 2012; 32(45):15902-12.

Hohlfeld, R;Kerschensteiner, M;Meinl, E. Dual role of inflammation in CNS disease. *Neurology.* 2007; 68 (Suppl 3):S58–S63.

Huang, H;Chen, L;Wang, H et al. Influence of patients' age on functional recovery after transplantation of olfactory ensheathing cells into injured spinal cord injury. *Chin. Med. J.* (Engl). 2003;116(10):1488-1491.

Huang, H;Chen, L;Xi, H;W et al. Olfactory ensheathing cells transplantation for central nervous system diseases in 1255 patients. Zhongguo Xiu Fu Chong Jian Wai Ke Za Zhi. 2009;23(1):14-20.

Hunt, CJ. Cryopreservation of Human Stem Cells for Clinical Application: A Review. *Transfus Med. Hemother.* 2011;38(2):107-123.

Hunt, DP;Jahoda, C;Chandran, S. Multipotent skin-derived precursors: from biology to clinical translation. *Curr. Opin. Biotechnol.* 2009;20(5):522-530.

Hunt, DP;Irvine, KA;Webber, DJ;Compston, DA;Blakemore, WF;Chandran, S. Effects of direct transplantation of multipotent mesenchymal stromal/stem cells into the demyelinated spinal cord. *Cell. Transplant.* 2008; 17(7):865-73.

Ii, M;Nishimura, H;Sekiguchi, H;Kamei, N;Yokoyama, A;Horii, M;Asahara, T. Concurrent vasculogenesis and neurogenesis from adult neural stem cells. *Circ. Res.* 2009;105(9):860-8.

Imaizumi, T;Lankford, KL;Burton, WV et al. Xenotransplantation of transgenic pig olfactory ensheathing cells promotes axonal regeneration in rat spinal cord. *Nat. Biotechnol.* 2000;18(9):949-953.

Jessen, KR;Brennan, A;Morgan, L;Mirsky, R;Kent, A;Hashimoto, Y;Gavrilovic, J. The Schwann cell precursor and its fate: a study of cell death and differentiation during gliogenesis in rat embryonic nerves. *Neuron.* 1994;12(3):509-527.

Jin, K;Galvan, V. Endogenous neural stem cells in the adult brain. *J Neuroimmune Pharmacol.* 2007;2(3):236-242.

Joannides, A;Gaughwin, P;Schwiening, C;Majed, H;Sterling, J;Compston, A;Chandran, S. Efficient generation of neural precursors from adult human skin: astrocytes promote neurogenesis from skin-derived stem cells. *Lancet.* 2004;364:172–178.

Kang, KS;Kim, SW;Oh, YH;Yu, JW;Kim, KY;Park, HK;Song, CH;Han, H. A 37-year-old spinal cord-injured female patient, transplanted of multipotent stem cells from human UC blood, with improved sensory perception and mobility, both functionally and morphologically: a case study. *Cytotherapy.* 2005;7(4):368-73.

Karussis, D;Kassis, I;Kurkalli, BG;Slavin, S. Immunomodulation and neuroprotection with mesenchymal bone marrow stem cells (MSCs): a proposed treatment for multiple sclerosis and other neuroimmunological/neurodegenerative diseases. *J. Neurol. Sci.* 2008;15; 265(1-2):131-5.

Kassem, M;Abdallah, BM. Human bone-marrow-derived mesenchymal stem cells: biological characteristics and potential role in therapy of degenerative diseases. *Cell. Tissue Res.* 2008;331:157–163.

Kerschensteiner, M;Gallmeier, E;Behrens, L;Leal, VV;Misgeld, T;Klinkert, WEF;Kolbeck, R;Hoppe, E;Oropeza-Wekerle, R-L;Bartke, I;Stadelmann, C;Lassman, H;Wekerle, H;Hohlfeld, R. Activated human T cells, B cells, and monocytes produce brain-derived neurotrophic factor in vitro and in inflammatory brain lesions: A neuroprotective role of inflammation? *J. Exp. Med.* 1999;189:865–870.

Kiefer, JC. Primer and interviews: Promises and realities of induced pluripotent stem cells. *Dev. Dyn.* 2011;240(8):2034-2041.

Kigerl, KA;Gensel, JC;Ankeny, DP;Alexander, JK;Donnelly, DJ;Popovich, PG. Identification of two distinct macrophage subsets with divergent effects causing either neurotoxicity or regeneration in the injured mouse spinal cord. *J Neurosci.* 2009 ;29(43):13435-44.

Kim, BG;Hwang, DH;Lee, SI;Kim, EJ;Kim, SU. Stem cell-based cell therapy for spinal cord injury. *Cell. Transplant.* 2007;16(4):355-64.

Kim, WS;Park, BS;Sung, JH. The wound-healing and antioxidant effects of adipose-derived stem cells. *Expert Opin. Biol. Ther.* 2009;9(7):879-887.

Knoepfler, PS. Deconstructing stem cell tumorigenicity: a roadmap to safe regenerative medicine. *Stem Cells.* 2009;27(5):1050-1056.

Knoller, N;Auerbach, G;Fulga, V;Zelig, G;Attias, J;Bakimer, R;Marder, JB;Yoles, E;Belkin, M;Schwartz, M;Hadani, M. Clinical experience using incubated autologous macrophages as a treatment for complete spinal cord injury: phase I study results. *J. Neurosurg.* 2005; 3:173–181.

Kopen, GC;Prockop, DJ;Phinney, DG. Marrow stromal cells migrate throughout forebrain and cerebellum, and they differentiate into astrocytes after injection into neonatal mouse brains. *Proc. Natl. Acad. Sci. U S A.* 1999;96:10711–10716.

Koshizuka, S;Okada, S;Okawa, A et al. Transplanted hematopoietic stem cells from bone marrow differentiate into neural lineage cells and promote functional recovery after spinal cord injury in mice. *J. Neuropathol. Exp. Neurol.* 2004;63(1):64-72.

Kotter, MR;Zhao, C;van Rooijen, N;Franklin, RJ. Macrophage-depletion induced impairment of experimental CNS remyelination is associated with a reduced oligodendrocyte progenitor cell response and altered growth factor expression. *Neurobiol. Dis.* 2005;18:166–175.

Lakatos, A;Barnett, SC;Franklin, RJ. Olfactory ensheathing cells induce less host astrocyte response and chondroitin sulphate proteoglycan expression than Schwann cells following transplantation into adult CNS white matter. *Exp. Neurol.* 2003;184(1):237-46.

Lamond, R;Barnett, SC. Schwann cells but not olfactory ensheathing cells inhibit CNS myelination via the secretion of connective tissue growth factor. *J. Neurosci.* 2013; 33(47):18686 –18697.

Lankford, KL;Sasaki, M;Radtke, C;Kocsis, JD. Olfactory ensheathing cells exhibit unique migratory, phagocytic, and myelinating properties in the X-irradiated spinal cord not shared by Schwann cells. *Glia.* 2008;56(15):1664-1678.

Lavdas, AA;Papastefanaki, F;Thomaidou, D;Matsas, R. Schwann cell transplantation for CNS repair. *Curr. Med. Chem.* 2008;15(2):151-60.

Lee, JH;Chung, WH;Kang, EH;C et al. Schwann cell-like remyelination following transplantation of human umbilical cord blood (hUCB)-derived mesenchymal stem cells in dogs with acute spinal cord injury. *J. Neurol. Sci.* 2011;300(1-2):86-96.

Leung, JY;Chapman, JA;Harris, JA et al. Olfactory ensheathing cells are attracted to, and can endocytose, bacteria. *Cell. Mol. Life Sci.* 2008;65(17):2732-2739.

Li, JY;Christophersen, NS;Hall, V;Soulet, D;Brundin, P. Critical issues of clinical human embryonic stem cell therapy for brain repair. *Trends Neurosci.* 2008;31(3):146-153.

Li, Y;Chen, J;Chen, XG;Wang, L;Gautam, SC;Xu, YX;Katakowski, M;Zhang, LJ;Lu, M;Janakiraman, N;Chopp, M. Human marrow stromal cell therapy for stroke in rat: Neurotrophins and functional recovery. *Neurology.* 2002;59:514–523.

Li, Y;Chen, L;Zhao, Y;Bao, J;Xiao, J;Liu, J;Jiang, X;Zhou, C;Wang, H;Huang, H. Intracranial transplant of olfactory ensheathing cells can protect both upper and lower motor neurons in amyotrophic lateral sclerosis. *Cell. Transplant.* 2013;22 Suppl 1:51-65.

Lipson, AC;Widenfalk, J;Linquist, E;Ebendal, T;Olson, L. Neurotrophic properties of olfactory ensheathing glia. *Exp. Neurol.* 2003;180:167–171.

Liu, S;Qu, Y;Stewart, TJ;Howard, MJ;Chakrabortty, S;Holekamp, TF;McDonald, JW. Embryonic stem cells differentiate into oligodendrocytes and myelinate in culture and after spinal cord transplantation. *Proc. Natl. Acad. Sci. U S A.* 2000;97(11):6126-6131.

Loh, YS;Hwang, WY;Ratnagopal, P. Autologous haematopoietic stem cell transplantation for the treatment of multiple sclerosis. *Ann. Acad. Med. Singapore.* 2007;36(6):421-426.

López-González, R;Kunckles, P;Velasco, I. Transient recovery in a rat model of familial amyotrophic lateral sclerosis after transplantation of motor neurons derived from mouse embryonic stem cells. *Cell. Transplant.* 2009;18(10):1171-1181.

Low, CB;Liou, YC;Tang, BL. Neural differentiation and potential use of stem cells from the human umbilical cord for central nervous system transplantation therapy. *J. Neurosci. Res.* 2008; 86(8):1670-9.

Lukovic, D;Stojkovic, M;Moreno-Manzano, V;Bhattacharya, SS;Erceg, S. Perspectives and Future Directions of Human Pluripotent Stem Cell-Based Therapies: Lessons from Geron's Clinical Trial for Spinal Cord Injury. *Stem Cells Dev.* 2014 ;23(1):1-4.

Luo, J;Bo, X;Wu, D;Yeh, J;Richardson, PM;Zhang, Y. Promoting survival, migration, and integration of transplanted Schwann cells by over-expressing polysialic acid. *Glia.* 2011;59(3):424-434.

Ma, L;Liu, Y;Zhang, SC. Directed differentiation of dopamine neurons from human pluripotent stem cells. *Methods Mol. Biol.* 2011;767:411-418.

Mackay-Sim, A. Olfactory ensheathing cells and spinal cord repair. *Keio. J. Med.* 2005;54(1):8-14.

Mandalfino, P;Rice, G;Smith, A et al. Bone marrow transplantation in multiple sclerosis. *J. Neurol.* 2000;247(9):691-695.

Marchetto, MC;Brennand, KJ;Boyer, LF;Gage, FH. Induced pluripotent stem cells (iPSCs) and neurological disease modeling: progress and promises. *Hum. Mol. Genet.* 2011;20(R2):R109-115.

Martin, GR. Isolation of a pluripotent cell line from early mouse embryos cultured in medium conditioned by teratocarcinoma stem cells. *Proc. Natl. Acad. Sci. U S A.* 1981;78(12):7634-7638.

McKenzie, IA;Biernaskie, J;Toma, JG;Midha, R;Miller, FD. Skin-derived precursors generate myelinating Schwann cells for the injured and dysmyelinated nervous system. *J. Neurosci.* 2006;26(24):6651-6660.

Meyer, M;Matsuoka, I;Wetmore, C;Olson, L;Thoenen, H. Enhanced synthesis of brain-derived neurotrophic factor in the lesioned peripheral nerve: different mechanisms are responsible for the regulation of BDNF and NGF mRNA. *J. Cell. Biol.* 1992;119:45–54.

Miron, VE;Kuhlmann, T;Antel, JP. Cells of the oligodendroglial lineage, myelination, and remyelination. *Biochim. Biophys. Acta.* 2011;1812(2):184-93.

Miron, VE. Dissecting the damaging versus regenerative roles of CNS macrophages: implications for the use of immunomodulatory therapeutics. *Regen. Med.* 2013;8(6): 673-6.

Mizuno, H. Adipose-derived stem cells for tissue repair and regeneration: ten years of research and a literature review. *J. Nippon. Med. Sch.* 2009;76(2):56-66.

Moalem, G;Gdalyahu, A;Shani, Y;Otten, U;Lazarovici, P;Cohen, IR;Schwartz, M. Production of neurotrophins by activated T cells: implications for neuroprotective autoimmunity. *J. Autoimmunity.* 2000; 15: 331-345.

Nakagami, H;Morishita, R;Maeda, K;Kikuchi, Y;Ogihara, T;Kaneda, Y. Adipose tissue-derived stromal cells as a novel option for regenerative cell therapy. *J. Atheroscler. Thromb.* 2006;13(2):77-81.

Nakajima, K;Kohsaka, S. Microglia: neuroprotective and neurotrophic cells in the central nervous system. *Curr. Drug Targets Cardiovasc. Haematol. Disord.* 2004; 4:65–84.

Nekanti, U;Mohanty, L;Venugopal, P;Balasubramanian, S;Totey, S;Ta, M. Optimization and scale-up of Wharton's jelly-derived mesenchymal stem cells for clinical applications. *Stem Cell Res.* 2010;5(3):244-54.

Newman, MB;Bakay, RA. Therapeutic potentials of human embryonic stem cells in Parkinson's disease. *Neurotherapeutics.* 2008;5(2):237-251.

Ng, TK;Fortino, VR;Pelaez, D;Cheung, HS. Progress of mesenchymal stem cell therapy for neural and retinal diseases. *World J. Stem Cells.* 2014;6(2):111-9.

Ogawa, R. The importance of adipose-derived stem cells and vascularized tissue regeneration in the field of tissue transplantation. *Curr. Stem Cell. Res. Ther.* 2006;1(1):13-20.

Ogawa, S;Tokumoto, Y;Miyake, J;Nagamune, T. Induction of oligodendrocyte differentiation from adult human fibroblast-derived induced pluripotent stem cells. *In Vitro Cell. Dev. Biol. Anim. 2011*;47(7):464-469.

Okano, H. Neural stem cells and strategies for the regeneration of the central nervous system. *Proc. Jpn. Acad. Ser. B. Phys. Biol. Sci.* 2010;86(4):438-50.

Okano, H. Stem cell biology of the central nervous system. *J. Neurosci. Res.* 2002;69(6):698-707.

Oudega, M;Xu, XM. Schwann cell transplantation for repair of the adult spinal cord. *J. Neurotrauma.* 2006;23(3-4):453-467.

Papadopoulos, KI;Karussis, D;Karageorgiou, C;Vaknin-Dembinsky, Aet al. Safety and immunological effects of mesenchymal stem cell transplantation in patients with multiple sclerosis and amyotrophic lateral sclerosis. *Arch. Neurol.* 2010;67(10):1187-1194.

Papadopoulos, KI;Low, SS;Aw, TC;Chantarojanasiri, T. Safety and feasibility of autologous umbilical cord blood transfusion in 2 toddlers with cerebral palsy and the role of low dose granulocyte-colony stimulating factor injections. *Restor. Neurol. Neurosci.* 2011;29(1):17-22.

Patel, AN;Park, E;Kuzman, M;Benetti, F;Silva, FJ;Allickson, JG. Multipotent menstrual blood stromal stem cells: isolation, characterization, and differentiation. *Cell. Transplant.* 2008; 17(3):303-11.

Pellitteri, R;Spatuzza, M;Russo, A;Stanzani, S. Olfactory ensheathing cells exert a trophic effect on the hypothalamic neurons in vitro. *Neurosci. Lett.* 2007;417(1):24-29.

Pellitteri, R;Spatuzza, M;Russo, A;Zaccheo, D;Stanzani, S. Olfactory ensheathing cells represent an optimal substrate for hippocampal neurons: an in vitro study. *Int. J. Dev. Neurosci.* 2009; 27(5):453-8.

Peng, J;Wang, Y;Zhang, L;Zhao, B;Zhao, Z;Chen, J;Guo, Q;Liu, S;Sui, X;Xu, W;Lu, S. Human umbilical cord Wharton's jelly-derived mesenchymal stem cells differentiate into a Schwann-cell phenotype and promote neurite outgrowth in vitro. *Brain Res. Bull.* 2011;84(3):235-43.

Peterson, DA. Umbilical cord blood cells and brain stroke injury: bringing in fresh blood to address an old problem. *J. Clin. Invest.* 2004;114(3):312-314.

Pluchino, S;Quattrini, A;Brambilla, E et al. Injection of adult neurospheres induces recovery in a chronic model of multiple sclerosis. *Nature.* 2003;422(6933):688-694.

Proulx, S;Fradette, J;Gauvin, R et al. Stem cells of the skin and cornea: their clinical applications in regenerative medicine. *Curr. Opin. Organ. Transplant.* 2011;16(1):83-9.

Radtke, C;Aizer, AA;Agulian, SK;Lankford, KL;Vogt, PM et al. Transplantation of olfactory ensheathing cells enhances peripheral nerve regeneration after microsurgical nerve repair. *Brain Res.* 2009;1254:10–17.

Radtke, C;Vogt, PM. Peripheral nerve regeneration: a current perspective. *Eplasty.* 2009;9:e47.

Ramer, LM;Au, E;Richter, MW et al. Peripheral olfactory ensheathing cells reduce scar and cavity formation and promote regeneration after spinal cord injury. *J. Comp. Neurol.* 2004;473(1):1-15.

Ramon y Cajal, S. Degeneration and regeneration of the nervous system. Volume 2. *New York, USA: Haffner Publishing Co.;1928.*

Ramos, AB;Vasconcelos-Dos-Santos, A;Lopes de Souza, SA;Rosado-de-Castro, PH;Barbosa da Fonseca, LM;Gutfilen, B;Cintra, WM;Mendez-Otero, R. Bone-marrow mononuclear cells reduce neurodegeneration in hippocampal CA1 layer after transient global ischemia in rats. *Brain Res.* 2013;1522:1-11.

Rapalino, O;Lazarov-Spiegler, O;Agranov, E;Velan, GJ;Yoles, E;Fraidakis, M;Solomon, A;Gepstein, R;Katz, A;Belkin, M;Hadani, M;Schwartz, M. Implantation of stimulated homologous macrophages results in partial recovery of paraplegic rats. *Nat. Med* 1998; 4:814–821.

Rende, M;Muir, D;Ruoslahti, E;Hagg, T;Varon, S;Manthorpe, M. Immunolocalization of ciliary neuronotrophic factor in adult rat sciatic nerve. *Glia.* 1992;5:25–32.

Reynolds, BA;Weiss, S. Clonal and population analyses demonstrate that an EGF-responsive mammalian embryonic CNS precursor is a stem cell. *Dev. Biol.* 1996; 175(1):1-13.

Riordan, NH;Ichim, TE;Min, WP et al. Non-expanded adipose stromal vascular fraction cell therapy for multiple sclerosis. *J. Transl. Med.* 2009;7:29.

Rogojan, C;Frederiksen, JL. Hematopoietic stem cell transplantation in multiple sclerosis. *ActaNeurol. Scand.* 2009;120(6):371-382.

Rosenkranz, K;Meier, C. Umbilical cord blood cell transplantation after brain ischemia-From recovery of function to cellular mechanisms. *Ann. Anat.* 2011;193(4):371-379.

Roszek, K;Komoszyński, M. Regulation and direction of umbilical cord blood stem cells differentiation and their therapeutic application. *Postepy Hig. Med. Dosw.* (Online). 2008;62:660-7.

Saberi, H;Moshayedi, P;Aghayan, HR et al. Treatment of chronic thoracic spinal cord injury patients with autologous Schwann cell transplantation: an interim report on safety considerations and possible outcomes. *Neurosci. Lett.* 2008;443(1):46-50.

Saccardi, R;Mancardi, GL;Solari, A et al. Autologous HSCT for severe progressive multiple sclerosis in a multicenter trial: impact on disease activity and quality of life. *Blood.* 2005;105(6):2601-2607.

Safford, KM;Rice, HE. Stem cell therapy for neurologic disorders: therapeutic potential of adipose-derived stem cells. *Curr. Drug Targets.* 2005;6(1):57-62.

Safford, KM;Safford, SD;Gimble, JM;Shetty, AK;Rice, HE. Characterization of neuronal/glial differentiation of murine adipose-derived adult stromal cells. *Exp. Neurol.* 2004; 187: 319-328.

Saito, T;Kuang, JQ;Bittira, B;Al-Khaldi, A;Chiu, RC. Xenotransplant cardiac chimera: Immune tolerance of adult stem cells. *Ann. Thorac. Surg.* 2002;74:19–24. discussion 24.

Salem H,Thiemermann, C. Mesenchymal stromal cells: current understanding and clinical status. *Stem Cells.* 2010;28 (3):585-96.

Sanberg, PR;Eve, DJ;Willing, AE et al. The treatment of neurodegenerative disorders using umbilical cord blood and menstrual blood-derived stem cells. *Cell. Transplant.* 2011;20(1):85-94.

Sanberg, PR;Willing, AE;Garbuzova-Davis, S;S et al. Umbilical cord blood-derived stem cells and brain repair. *Ann. N. Y. Acad. Sci.* 2005;1049:67-83.

Santos-Silva, A;Fairless, R;Frame, MC;Montague, P;Smith, GM;Toft, A;Riddell, JS;Barnett, SC. FGF/heparin differentially regulates Schwann cell and olfactory ensheathing cell interactions with astrocytes: a role in astrocytosis. *J. Neurosci.* 2007;27(27):7154-67.

Sasaki, M;Honmou, O;Akiyama, Y et al. Transplantation of an acutely isolated bone marrow fraction repairs demyelinated adult rat spinal cord axons. *Glia.* 2001;35(1):26-34.

Sasaki, M;Li, B;Lankford, KL;Radtke, C;Kocsis, JD. Remyelination of the injured spinal cord. *Prog. Brain Res.* 2007;161:419-433.

Sendtner, M. Therapy development in spinal muscular atrophy. *Nat. Neurosci.* 2010;13(7):795-799.

Shechter, R;London, A;Varol, C;Raposo, C;Cusimano, M;Yovel, G;Rolls, A;Mack, M;Pluchino, S;Martino, G;Jung, S;Schwartz, M. Infiltrating blood-derived macrophages are vital cells playing an anti-inflammatory role in recovery from spinal cord injury in mice. *PLoS Medicine.* 2009; 6: 1–16.

Shih, CC;Fu, L;Zhu, L;Huang, Y;Lee, TD;Forman, SJ. Derivation of neural stem cells from mesenchymal stem cells: evidence for a bipotential stem cell population. *Stem Cells Dev.* 2008;17:1109–1122.

Souayah, N;Coakley, KM;Chen, R et al. Defective Neuromuscular Transmission in the SOD1(G93A) Transgenic Mouse Improves After Administration of Human Umbilical Cord Blood Cells. *Stem Cell. Rev.* 2012;8(1):224-8.

Tabakow, P;Jarmundowicz, W;Czapiga, B;Fortuna, W;Miedzybrodzki, R;Czyz, M;Huber, J, Szarek, D;Okurowski, S;Szewczyk, P;Gorski, A;Raisman, G. Transplantation of autologous olfactory ensheathing cells in complete human spinal cord injury. *Cell. Transplant.* 2013;22(9):1591-612.

Takahashi, K;Tanabe, K;Ohnuki, M;Narita, M;Ichisaka, T;Tomoda, K;Yamanaka, S. Induction of pluripotent stem cells from adult human fibroblasts by defined factors. *Cell.* 2007;131(5):861-72.

Takahashi, K;Yamanaka, S. Induction of pluripotent stem cells from mouse embryonic and adult fibroblast cultures by defined factors. *Cell.* 2006;126(4):663-676.

Takizawa, S. Differentiation of adult bone marrow cells into neurons and endothelial cells in rat brain after stroke in the presence of cytokines. *Rinsho Shinkeigaku.* 2003;43(11):830-831.

Teng, YD;Lavik, EB;Qu, X et al. Functional recovery following traumatic spinal cord injury mediated by a unique polymer scaffold seeded with neural stem cells. *Proc. Natl. Acad. Sci. USA.* 2002;99:3024–9.

Thomson, JA;Itskovitz-Eldor, J;Shapiro, SS;Waknitz, MA;Swiergiel, JJ;Marshall, VS;Jones, JM. Embryonic stem cell lines derived from human blastocysts. *Science.* 1998;282(5391):1145-7.

Toft, A;Scott, DT;Barnett, SC;Riddell, JS. Electrophysiological evidence that olfactory cell transplants improve function after spinal cord injury. *Brain.* 2007; 130(Pt 4):970-84.

Toma, JG;McKenzie, IA;Bagli, D;Miller, FD. Isolation and characterization of multipotent skin-derived precursors from human skin. *Stem Cells.* 2005;23(6):727-737.

Tomaskovic-Crook, E;Crook, JM. Human embryonic stem cell therapies for neurodegenerative diseases. *CNS Neurol. Disord. Drug Targets.* 2011;10(4):440-448.

Torrente, Y;Polli, E. Mesenchymal stem cell transplantation for neurodegenerative diseases. *Cell. Transplant.* 2008;17(10-11):1103-1113.

Trujillo, CA;Schwindt, TT;Martins, AH et al. Novel perspectives of neural stem cell differentiation: from neurotransmitters to therapeutics. *Cytometry A.* 2009;75(1):38-53.

Tyndall, A;Koike, T. High-dose immunoablative therapy with hematopoietic stem cell support in the treatment of severe autoimmune disease: current status and future direction. *Intern. Med.* 2002;41(8):608-612.

Uccelli, A;Pistoia, V;Moretta, L. Mesenchymal stem cells: a new strategy for immunosuppression? *Trends Immunol.* 2007;28(5):219-26.

Vallières, N;Berard, JL;David, S;Lacroix, S. Systemic injections of lipopolysaccharide accelerates myelin phagocytosis during Wallerian degeneration in the injured mouse spinal cord. *Glia.* 2006; 53:103–113.

Vincent, AJ;Lau, PW;Roskams, AJ. SPARC is expressed by macroglia and microglia in the developing and mature nervous system. *Dev. Dyn.* 2008;237(5):1449-1462.

Wang, A;Tang, Z;Park, IH et al. Induced pluripotent stem cells for neural tissue engineering. *Biomaterials.* 2011;32(22):5023-5032.

Wewetzer, K;Brandes, G. Axonal signalling and the making of olfactory ensheathing cells: a hypothesis. *Neuron. Glia Biol.* 2006;2(3):217-224.

Wewetzer, K;Kern, N;Ebel, C;Radtke, C;Brandes, G. Phagocytosis of O4+ axonal fragments in vitro by p75- neonatal rat olfactory ensheathing cells. *Glia.* 2005;49(4):577-587.

Widenfalk, J;Lundstromer, K;Jubran, M;Brene, S;Olson, L. Neurotrophic factors and receptors in the immature and adult spinal cord after mechanical injury or kainic acid. *J. Neurosci.* 2001;21:3457–3475.

Wislet-Gendebien, S;Hans, G;Leprince, P;Rigo, JM;Moonen, G;Rogister, B. Plasticity of cultured mesenchymal stem cells: switch from nestin-positive to excitable neuron-like phenotype. *Stem Cells.* 2005;23:392–402.

Yanai, J;Doetchman, T;Laufer, N et al. Embryonic cultures but not embryos transplanted to the mouse's brain grow rapidly without immunosupression. *Int. J. Neurosci.* 1995;81:21–26.

Yang, LY;Liu, XM;Sun, B;Hui, GZ;Fei, J;Guo, LH. Adipose tissue-derived stromal cells express neuronal phenotypes. *Chin Med J* (Engl). 2004;117(3):425-429.

Yang, WZ;Zhang, Y;Wu, F et al. Human umbilical cord blood-derived mononuclear cell transplantation: case series of 30 subjects with hereditary ataxia. *J Transl Med.* 2011;9:65.

Yang, YC;Liu, BS;Shen, CC;Lin, CH;Chiao, MT;Cheng, HC. Transplantation of adipose tissue-derived stem cells for treatment of focal cerebral ischemia. *Curr. Neurovasc. Res.* 2011;8(1):1-13.

Yin, Y;Cui, Q;Li, Y;Irwin, N;Fischer, D;Harvey, AR;Benowitz, LI. Macrophage-derived factors stimulate optic nerve regeneration. *J. Neurosci.* 2003; 23:2284–2293.

Yu, J;Vodyanik, MA;Smuga-Otto, K;Antosiewicz-Bourget, J;Frane, JL;Tian, S;Nie, J;Jonsdottir, GA;Ruotti, V;Stewart, R;Slukvin, II;Thomson, JA. Induced pluripotent stem cell lines derived from human somatic cells. *Science.* 2007;318(5858):1917-20.

Yu, JM;Bunnell, BA;Kang, SK. Neural differentiation of human adipose tissue-derived stem cells. *Methods Mol. Biol.* 2011;702:219-231.

Yu, XD;Luo, ZJ;Zhang, L;Gong, K. Effects of olfactory ensheathing cells on hydrogen peroxide -induced apoptosis in cultured dorsal root ganglion neurons. *Chin. Med. J.* (Engl). 2007;120(16):1438-1443.

Zavan, B;Michelotto, L;Lancerotto, L et al. Neural potential of a stem cell population in the adipose and cutaneous tissues. *Neurol. Res.* 2010;32(1):47-54.

Zhang, C;Zhang, X;Chen, XH. Granulocyte-colony stimulating factor-mobilized mesenchymal stem cells: A new resource for rapid engraftment in hematopoietic stem cell transplantation. *Med. Hypotheses.* 2011;76(2):241-243.

Zhang, WC;Ding, YJ;Cao, JK et al. Intracerebral co-grafting of Schwann's cells and fetal adrenal medulla in the treatment of Parkinson's disease. *Chin. Med. J.* (Engl). 1994;107(8):583-588.

Ziegler, MD;Hsu, D;Takeoka, A;Zhong, H;Ramón-Cueto, A;Phelps, PE;Roy, RR;Edgerton, VR. Further evidence of olfactory ensheathing glia facilitating axonal regeneration after a complete spinal cord transection. *Exp. Neurol.* 2011;229(1):109-119.

Ziv, Y;Avidan, H;Pluchino, S;Martino, G;Schwartz, M. Synergy between immune cells and adult neural stem/progenitor cells promotes functional recovery from spinal cord injury. *Proc. Natl. Acad. Sci. USA*. 2006; 103:13174–13179.

Zuk, PA;Zhu, M;Ashjian, P;De Ugarte, DA;Huang, JI;Mizuno, H;Alfonso, ZC;Fraser, JK;Benhaim, P;Hedrick, MH. Human adipose tissue is a source of multipotent stem cells. *Mol. Biol. Cell.* 2002; 13: 4279–4295.

Zupanc, GK;Clint, SC;Takimoto, N;Hughes, AT;Wellbrock, UM;Meissner, D. Spatio-temporal distribution of microglia/macrophages during regeneration in the cerebellum of adult teleost fish, Apteronotus leptorhynchus: a quantitative analysis. *Brain Behav. Evol.* 2003;62(1):31-42.

In: Neurorestoratology, volume 1
Editors: H. Huang, G. Raisman, P. R. Sanberg et al.
ISBN: 978-1-63463-599-8


*Chapter 5*

# Procedures of Cell Therapy

***Lin Chen*[1,2]*, Hongyun Huang*[3,4]*, Miroslaw Janowski*[5]**
***and Krystyna Domanska-Janik*[5]**
[1]Tsinghua University Yuquan Hospital, Beijing, China
[2]Medical Center, Tsinghua University, Beijing, China
[3]Beijing Rehabilitation Hospital of Capital Medical University, Beijing, China
[4]Beijing Hongtianji Neuroscience Academy, Beijing, China
[5]Mossakowski Medical Research Centre, Polish Academy of Sciences, Warsaw, Poland

## 1. Cell Preparation

***Lin Chen, Hongyun Huang***

There are many kinds of cells which have being used in the clinic; here we simply introduce those most frequently used. If cells are from abortion source, they must have signed proper written informed consent from the donors.

### 1.1. Olfactory Ensheathing Cells

Outer layer of olfactory bulbs was divided into small pieces, cultured in Dulbecco's modified Eagle's medium/Ham's F12 (DMEM/F12) (Hyclone) with 10% fetal bovine serum (FBS) (Hyclone) and propagated for 14-21 days and then characterized by immunostaining with antibodies against p75 (Sigma).

These cells were detached with trypsin-EDTA, and resuspended at a density of 20,000 cells/μliter.

* Corresponding author: Lin Chen chenlin_china@163.com.

## 1.2. Schwann Cells

Taking human fetal sciatic nerve (for example), the specimen was sliced, digested in trypsin (Invitrogen) and dispersed into a single-cell suspension. Cells were cultured in DMEM/F12 (Hyclone) with 15% FBS (Hyclone) and harvested after 7 days. Double-label immunofluorescence staining of S100 (Sigma) and Hoechst (Sigma) was used to calculate the purity of the SCs.

## 1.3. Neural Progenitor Cells

Under aseptic conditions, tissue from the subependymal zone of fetal human brain was collected and a cell suspension prepared after repeated gentle mechanical trituration by pushing the medium through suction tube.

The cells were cultured in DMEM/F12 (Hyclone) with 20% FBS (Hyclone) and passaged by plating on poly-L-lysine (PLL)-coated dishes (Corning) and immunostained for nestin reactivity (Chemicon).

## 1.4. Umbilical Cord Mesenchymal Stromal Cells

Tissues of umbilical cord from human fetus were harvested and tissue blocks were implanted into dishes (Corning) with DMEM/F12 (Hyclone) with 10% FBS (Hyclone), then incubated in a 37°C 5% $CO_2$ incubator. After 10 days, cells which had migrated from the tissue block were digested using 0.25% EDTA/trypsin (Invitrogen), then passed gradually from 1 to 5 passages.

## 1.5. Bone Marrow Mononuclear Cells

Autologous bone marrow was harvested from the iliac crest. Bone marrow mononuclear cells were separated into adherent and non-adherent cells by culturing overnight at 37℃ in an atmosphere of 5% $CO_2$/95% air. Adherent and non-adherent cells were then re-suspended in physiological saline (2 ml and 100 ml, respectively), and delivered into the cystic cavity or around atrophic/scar degenerative area during surgery (adherent cells) and intravenously (non-adherent cells). Cell viability determined by trypan blue staining was never less than 95%.

# 2. Routes of Cell Transplant to Brain or Cord Parenchyma

*Lin Chen and Hongyun Huang*

There are three routes to deliver cells for patients with CNS disease or damage, which include brain parenchyma or • spinal cord, cerebrospinal fluid (ventricle and subarachnoid space) and intravenous (IV) or intra artery (IA).

## 2.1. Brain Parenchyma Cell Transplants

Stereotactic injection with local anesthesia is used to deliver cells into the brain. Children or nervous adults should receive basic anesthesia. Preoperative brain magnetic resonance imaging (MRI) scan or computed tomography (CT) scan is performed.

According to disease or damage, transplanted cells can be injected into two sites. One is the key point for neural network restoration (KPNNR) (detailed explanation can be found at the paragraph of chapter 1 of first section "*Key point for neural network restoration (KPNNR)*") which is suitable for cerebral palsy, amyotrophic lateral sclerosis, ataxia, multiple sclerosis, dementia, and epilepsy (Figure 1).

Another is the junction at the edge between normal brain and injured area which fits for stroke, brain injury or some local pathological changes (Figure 2).

*Procedure of Intracranial cell transplantation:*

1) Local anesthesia and intravenous sedation if necessary.
2) The patient is placed in a prone position with multi-function electrocardiogram.
3) According to MRI films or CT images, to calculate three-dimensional coordinates of the targets where the KPNNR or edge of lesion area are.
4) Draw the head-lines.
5) Disinfect head skin and overlay sterile towels.
6) Two incisions 5 mm in length are made, which are located 1.5-2.5 cm within the hair, 2.2-2.7 cm midline.
7) Drill bone holes 3 mm in diameter in the front bilaterally.
8) Fine needle (1.1 mm) punctures are made along a predetermined path to the target in accordance with the coordinates mentioned above.
9) The cells are implanted into the brain target.
10) Ten minutes later suture the incision.

*Key points:*

1) Sedation and anesthesia usually are given to children and patients who do not cooperate or who move restlessly.

2) Intraoperative vital signs are monitored, i.e., multifunctional monitoring equipment is used.
3) Continuous cooling with cold saline infusion during cranial skull drilling, to prevent heat burns to the scalp.
4) The needle is implanted into the brain softly and slowly to prevent damage to blood vessels and brain tissue.
5) The injection of cells should be performed slowly.
6) After suturing the incision thick gauze is used to cover the incisions for 2 to 3 days to prevent possible seroma.

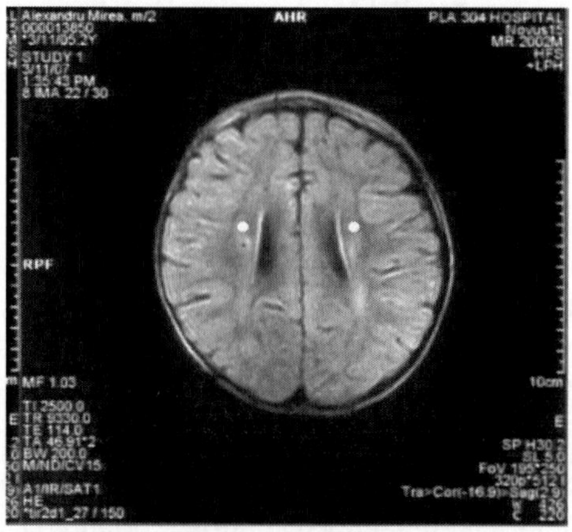

Figure 1. MRI films showing the targets of cell transplantation: two injection sites of OECs in the corona radiate of both-sided frontal lobes (i.e., the key point for neural network restoration (KPNNR)). [Reprinted from Cell Transplantation 19, Chen L, Huang H, Xi H, Xie Z, Liu R, Jiang Z, Zhang F, Liu Y, Chen D, Wang Q, Wang H, Ren Y, Zhou C. Intracranial transplant of olfactory ensheathing cells in children and adolescents with cerebral palsy: a randomized controlled clinical trial, 185-191 (Fig. 2), Copyright (2010), with permission from Cognizant Comm. Corp.].

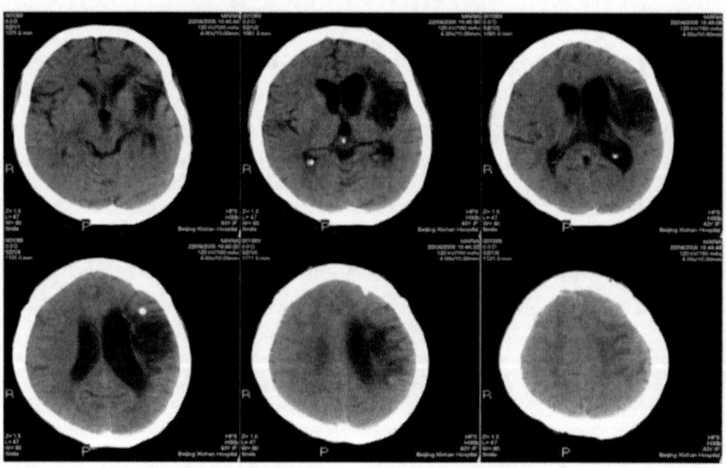

Figure 2. CT films showing the sites of cell transplantation locate at the edge between normal brain and injured area (stoke) [Reprinted from Cell Transplantation 22(S1), Chen L, Xi H, Huang H, Zhang F, Liu Y, Chen D, Xiao J. Multiple cell transplantation based on an intraparenchymal approach for patients with chronic phase stroke, S83-S91 (Fig. 1), Copyright (2013), with permission from Cognizant Comm. Corp.]

*Sedation and anesthesia for children:*

1) Non per os (NPO) for four hours.
2) Venous access is established and intraoperative transfusion appropriately done to avoid hypovolemia.
3) Conventional intravenous diazepam prescription: ① For children of 30 days to 5 years of age: 0.2-0.5 mg every 2 to 5 minutes, the maximum dose of 5 mg; ② For children who are 5 years of age and older: 1mg every 2 to 5 minutes with the maximum dosage of 10mg.
4) Children >2 years of age with ineffective conventional sedation, the following options are recommended: 1) Atropine 0.05-0.2 mg im for reducing secretions; dexamethasone 2-4 mg IV (150 μg/kg); 2) Intravenous administration: 0.9% normal saline, 5% or 10% GS (define), RS (define) dilution midazolam 0.05-0.3 mg/kg, injection should be done slowly. Usually within, about 1 minute children enter light sleep; midazolam continuous infusion, 0.05 mg/kg/h by micro pump; 3) Slow intravenous injection of propofol 1.5-4.0 mg/kg (1.5-2 ml within 30-60 seconds); neurosurgical operation starts after the disappearance of responses in children; 4) At the end of surgery, promethazine 12.5 mg IV and diphenhydramine 0.5 mg/kg should be given to prevent possible postoperative vomiting.
5) Note: 1) Common dangerous complications: regurgitation and aspiration, respiratory depression, hypotension, and laryngospasm; 2) Electrocardiogram monitor and pediatric cardiopulmonary resuscitation equipment (including masks, balloons, laryngoscope, and endotracheal intubation), emergency medicine (including atropine, dopamine, etc.), and oxygen should be ready; 3) Emergency Prescription: for the treatment of laryngospasm, dexamethasone 2-5 mg, deep anesthesia+oxygen+ succinylcholine; for decreased heart rate, atropine subcutaneously: 0.01-0.02 mg/kg; when blood pressure drops, dopamine 2-5 μg/kg/min are used and can be increased to 5-10 μg/kg/min.

## 2.2. Intraspinal Parenchymal Cell Transplant

Minimally invasive keyhole approach is commonly used for intraspinal parenchymal cell transplantation. The operation is performed most frequently under general anesthesia. In any patient who has multiple spinal surgeries, poor wound healing, or cannot tolerate general anesthesia, the procedure of myelography CT-guided percutaneous puncture under local general anesthesia is recommended.

### *Procedure of Intraspinal Cell Transplantation*

Positioning: The patient is placed in a prone or lateral position.

A small midline incision is made over the injury and a laminectomy performed. Self-retaining retractors are placed after incision and the muscles retracted. Posterior elements are excised with the use of Kerrison rongeurs. The spinous processes at the levels involved are removed. With the use of a high-speed burr, a drill hole is placed into the laminae in the segments with half of the vertebral segment above and below the lesion for spinal cord trauma or the involved area of neurological impairment, usually of dimensions 1.0cm×1.5cm. The epidural space is entered. Epidural venous bleeding is controlled with bipolar cautery, packing, and coagulating agents.

Dural incision was done carefully for intraspinal cell transplantation (China Beijing Hongtianji Neuroscience Academy with Beijing Beiqi Medical Technology Co., Ltd., using the 4.5 # thin needle (Figure 3). Two sites for injection with no vessels are routinely selected, but often one site for the cone injury (T12-L1) (Figure 4). The volume of cells is less than 25 μl per site. A piece of cotton is used to gently press the injected point in the cord for 3 min. A final check is made for bleeding and the laminotomy is then covered with a fat graft or cellulose. A suction drain is usually not necessary as drainage is minimal. The wound is then closed in layers to include the dura, fascia, subcutaneous tissue, and skin.

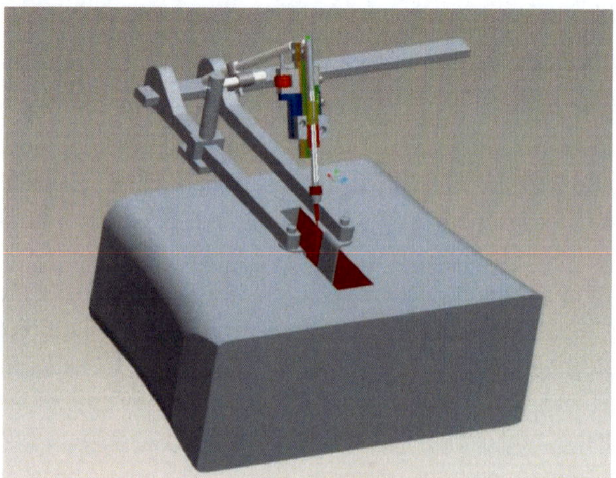

Figure 3. Intraspinal cell transplantation system (BQ-HTJ-I). [Reprinted from CNS Neurorestoratology, Huang H. 238 (Fig. 4-25), Copyright (2009), with permission from Science Press.]

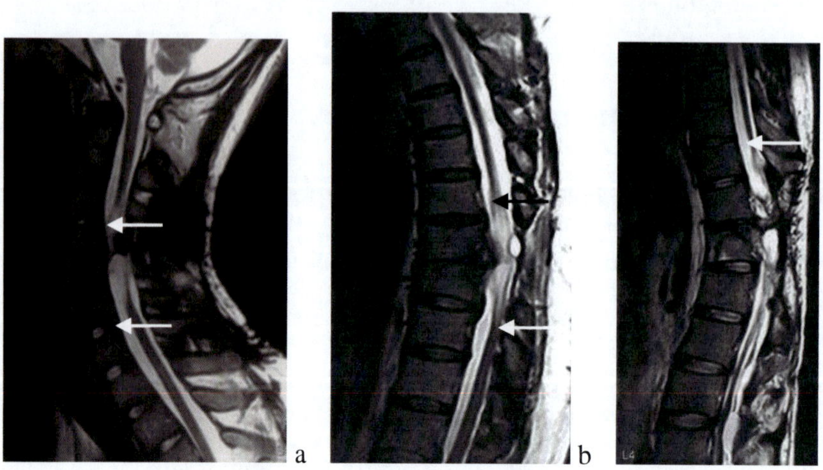


Figure 4. The sites of cell transplantation in the patient with spinal cord trauma (arrows).
a) Cervical; b) Thoracic; c) Thoraolumbar. [Reprinted from CNS Neurorestoratology, Huang HY. 238 (Fig. 4-26), Copyright (2009), with permission from Science Press.]

### *Postoperative Care*

Take care of patients by routine rules as for general spinal surgery.

### *Complications*

The main severe complication of this operation is leakage of cerebrospinal fluid (approaches 3%). The likelihood of fever, headache, and infection are approximately 5%.

### *Key Points*

1) Neurological status must be checked related to the neck flexion-extension before surgery in patients with severe cervical unstablility. Intubation under fiber light microscopy while awake and monitoring of neurological status should be considered.
2) Intravenous antibiotics are used 30 min before surgery.
3) Intravenous infusion of methylprednisolone is used at 30 mg/kg body weight within 30 min before cell implant.
4) Care should be taken not to damage the cord and nerve roots.
5) Suction should not be by direct contact with the spinal cord, but with a cotton pad.
6) Cells should be implanted into the avascular zone, avoiding a too deep needle puncture - usually within 3-4 mm.
7) Intraoperative bleeding should be controlled thoroughly to prevent blood flow into the subarachnoid space, which may lead to postoperative fever, headache, and arachnoid adhesions.

Functional changes should be closely observed, if necessary, MRI of spinal cord is required to exclude spinal cord hemorrhage and other serious complications (Huang H et al., 2003, 2006a, 2006b, 2009).

## 3. Routes of Cell Delivery to the Cerebrospinal Fluid

***Miroslaw Janowski and Krystyna Domanska-Janik***

The cerebrospinal fluid (CSF) plays a vital role for the CNS homeostasis. Mechanical function of CSF as a buffer to prevent primary CNS injury has known for centuries. The impact of CSF on cellular metabolism and growth has been highlighted more recently (Buddensiek et al., 2010). Choroid plexus is known for production of CSF but is also responsible for secretion of various regulatory factors integrating function of CNS at the level of single cell responses (Skinner et al., 2009). Additionally, it has been shown that secretion of numerous neurotrophic factors by choroid plexus is enhanced by brain injury (Johanson et al., 2011).

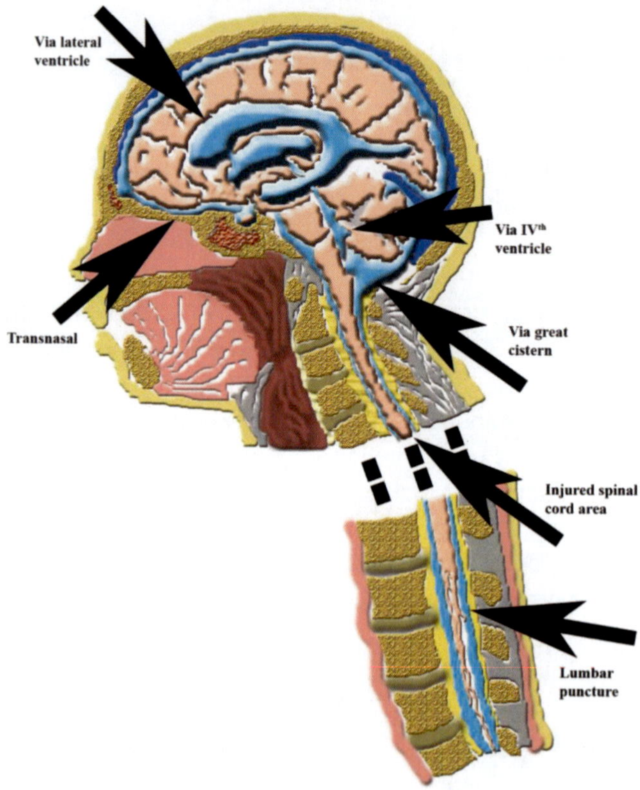


Figure 5. The routes of CSF-targeted cell delivery.

The supportive role of CSF for CNS function in physiological and pathological conditions is well known. Thus, it was hypothesized that choroid plexus and CSF form an additional organ regulating CNS function not only under physiological conditions but also supporting brain repair processes and advancing functional recovery after injury.

In effect the CSF has been recognized as a valuable compartment for transplanted therapeutic cells. Cells deposited in CSF may enter the parenchyma and/or secrete soluble factors able to penetrate the entire CNS. It allows not only for delivery of cells beyond the blood-brain barrier but also enables wide exposure of various CNS regions to transplanted material and products of their secretion. There are several cell delivery routes though CSF, such as, lateral ventricles, IVth ventricle, great cistern, lumbar puncture, injured spinal cord area and transnasal route (Figure 5).

## 3.1. Lateral Ventricles

Most of the CSF is produced in lateral ventricles and then circulates throughout the entire ventricular system to leave the CNS through the subarachnoid space. Importantly, both neurogenic niches (subventricular zone and dentate gyrus) are adjacent to lateral ventricles. Thus deposition of cells in lateral ventricles is most justified for brain diseases but also may be considered for spinal cord disorders. This location facilitates cell incorporation into brain parenchyma within neurogenic zones and at the same time gives an access to soluble factors secreted by cells to the entire surface of CNS in contact with the ventricular system (Kim et al., 2004). Additionally, ependymal lining ventricles are more penetrable to soluble factors than the outer surface of the CNS, which is covered by pia mater.

Although cell injection into the lateral ventricles is a rather invasive procedure and may cause injury of brain parenchyma, the procedure itself is widely used for other neurosurgical purposes and considered as minimally harmful with less than 2% of serious complications. The injection procedure consists in stereotaxic or free hand puncture of the lateral ventricle in the frontal or occipital brain area. Cells can be injected to the ventricle via stereotaxic needle or ventricular catheter taken from a shunt system kit. Either general or local anesthesia can be employed during surgery. This procedure is also routinely performed in small animals by stereotaxic injection of cells via Hamilton needle or glass capillary (Ohta et al., 2004).

## 3.2. Great Cistern

Previously a great cistern puncture in local anesthesia was routinely used in the clinic. Now it still can be performed safely for cell therapy (Chen L et al., 2013; Xi H et al., 2013). A advantage of this route of cell delivery is that CNS parenchyma is left intact. One should take into account that the great cistern is located relatively downstream to CSF circulation. Thus, this procedure can be preferred for disorders with major involvement of spinal cord pathology. The same procedure is also easily applicable to most animal models (Zhang et al., 2003) the only exception being smaller rodents such as mice. Even these difficulties in small animals can be overcome by the use of new procedures as reported recently (Janowski et al., 2008; Zhang et al., 2009).

## 3.3. Injured Spinal Cord Area Delivery

The closer the site of cell transplantation is to the lesion of spinal cord, the better result will generally be. For CSF delivery pathways, the ideal solution is to inject the cells by puncture into the CSF close to the area surrounding the spinal cord injury. The main risk is spinal cord secondary injury caused by puncture. There are two surgical methods: direct puncture and CT-guided operation (Chinese Branch of IANR, 2013). Regarding advantages and disadvantages, the former is fast, but sometimes fails; for the latter, CT guidance operation under direct vision has a higher success rate, although it is time-consuming.

## 3.4. Lumbar Puncture

Due to its simplicity and safety lumbar puncture is the procedure of choice to access CSF in patients. It does not require surgery and can be easily performed by any physician without sedation. A catheter can also be placed in the spinal canal via lumbar puncture for prolonged or repeated and well-controlled injections with the use of an infusion pump. In large animals this route is equally simple, but is possible even in small animals. The drawback of this approach is related to restrained CSF circulation caused by extreme downstream location of the lumbar vertebral canal. Patient positioning during and after infusion may facilitate access of cells to more proximal parts of the spinal cord but even then, retrograde inflow into the ventricular system is not sufficient to efficiently deliver cells as well as their secreted trophic factors. It was shown experimentally that spinal cord injury in its acute phase leads to homing of cells transplanted via lumbar puncture (Paul et al., 2009). This approach was used also in clinical setting (Callera and de Melo, 2007).

### 3.5. Transnasal Route

The efficiency of transnasal cell delivery to the CSF has been revealed recently. Transplanted mesenchymal stem cells migrate from the nasal mucosa, through the cribriform plate to brain and CSF (Danielyan et al., 2009). Intranasal pre-treatment with hyaluronidase facilitated migration of mesenchymal stem cells. This route seems to be promising but still needs to be validated in more studies.

As the mechanisms of cell migration within CSF have not been determined yet, there is a scientific duty to follow cell fate by means of non-invasive in vivo imaging and is a very attractive target for cell transplantation.

## 4. Cell Infusion Procedures

1) Doctors and nurses should be present during the procedure.
2) Emergency equipment and emergency medicine should be ready.
3) In the dispensing sterile operating room, extract 8 ml saline with a 10 ml syringe, and then slowly extract cells, repeat 3 times.
4) Cells are slowly injected into 100 ml of normal saline (bag), and the syringe rinsed three times.
5) Liquids are mixed gently 5 times and then are brought to the ward, standing upside down after 5 min.
6) Blood pressure, heart rate, respiration, and body temperature are monitored.
7) Dexamethasone infusion into the pot with the dosage of 5 mg.
8) Fluid containing cells is connected with transfusion apparatus with assurance of closed connection.
9) Infusion starts slowly for the initial 5 min and is then raised to 70 drops of liquid/min. Flip filter regularly.
10) Refill bags with 100 ml of normal saline infusion. At the same time, fill liquid pipeline with gas. Meanwhile, rapid infusion of 20% mannitol 250 ml is completed within 30 min in adult.
11) Infusion of 150 ml of normal saline at the conventional rate. Flip filter regularly.
12) Intensive bedside care is required with watching for allergic, hemolytic reactions. Blood pressure, heart rate, respiration, and body temperature should be continuous observed for the next 3 hours.

# References

Buddensiek, J; Dressel, A; Kowalski, M; Runge, U; Schroeder, H; Hermann, A; Kirsch, M; Storch, A; Sabolek, M. Cerebrospinal fluid promotes survival and astroglial differentiation of adult human neural progenitor cells but inhibits proliferation and neuronal differentiation. *BMC Neurosci.* 2010;11:48.

Callera, F; de Melo, CM. Magnetic resonance tracking of magnetically labeled autologous bone marrow CD34+ cells transplanted into the spinal cord via lumbar puncture technique in patients with chronic spinal cord injury: CD34+ cells' migration into the injured site. *Stem Cells.* 2007; 461-466.

Chen, L; Xi, H; Huang, H; Zhang, F; Liu, Y; Chen, D; Xiao, J. Multiple cell transplantation based on an intraparenchymal approach for patients with chronic phase stroke. *Cell Transplant.* 2013;22 Suppl 1:S83-91.

Chinese Branch of International Association of Neurorestoratology (IANR); Preparatory Committee of Chinese Association of Neurorestoratology. Standard recommendations for the application of Chinese clinical cell therapy for neurorestoration (2012). *Cell Transplant.* 2013; 22 Suppl 1:S5-10.

Danielyan, L; Schafer, R; von Ameln-Mayerhofer, A; Buadze, M; Geisler, J; Klopfer, T; Burkhardt, U; Proksch, B; Verleysdonk, S; Ayturan, M et al. Intranasal delivery of cells to the brain. *Eur. J. Cell Biol.* 2009; 88: 315-324.

Huang, H; Chen, L; Wang, H; Xi, H; Gou, C; Zhang, J; Zhang, F; Liu, Y. Safety of fetal olfactory ensheathing cell transplantation in patients with chronic spinal cord injury. A 38-month follow-up with MRI. *Zhongguo Xiu Fu Chong Jian Wai Ke Za Zhi.* 2006a; 20(4):439-43.

Huang, H; Chen, L; Wang, H; Xiu, B; Li, B; Wang, R; Zhang, J; Zhang, F; Gu, Z; Li, Y; Song, Y; Hao, W; Pang, S; Sun, J. Influence of patients' age on functional recovery after transplantation of olfactory ensheathing cells into injured spinal cord injury. *Chin. Med. J. (Engl).* 2003;116(10):1488-91.

Huang, H; Chen, L; Xi, H; Wang, Q; Zhang, J; Liu, Y; Zhang, F. Olfactory ensheathing cells transplantation for central nervous system diseases in 1255 patients. *Zhongguo Xiu Fu Chong Jian Wai Ke Za Zhi.* 2009;23(1):14-20.

Huang, H; Wang, H; Chen, L; Gu, Z; Zhang, J; Zhang, F; Song, Y; Li, Y; Tan, K, Liu Y, Xi H. Influence factors for functional improvement after olfactory ensheathing cell transplantation for chronic spinal cord injury. *Zhongguo Xiu Fu Chong Jian Wai Ke Za Zhi.* 2006b; 20(4):434-8.

Janowski, M; Kuzma-Kozakiewicz, M; Binder, D;Habisch, HJ; Habich, A; Lukomska, B; Domanska-Janik, K; Ludolph, AC; Storch, A. Neurotransplantation in mice: the concorde-like position ensures minimal cell leakage and widespread distribution of cells transplanted into the cisterna magna. *Neurosci. Lett.* 2008;430:169-174.

Johanson, C; Stopa, E; Baird, A; Sharma, H. Traumatic brain injury and recovery mechanisms: peptide modulation of periventricular neurogenic regions by the choroid plexus-CSF nexus. *J. Neural. Transm.* 2011;118(1):115-33.

Kim, DE; Schellingerhout, D; Ishii, K; Shah, K; Weissleder, R. Imaging of stem cell recruitment to ischemic infarcts in a murine model. *Stroke.* 2004; 35: 952-957.

Ohta, M; Suzuki, Y; Noda, T; Ejiri, Y; Dezawa, M; Kataoka, K; Chou, H; Ishikawa, N; Matsumoto, N; Iwashita, Y et al. Bone marrow stromal cells infused into the cerebrospinal fluid promote functional recovery of the injured rat spinal cord with reduced cavity formation. *Exp. Neurol.* 2004;187: 266-278.

Paul, C; Samdani, AF; Betz, RR; Fischer, I; Neuhuber, B. Grafting of human bone marrow stromal cells into spinal cord injury: a comparison of delivery methods. *Spine.* (Phila Pa 1976). 2009;34: 328-334.

Skinner, SJ; Geaney, MS; Lin, H; Muzina, M; Anal, AK; Elliott, RB; Tan, PL. Encapsulated living choroid plexus cells: potential long-term treatments for central nervous system disease and trauma. *J. Neural. Eng.* 2009;6: 065001.

Xi, H; Chen, L; Huang, H; Zhang, F; Liu, Y; Chen, D; Xiao, J. Preliminary report of multiple cell therapy for patients with multiple system atrophy. *Cell Transplant.* 2013;22 Suppl 1:S93-9.

Zhang, C; Zhou, C; Teng, JJ; Zhao, RL; Song, YQ; Zhang, C. Multiple administrations of human marrow stromal cells through cerebrospinal fluid prolong survival in a transgenic mouse model of amyotrophic lateral sclerosis. *Cytotherapy.* 2009;11: 299-306.

Zhang, ZG; Jiang, Q; Zhang, R; Zhang, L; Wang, L; Zhang, L; Arniego, P; Ho, KL; Chopp, M. Magnetic resonance imaging and neurosphere therapy of stroke in rat. *Ann. Neurol.* 2003;53: 259-263.

In: Neurorestoratology, volume 1
Editors: H. Huang, G. Raisman, P. R. Sanberg et al.
ISBN: 978-1-63463-599-8


*Chapter 6*

# Neuromodulation

***Junming Zhu, Ph.D., M.D.[1,*], Jianmin Zhang, Ph.D., M.D.[1], and Hongyun Huang, Ph.D., M.D.[2,3,†]***
[1]Department of Neurosurgery, the Second Affiliated Hospital, Zhejiang University, School of Medicine, Zhejiang, China
[2]Center of Neurorestoratology, Beijing Rehabilitation Hospital of Capital Medical University, Beijing, China
[3]Beijing Hongtianji Neuroscience Academy, Beijing, China

## Introduction

Neuromodulation is a very complex term, as a physiological process, it refers to regulate diverse populations of neurons by one or more neurotransmitters; as a medical therapy, it targets the nervous system for restoring function, relieving pain, or controlling symptoms by electrical or magnetic stimulation, or infusing medications into the cerebrospinal fluid using intrathecal drug delivery (http://en.wikipedia.org/wiki/Neuromodulation) and neuroprosthetics. Here briefly describe its main methods as medical therapies.

## 1. Transcranial Magnetic Stimulation

Transcranial magnetic stimulation (TMS) entails stimulation of the brain through the intact skull by using a pulse generator to produce a rapidly cycling magnetic field which induces electrical currents intracranially (Zimmerman M and Hummel FC, 2010). TMS of the cortex can result in depolarization of neurons and production of an action potentia. Repetitive TMS (rTMS) may produce effects which persist for longer periods (possibly days or weeks), presumably changes in synaptic function or thresholds (e.g. long-term potentiation (LTP) or

* Corresponding author: Junming Zhu. E-mail: dr.zhujunming@gmail.com.
† Corresponding author: Hongyun Huang. E-mail: hongyunh@gmail.com.

long-term depression (LTD). The rapidity with which TMS can be performed allows it to be used to investigate ipsilateral vs contralateral effects and the role of the corpus callosum (Premji A et al., 2010; Voineskos AN et al., 2010). Various methods have been used to study the effects of rTMS: EEG, fMRI, MR spectroscopy, near infrared spectroscopy (NIRS), and PET (Platz T and Rothwell JC, 2010; Thomson RH et al., 2011; Zheng H et al., 2010). A major recent refinement is the development of deep TMS (DTMS), which can result in stimulation to a depth of up to 3 cm in the brain (Isserles M et al., 2011). Another procedural development is accelerated TMS (aTMS) (Holtzheimer PE et al., 2010). Additional new techniques for delivering TMS include paired-pulse TMS and dual-site TMS (Chouinard PA and Paus T, 2010), and quadripulse stimulation (Hamada M and Ugawa Y, 2010).

The US Food and Drug Administration (FDA) has only cleared rTMS for the treatment of refractory depression (in late 2008) - noting that although the benefit of rTMS appears to be modest based on the studies available with less risks. There are more other disorders, such as, stroke, pain, and Parkinson's disease to be treated by rTMS.

## 1.1. rTMS for Depression

The vast majority of studies of rTMS for depression have utilized either excitatory stimulation (5 Hz or greater) of the left dorsolateral prefrontal cortex (DLPFC) or inhibitory stimulation (1 Hz or less) of the right DLPFC (Schönfeldt-Lecuona C et al., 2010). The site of stimulation has traditionally been defined as 5 cm anterior to the motor cortex, although clearly this type of localization fails to have good reproducibility nor does it take into account individual variations in cortical organization/localization (Nauczyciel C et al., 2011). Most reports are positive by rTMS for patients with depression (O'Reardon JP et al., 2007), (Frank E et al., 2011), (Zheng H et al., 2010); a few is negative (Herwig U et al., 2007).

## 1.2. rTMS for Stroke

The goal with rTMS is to inhibit the contralateral unaffected hemisphere and excite the remaining neurons in the affected hemisphere. Improvement in motor function of up to 30% has been reported (Khedr EM and Abo-El Fatoh, 2010). Improvements in post-stroke swallowing disorders (dysphagia) have also been noted following rTMS; the mechanism of improvement is likely different in cortical versus brainstem stroke that results in dysphagia (Khedr EM and Abo-El Fatoh, 2010; Platz T and Rothwell JC, 2010). The treatment of post-stroke aphasia with rTMS had led to involved protocols in light of the various regions in the brain involved in language (Naeser MA et al., 2010).

## 1.3. rTMS for Pain

One recent study found rTMS of benefit in the treatment of chronic pancreatitis pain; although the number of subjects was small (8 sham rTMS, 9 real rTMS), the improvement in pain was correlated with increases in the excitatory neurotransmitters glutamate and N-acetylaspartate on magnetic resonance spectroscopy (MRS) (Fregni F et al., 2011). Guidance regarding the most effective rTMS protocols may be gained by studying the effect of rTMS on pain perception in normal individuals who have pain induced in a controlled fashion (Platz T and Rothwell JC, 2010; Antal A and Paulus W, 2010).

### 1.4. rTMS for Parkinson's Disease

Two aspects of Parkinson's disease have been addressed with rTMS: (1) primary motor symptoms and (2) levodopa-induced dyskinesias. There may be benefit for Parkinsonian bradykinesia from 5 Hz rTMS over the supplementary motor area (Hamada M, 2009). For levodopa-induced dyskinesias, it is likely that rTMS over the lateral cerebellum is more beneficial than rTMS over the primary or supplementary motor cortex (Koch G, 2010).

## 2. Electrical Neurostmulation

### 2.1. Deep Brain Stimulation (DBS)

DBS is now an established symptomatic treatment modality for movement disorders, especially Parkinson's disease; DBS devices apply electricity via stereotactic implantation of electrodes in specific areas of the brain such as the thalamus. The electrodes are attached to a neurostimulator placed subcutaneously. Food and Drug Administration in USA (FDA) approval was granted in 1997 for thalamic DBS for essential tremor and Parkinson's disease-related tremor, followed in 2003 by approval for subthalamic nucleus (STN) (Limousin P et al., 1998) and globus pallidus internus (GPi) DBS for PD (Siegfried J et al., 1994). There is a great deal of research showing successful DBS use in epilepsy (Fisher R et al., 2010), depression (Holtzheimer PE and Mayberg HS, 2011), headache (Jenkins B and Tepper SJ, 2011), pain and dystonia (VercueilL et al., 2002).

### 2.2. Spinal Cord Stimulation (SCS)

SCS is also an accepted method of pain control (Pain SA et al., 2013). Recently, there have been a number of other implantable devices developed for epilepsy.

### 2.3. Vagus Nerve Stimulation (VNS)

VNS was approved as adjunctive therapy for patients >12 years of age with partial onset seizures refractory to antiepileptic medications by FDA in 1997 (DeGiorgio CM et al., 2000). After demonstrating antidepressant properties, VNS received FDA approval in 2005 as an adjunctive long-term treatment for patients age >18 with treatment-resistant depression (TRD) (Cyberonics Inc, 2011-2012). It is presumed that stimulation of the vagus nerve results in alterations of activity in the brain, resulting in a decrease in seizures or improvement in mood.

Recently VNS was recommended to be considered for seizures in children, for Lennox-Gastaut syndrome (LGS)-associated seizures, and for improving mood in adults with epilepsy (George L et al., 2013).

## 2.4. Closed-Loop Neuromodulation

While the above treatments provide stimulation regardless of neuronal activity, a closed-loop system (Morrell MJ et al., 2008; Smith JR et al., 2010) aims to suppress epileptiform activity by delivering stimulation directly in response to electrographic activity. The system is comprised of invasive electrodes, a cranially implanted neurostimulator, a programmer, patient data transmitter and a web-based database for upload and review of intracranial EEG recordings instead of targeting a predetermined target in all patients, however, the target of stimulation depends on each patient's seizure focus.

In a multicenter, double-blind, randomized controlled trial assessed the safety and effectiveness of responsive cortical stimulation, 191 patients with medically intractable partial epilepsy were implanted with the responsive neurostimulation system (RNS). Seizures were significantly reduced in the treatment (−37.9%, n = 97) compared to the control group (−17.3%, n = 94; $p = 0.012$) in the blind period and there was no difference between the treatment and control groups in adverse events (Morrell MJ and RNSSiES Group, 2011). The median percent reduction in seizures in the open label period was 44% at 1 year and 53% at 2 years, which represents a progressive and significant improvement with time ($p < 0.0001$) (Heck CN et al., 2014).

The RNS system has recently received FDA approval for the treatment of refractory epilepsy. The closed-loop neuromodulation have also been taken: researchers at Stanford University in California have recorded brain electrical activity in a patient with Parkinson's disease through the DBS stimulation electrode previously implanted; researchers at the Mayo Clinic in Minnesota have developed an electrode that can record both brain electrical activity and brain chemical activity (Shen H, 2014).

Moreover, closed-loop stimulation (i.e. feedback-guided) can offer advantages in efficacy and efficiency, with effects lasting days to weeks after the stimulation has been discontinued (Hauptmann C et al., 2007; Popovych O et al., 2008; Tass PA et al., 2012; Adamchic I et al., 2014; Chang SY et al., 2013).

# 3. Neuroprosthetics

Neuroprosthetics is a discipline related to neuroscience and biomedical engineering concerned with developing neural prostheses (a series of implantable devices), which can substitute or monitor a motor, sensory or cognitive modality that might have been damaged as a result of an injury or a disease (http://en.wikipedia.org/wiki/Neuroprosthetics).

Here we mainly focus on brain-machine interface technology which is an important strategy of neurorestoration.

## 3.1. Brain Machine Interface (BMI)

The BMI is also known as brain-computer interface, or neuroprosthetics. The BMI system consist of hardware and software that communicates with the brain. The hardware component of the interface records brain signals, while the software component decodes the signals and converts them into a command that controls a device (a computer cursor or robotic limb) or sends a feedback signal to the brain. The brain receives feedback, which in turn affects the brain activity and influences subsequent output.

Therefore, the BMI system can be conceptually separated into 3 distinct parts: (1) a sensor to record electrical signals from the brain, (2) a signal processor of the neural signals to decode intended movement or action, and (3) an effector such as a cursor or robotic limb. Signal acquisition is the fundamental design-point in a BMI. Using different kinds of electrodes, neural signals can be recorded at the scalp (EEG activity), at the cortical surface (electrocorticographic (ECoG) activity), or within the brain (local field potentials (LFP) or neuronal action potentials (spikes). The next step is signal analysis (Shaomin Z et al., 2011), a complex process of decoding the motor plan and intention of the patient into machine commands. This process involves numerous mathematical algorithms and is highly dependent on the quality of the signal recorded. The more accurately the algorithm can decode the intended movement from neural signals, the easier it will be to generate natural movement. In the output step, motor execution can take many forms such as a cursor on a computer screen, a keyboard, maneuver of wheelchair or a robotic limb. Some have even tested the integrated BMI/functional electrical stimulation (FES) systems. In addition to the three fundamental components of a BMI system listed above, some form of a feedback mechanism is also essential.

BrainGate (one kind of BMI) allows paralyzed humans to use neural signals ordinarily used to control the arm to operate devices such as computer software or robotic assistants. Control signals are derived from the neural activity in arm area of motor cortex, through a 100 chronically implanted microelectrode array that enables recordings of action and field potentials, both of which can provided useful command signals. Preliminary experience from five tetraplegia participants, including one for more than 5 years, demonstrate that arm-related motor cortical signals remain in motor cortex long after injury or disease onset and can record for extended durations. Participants are able to move and click a computer cursor and to control physical device (Donoghue JP et al., 2006; Truccolo W et al., 2008; Simeral JD et al., 2011). In the further study, participants controlled the arm to perform three-dimensional reach and grasp movements without explicit training (Hochberg LR et al., 2012). One of the study participants, implanted with the sensor for 5 years, also used a robotic arm to drink coffee from a bottle.

Functional electrical stimulation (FES) can be used to restore movement control following paralysis by the application of electrical stimuli to the nerves innervating the muscles. In existing clinical systems, the patient uses residual proximal muscle movements to trigger pre-programmed stimulation that causes the paralyzed muscles to contract, providing basic hand grasp. In an early study, a BMI integrated FES system in primates had restored to the monkeys voluntary movement of their paralyzed muscles, using neural signals recorded from a multi-electrode array implanted in the motor cortex (Ethier C et al., 2012). Then it was proved that such a system could also benefit paralyzed patients (Chadwick EK et al., 2011).

Recently, a device named Neurobridge designed by Collinger JL and coworkers shows that FES can be controlled using cortical activity in paralyzed patients to passes damaged areas of the nervous system so the brain can communicate directly with the muscles. The Neurobridge system could decode the neural signals and sends them to a computer that recodes them as signals that the muscles can pick up. The computer then sends those signals to the sleeve, which is covered with about 200 electrodes, which stimulate the muscles and make the patient regain conscious control of their fingers, hands, wrists and arms. Then they reported that a 52-year old woman paralyzed from the neck down and suffering from tetraplegia had been able to guide a robotic arm with her thoughts with a level of agility closer to normal. This technology may offer even greater advantages to patients affected by paralysis resulting from SCI, traumatic brain injury (TBI), stroke, and other severe neurological disorders, who have a greater need for replaced function but possess even fewer available sources of control (Collinger JL et al., 2013).

EEG is probably an alternative method to enable patients with tetraplegia to control robotic arm prostheses. Real or imagined movements of the limbs are associated with desynchronization of 10–20-Hz rhythms recorded over sensorimotor cortical areas. The detection of power changes at these frequencies has enabled impressive control of 1D (Wolpaw JR et al., 1991), 2D (Wolpaw JR and McFarland DJ, 2004) and 3D (McFarland DJ et al., 2010) computer cursors. Unfortunately, as any imagined movement of a given limb produces the same general pattern of desynchronization over a wide area of cortex, it's very difficult to decode the accurate movement plan.

The P300-BMI appears to be the most commonly used BMI system, and the only system for which regular home use by locked-in patients has been reported (Neumann N and Kubler A, 2003). The P300 signal appears in the EEG recording over central cortical areas about 300 ms after a salient or attended stimulus.

In most P300-based BMI technologies described so far, the stimulus is visual. In the typical P300 BMI format, letters, numbers, or other visual stimuli are arranged in a matrix, and the rows and columns of the matrix flash in rapid succession while the user focuses attention on the item that he or she wishes to select.

Only the row and column that contain the specific item will produce a P300 potential. By recognizing this P300 potential, the BMI system can determine the user's selection. Based on that approach, three kinds of P300-BMI systems have been tested in human beings (Birbaumer N and Cohen LG, 2007; Daly JJ and Wolpaw JR, 2008), including BMI for languages with logographic writing system, BMI as a switch and BMI as an environmental control.

## 3.2. Auditory Neuroprosthetics

Currently implanted in more than 220,000 individuals' world worldwide, cochlear implants (CIs) are thought to be the most successful neuroprosthetic to date (Cosetti MK and Waltzman SB, 2011).

A CI receives acoustic information and converts it to electrical impulses and transmits the electric signal to the cochlea. Using a variety of speech-coding strategies and programming techniques, the implant can be customized to maximize each patient's understanding of speech. Multichannel CIs have become an accepted, well-recognized treatment for severe-to-profound sensorineural hearing loss (SNHL) in adults and children.

## 3.3. Visual Neuroprosthetics

In ophthalmology, visual neuroprosthetics are designed to provide prosthetic vision to the blind by stimulating localized neural populations in one of the retinotopically organized structures of the visual pathway – typically the retina or visual cortex. But the effectiveness of visual neuroprosthetics has not been well demonstrated (Shepherd RK et al., 2013).

In summary, the development of neuromodulation including functional magnetic stimulation, electrical neurostimulation, and neuroprosthetics has taken an extraordinary amount of effort from a vast number of scientific and clinical disciplines. Especially incremental improvements in numerous areas of BMI technology are occurring. The attractiveness of this promising treatment will no doubt keep neuromodulation on the forefront as a neurorestorative therapeutic option with a robust future for many nervous system disorders.

## References

Adamchic, I., Hauptmann, C., Barnikol, U. B., Pawelczyk, N., Popovych, O., Barnikol, T. T., Silchenko, A., Volkmann, J., Deuschl, G., Meissner, W. G., Maarouf, M., Sturm, V., Freund, H.-J., Tass, P. A. Coordinated reset neuromodulation for Parkinson's disease: a proof-of-concept study. *Mov. Disord.* 2014. doi: 10.1002/mds.25923 (Epub. ahead of print).

Antal, A., Paulus, W. Effects of transcranial theta-burst stimulation on acute pain perception. *Restor. Neurol. Neurosci.* 2010;28:477-484.

Birbaumer, N., Cohen, L. G. Brain-computer interfaces: communication and restoration of movement in paralysis. *J. Physiol.* 2007; 579: 621-636.

Chadwick, E. K., Blana, D., Simeral, J. D., et al. Continuous neuronal ensemble control of simulated arm reaching by a human with tetraplegia. *J. Neural Eng.* 2011;8(3):034003.

Chang, S.-Y., Kimble, C. J., Kim, I., Paek, S. B., Kressin, K. R., Boesche, J. B., Whitlock, S. V., Eaker, D. R., Kasasbeh, A., Horne, A. E., Blaha, C. D., Bennet, K. E., Lee, K. H. Development of the Mayo Investigational Neuromodulation Control System: toward a closed-loop electrochemical feedback system for deep brain stimulation. *J. Neurosurg.* 2013;119:1556-1565.

Chouinard, P. A., Paus, T. What have we learned from "perturbing" the human cortical motor system with transcranial magnetic stimulation? *Front. Human Neurosci.* 2010;4:1-14.

Collinger, J. L., Wodlinger, B., Downey, J. E., Wang, W., Tyler-Kabara, E. C., Weber, D. J., McMorland, A. J., Velliste, M., Boninger, M. L., Schwartz, A B. High-performance neuroprosthetic control by an individual with tetraplegia. *Lancet.* 2013; 381(9866):557-64.

Cosetti, M. K., Waltzman, S. B. Cochlear implants: current status and future potential. *Expert Rev. Med. Devices.* 2011; 8(3):389-401.

Cyberonics Inc. Physician's manual. VNS therapy™ AspireHC™ Model 105 Generator. Houston, TX: Cyberonics, Inc; 2011-2012.

Daly, J. J., Wolpaw, J. R. Brain-computer interfaces in neurological rehabilitation. *Lancet Neurol.* 2008; 7:1032-1043.

DeGiorgio, C. M., Schachter, S. C., Handforth, A., et al. Prospective long-term study of vagus nerve stimulation for the treatment of refractory seizures. *Epilepsia.* 2000; 41: 1195-1200.

Donoghue, J. P., Penn, R. D., Chen, D., et al. Neuronal ensemble control of prosthetic devices by a human with tetraplegia. *Nature.* 2006; 442: 164-171.

Ethier, C., Oby, E. R., Bauman, M. J., Miller, L. E. Restoration of grasp following paralysis through brain-controlled stimulation of muscles. *Nature.* 2012; 485(7398): 368-71.

Fisher, R., Salanova, V., Witt, T., et al. SANTE Study Group. Electrical stimulation of the anterior nucleus of thalamus for treatment of refractory epilepsy. *Epilepsia.* 2010; 51 (5):899-908.

Frank, E., Eichhammer, P., Burger, J., Zowe, M., Landgrebe, M., Hajak, G., Langguth, B. Transcranial magnetic stimulation for the treatment of depression: feasibility and results under naturalistic conditions: a retrospective analysis. *Eur. Arch. Psychiatry Clin. Neurosci.* 2011; 1:261-266.

Fregni, F., Potvin, K., DaSilva, D., Wang, X., Lenkinski, R. E., Freedman, S. D., Pascual-Leone, A. Clinical effects and brain metabolic correlates in non-invasive cortical neuromodulation for visceral pain. *Eur. J. Pain.* 2011; 15:53-60.

George, L., Morris, I. I. I., David, Gloss; Jeffrey, Buchhalter et al. Evidence-based guideline update: Vagus nerve stimulation for the treatment of epilepsy: Report of the Guideline Development Subcommittee of the American Academy of Neurology. *Neurology.* 2013; 81;1453-1459.

Hamada, M., Ugawa, Y., Tsuji, S. The Effectiveness of rTMS on Parkinson's Disease Study Group, Japan. High frequency rTMS over the supplementary motor area improves bradykinesia in Parkinson's disease: sub-analysis of doubleblind sham controlled study. *J. Neurol. Sci.* 2009;287:143-146.

Hamada, M., Ugawa, Y. Quadripulse stimulation - a new patterned rTMS. *Restor. Neurol. Neurosci.* 2010;28:419-424.

Hauptmann, C., Popovych, O., Tass, P. A. Desynchronizing the abnormally synchronized neural activity in the subthalamic nucleus: A modeling study. *Exp. Rev. Med. Devices.* 2007;4:633-650.

Heck, C. N., King-Stephens, D., Massey, A. D., Nair, D. R., Jobst, B. C., Barkley, G. L., Salanova, V., Cole, A. J., Smith, M. C., Gwinn, R. P., et al. Two-year seizure reduction in adults with medically intractable partial onset epilepsy treated with responsive neurostimulation: final results of the RNS System Pivotal trial. *Epilepsia.* 2014;55: 432-441.

Herwig, U., Fallgatter, A. J., Höppner, J., Eschweiler, G. W., Kron, M. H. G., Padberg, F., Naderi-Heiden, A., Abler, B., Eichhammer, P., Grossheinrich, N., Hay, B., Kammer, T., Langguth, B., Laske, C., Plewnia, C., Richter, M. M., Schulz, M., Unterecker, S., Zinke, A., Spitzer, M., Schönfeldt-Lecuona, C. Antidepressant effects of augmentative transcranial magnetic stimulation: randomised multicentre trial. *Brit. J. Psychiatry.* 2007; 191:441-448.

Hochberg, L. R., Bacher, D., Jarosiewicz, B., Masse, N. Y., Simeral, J. D., Vogel, J., Haddadin, S., Liu, J., van der Smagt, P., Donoghue, J. P. Reach and grasp by people with tetraplegia using a neurally controlled robotic arm. *Nature*. 2012; 485 (7398): 372-5.

Holtzheimer, P. E., McDonald, W. M., Mufti, M., Kelley, M. E., Quinn, S., Corso, G., Epstein, C. M. Accelerated repetitive transcranial magnetic stimulation for treatment-resistant depression. *Depression Anxiety*. 2010;27:960-963.

Holtzheimer, P. E., Mayberg, H. S. Deep brain stimulation for psychiatric disorders. *Annu. Rev. Neurosci*. 2011, 34:289-307.

Isserles, M., Rosenberg, O., Dannon, P., Levkovitz, Y., Kotler, M., Deutsch, F., Lerer, B., Zangen, M. Cognitive-emotional reactivation during deep transcranial magnetic stimulation over the prefrontal cortex of depressive patients affects antidepressant outcome. *J. Affect. Disord*. 2011; 128:125-132.

Jenkins, B., Tepper, S. J. Neurostimulation for primary headache disorders: part 2, review of central neurostimulators for primary headache, overall therapeutic efficacy, safety, cost, patient selection, and future research in headache neuromodulation. *Headache*. 2011; 51(9):1408-1418.

Khedr, E. M., Abo-El Fetoh, N. Short- and long-term effect of rTMS on motor function recovery after ischemic stroke. *Restor. Neurol. Neurosci*. 2010;28:545-559.

Koch, G. rTMS effects on levodopa induced dyskinesias in Parkinson's disease patients: searching for effective cortical targets. *Restor. Neurol. Neurosci*. 2010; 28: 561-568.

Limousin, P., Krack, P., Pollak, P., et al. Electrical stimulation of the subthalamic nucleus in advanced Parkinson's disease. *N. Engl. J. Med*. 1998;39(16):1105-1111.

McFarland, D. J., Sarnacki, W. A., Wolpaw, J. R. E;ectroencephalographic (EEG) control of three-dimensional movement. *J. Neural. Eng*. 2010;7(3):036007.

Morrell, M. J., Sun, F. T., Wharen, R. E. Responsive cortical stimulation for the treatment of epilepsy. *Neurotherapeutics*. 2008; 5:68-74.

Morrell, M. J., RNSSiES Group. Responsive cortical stimulation for the treatment of medically intractable partial epilepsy. *Neurology*. 2011;77: 1295-1304.

Naeser, M. A., Martin, P. I., Treglia, E., Ho, M., Kaplan, E., Bashir, S., Hamilton, R., Branch Coslett, H., Pascual-Leone, A. Research with rTMS in the treatment of aphasia. *Restor. Neurol. Neurosci*. 2010;28:511-529.

Nauczyciel, C., Hellier, P., Morandi, X., Blestel, S., Drapier, D., Ferre, J. C., Barillot, C., Millet, B. Assessment of standard coil position in transcranial magnetic stimulation in depression. *Psychiatry Res*. 2011; 186:232-238.

Neumann, N., Kubler, A. Training locked-in patients: a challenge for the use of brain-computer interfaces. *IEEE Trans. Neur. Sys. Rehab. Engin*. 2003; 11(2):169-72.

O'Reardon, J. P., Solvason, H. B., Janicak, P. G., Sampson, S., Isenberg, K. E., Nahas, Z., McDonald, W., Avery, D., Fitzgerald, P. B., Loo, C., Demitrack, M. A., George, M. S., Sackeim, H. A. Efficacy and safety of transcranial magnetic stimulation in the acute treatment of major depression: a multisite randomized controlled trial. *Biol. Psychiatry*. 2007;62:1208-1216.

Pain, S. A., Raff, M., Melvill, R., Coetzee, G., Smuts, J. Spinal cord stimulation for the management of pain: Recommendations for best clinical practice. *S. Afr. Med. J*. 2013; 26; 103(6 Pt 2):423-30.

Platz, T., Rothwell, J. C. Brain stimulation and brain repair - rTMS: from animal experiement to clinical trials - what do we know? *Restor. Neurol. Neurosci*. 2010;28:387-398.

Popovych, O., Hauptmann, C., Tass, P. A. Impact of delayed nonlinear feedback on synchronized oscillators. *J. Biol. Physics.* 2008;34:367-379.

Premji, A., Ziluk, A., Nelson, A. J. Bilateral somatosensory evoked potentials following intermittent theta-burst repetitive transcranial magnetic stimulation. *BMC Neurosci.* 2010;11:91-97.

Schönfeldt-Lecuona, C., Cardenas-Morales, L., Freudenmann, R. W., Kammer, T., Herwig, U. Transcranial magnetic stimulation in depression - lessons from the multicentre trials. *Restor. Neurol. Neurosci.* 2010; 28:569-576.

Shaomin, Z., Bo, J., Junming, Z., Qiaosheng, Z., Weidong, C., Xiaoxiang, Z., Ting, Z. A Study on Combining Local Field Potential and Single Unit Activity for Better Neural Decoding. *Int. J. Imaging Systems and Technology.* 2011; 21(2):165-72.

Shen, H. Tuning the brain. *Nature.* 2014; 507:290-292.

Shepherd, R. K., Shivdasani, M. N., Nayagam, D. A., Williams, C. E., Blamey, P. J. Visual prostheses for the blind. *Trends Biotechnol.* 2013; 31(10): 562-71.

Siegfried, J., Lippitz, B. Bilateral chronic electrostimulation of ventroposterolateral pallidum: a new therapeutic approach for alleviating all parkinsonian symptoms. *Neurosurgery.* 1994; 35(6):1126-1129,

Simeral, J. D., Kim, S. P., Black, M. J., et al. Neural control of cursor trajectory and click by a human with tetraplegia 1000 days after implant of an intracortical microelectrode array. *J. Neural Eng.* 2011; 8(2): 025027.

Smith, J. R., Fountas, K. N., Murro, A. M., et al. Closed-Loop Stimulation in the Control of Focal Epilepsy of Insular Origin. *Stereotact. Funct. Neurosurg.* 2010; 88: 281-287.

Tass, P. A., Qin, L., Hauptmann, C., Dovero, S., Bezard, E., Boraud, T., Meissner, W. G. Coordinated reset has sustained aftereffects in Parkinsonian monkeys. *Ann. Neurol.* 2012; 72:816-820.

Thomson, R. H., Daskalakis, Z. J., Fitzgerald, P. B. A near infra-red spectroscopy study of the effects of pre-frontal single and paired pulse transcranial magnetic stimulation. *Clin. Neurophysiol.* 2011; 122:378-382.

Truccolo, W., Friehs, G. M., Donoghue, J. P., Hochberg, L. R. Primary motor cortex tuning to intended movement movement kinematics in humans with tetraplegia. *J. Neurosci.* 2008; 28:1163-1178.

Vercueil, L., Krack, P., Pollak, P. Results of deep brain stimulation for dystonia: a critical reappraisal. *Mov. Disord.* 2002;17(suppl. 3):S89-S93.

Voineskos, A. N., Farzan, F., Barr, M. S., Lobaugh, N. J., Mulsant, B. H., Chen, R., Fitzgerald, P. B., Daskalakis, Z. J. The role of the corpus callosum in transcranial magnetic stimulation induced interhemispheric signal propagation. *Biol. Psychiatry.* 2010; 68:825-831.

Wolpaw, J. R., McFarland, D. J., Neat, G. W., Forneris, C. A. An EEG-based brain–computer interface for cursor control. Electroencephalogr. *Clin. Neurophysiol.* 1991; 78: 252-259.

Wolpaw, J. R., McFarland, D. J. Control of a two-dimensional movement signal by a noninvasive brain-computer interface in humans. *Proc. Natl Acad. Sci. US.* 2004; 101:17849-17854.

Zheng, H., Zhang, L., Li, L., Liu, P., Gao, J., Liu, X., Zou, J., Zhang, Y., Liu, J., Zhang, Z., Li, Z., Men, W. High-frequency rTMS increases left prefrontal myo-inositol in young patients with treatment-resistant depression. *Prog. Neuro-Psychopharmacol. Biol. Psychiatry*. 2010; 34:1189-1195.

Zimmerman, M., Hummel, F. C. Non-invasive brain stimulation: enhancing motor and cognitive functions in healthy old subjects. *Front. Aging Neurosci*. 2010; 2:1-12.

In: Neurorestoratology, volume 1
Editors: H. Huang, G. Raisman, P. R. Sanberg et al.
ISBN: 978-1-63463-599-8


*Chapter 7*

# Medicines

***Dafin F. Muresanu*[1,2,*]*, Dana Slavoaca*[2]*, Yi-Lin Chen*[3]*,***
***Horng-Jyh Harn*[4,5]*, Shinn-Zong Lin,*[6,7,8]*, Stephen D. Skaper*[9]***
***and Hongyun Huang*[10,11]**

[1]Department of Clinical Neurosciences, "Iuliu Hatieganu"
University of Medicine and Pharmacy, Cluj-Napoca, Romania
[2]"RoNeuro" Institute for Neurological Research and Diagnosis, Cluj-Napoca, Romania
[3]Graduate Institute of Biotechnology and Department of Life Science,
National Ilan University, Ilan, Taiwan, China
[4]Department of Pathology, China Medical University and Hospital,
Taichung, Taiwan, China
[5]Department of Stem Cell Applied Technology,
Gwo Xi Stem Cell Applied Technology, Hsinchu, Taiwan, China
[6]Center for Neuropsychiatry, China Medical University Hospital,
Taichung, Taiwan, China
[7]Department of Neurosurgery, China Medical University Beigang Hospital,
Yunlin, Taiwan, China
[8]Department of Neurosurgery, China Medical University-An Nan Hospital,
Tainan, Taiwan, China
[9]Department of Pharmaceutical and Pharmacological Sciences,
University of Padua, Padua, Italy
[10]Beijing Rehabilitation Hospital of Capital Medical University, Beijing, China
[11]Beijing Hongtianji Neuroscience Academy, Beijing, China

[*] Corresponding author: Dafin F. Muresanu dafinm@ssnn.ro.

# 1. Chemical and Biological Medicines

*Dafin F. Muresanu, Dana Slavoaca*

## 1.1. Introduction

There are several limitations to the current way of thinking about brain protection and recovery.

### 1.1.1.

The general perception of the effects of brain lesions is that they are the linear sum of independent events, such as excitotoxicity, inflammation, apoptosis-like and oxidative stress, which generate the pathways of pathological cascades. This vision has developed the *subtractive suppressive strategy* for neurorestorative therapies. The backbone of this therapeutic strategy is the presumption that if we pharmacologically suppress a certain pathophysiological mechanism, we will simply subtract that specific amount of damage from the total amount created by all pathophysiological mechanisms.

Then, it can be supposed that the remaining extent of damage will be below the death threshold. Consequently, it can be assumed that the rest of the system remains unchanged. The expectation of discovering a key cell death pathway has affected the experimental design of neurorestorative studies. However, what is clear from clinical trials in neurorestoration is that the suppression subtractive strategy does not work.

The historical concept that neuroprotection means the suppression of pathophysiological processes (i.e., the idea that a single mechanism/molecule might be effective in clinical practice) is obsolete today and represents the root cause of failure of clinical neurorestoration.

This failure is a measurement of the failure of the reductionist approach to the problem (Ahn et al. 2006). In fact, as explained below, when one acute pathophysiological process (e.g., excitotoxicity or inflammation) is pharmacologically suppressed, the long-term endogenous drivers of restoration (e.g., plasticity and trophicity) are disturbed.

### 1.1.2.

Evaluations of the therapeutic effects of the suppressive single mechanism as applied to drugs in large randomized control trials (RCTs) of neurorestoration in stroke, traumatic brain injury (TBI) or degenerative disorders uses endpoints of 90 or 180 days (Labiche and Grotta, 2004; Maas et al., 2010; Saver et al., 2014). In most cases, we expect positive clinical results in neurorestoration, which is a long-term outcome, sustained by long-term processes (e.g., neuroplasticity) using molecules that often negatively interfere with plasticity. Because endogenous post-lesion brain patterns are based on the early switch from neuroprotection to neuroplasticity, the inconsistency lays in the evaluation of therapeutic effect of a drug's short-term therapeutic effect using long-term outcomes.

### 1.1.3.

It is not appropriate to approach neuroprotection and neurorestoration separately. This dichotomy might mislead the basic and clinical research in the field. In fact, in clinical practice, a complex restoration outcome is evaluated by all of the protection and restoration processes of endogenous defense activity (EDA) in an inseparable way.

### 1.1.4.

RCTs must be internally valid (i.e., the design and conduct must minimize the possibility of bias), but to be clinically useful, the result must also be relevant to a definable group of patients in a particular clinical setting.

This relevance is generally termed external validity, applicability or generalizability (Pocock, 1983; Friedman et al., 1998). There is compelling evidence that RCTs often lack external validity. However, the assessment of external validity is complex and requires clinical rather than statistical expertise (Rothwell, 2007).

The proper design of RCTs is difficult, particularly in neurorehabilitation, due to several significant limitations: RCTs results are not applicable to small heterogeneous samples, which is similar to most neurorehabilitation studies; difficulties in subgroup analyses; not all relevant information is used in meta-analyses (e.g., language); individual (e.g., genetic) dispositions for treatment (i.e., responsivity) are often not addressed; difficulty in approaching "complex situations", which are frequent in neurorehabilitation; and the high costs of properly running RCTs.

### 1.1.5.

Not many RCTs or systematic reviews have analyzed the deleterious effects of different drugs used as concomitant treatments in patients during the restoration phase and in neurorehabilitation in various pathologies.

## 1.2. Understanding the Neurobiology of Neurorestoration and Related Concepts

### 1.2.1. Cell Death Pathways

Two main types of cell death, passive and active, have been described. *Necrosis* is a process caused by almost any pathological insult, including physical, chemical and biological agents. The sequence of events leading to necrotic cell death is the same every time: osmolysis, which is caused by cellular edema, leads to the passive death of the damaged cell. Necrosis not only affects the dying cell itself, but inflammation is also triggered by the release of the cell's contents as a secondary effect, which is accompanied by cytokine discharge.

The other mechanism of cell death is *apoptosis*, which, in contrast to necrosis, requires adenosine triphosphate (ATP). Derived from an ancient Greek word, the term "apoptosis" in modern terminology designates a form of cell death with specific morphological characteristics, which is used by the organism to control the number and quality of cells to maintain functioning organs. The nervous system is one of the best examples where developmental cell death shapes its structure.

In addition to providing support to neurons throughout their lifetime, neurotrophic factors regulate apoptotic cell death and, therefore, form an important protective mechanism (Zhou S and Zhou J, 2014). Events similar to this form of cell death, including cellular signaling, have been observed in both neurodegenerative diseases and acute injury processes, such as trauma or stroke, in which neurons degenerate and die. There are clear differences between the two processes, the most evident being the time span involved. Apoptosis-like cell death takes longer, whereas necrosis is usually faster. However, dying cells occasionally display characteristics of both necrosis and apoptosis. In neurons, membrane rupture and DNA fragmentation, which indicate necrosis and apoptosis respectively, can sometimes affect the same cell. Thus, it is clear that the current vocabulary of cell death is inadequate. The term "active cell death" (ACD) has been suggested to designate cell death involving the activation of intracellular mechanisms regardless of cellular morphology. In contrast, "passive cell death" (PCD) should replace the historical term necrosis (Sloviter, 2002). The relationship between some pathophysiological mechanisms and the types of cell death can be briefly summarized as follows: excitotoxicity can lead to both necrosis and apoptosis-like death. Inflammation can also result in necrosis and apoptosis-like death, whereas protein misfolding usually induces only apoptosis-like death.

Novel mechanisms of cell death, beyond the traditional concepts of necrosis and apoptosis, include autophagy, phagoptosis, necroptosis, and pyroptosis (Dingledine et al., 2014). Axonal degeneration, which is characteristic for neurodegenerative disorders, represents the process of axonal self-destruction. It usually occurs earlier than neuronal cell body and has a distinctive active program from apoptosis. (Yan, 2010; Conforti, 2014).

The concept of a neurovascular unit was recently described. This unit consists of endothelial cells, pericytes, neurons, glial cells and matrix proteins that function together using biochemical signaling (Hawkins and Davis, 2005). This unit exists everywhere in the brain, including both the grey and white matter. Neurovascular unit dysfunction can explain the occurrence and evolution of several brain diseases, such as stroke, vascular dementia, migraine, trauma, all neurodegenerative disorders and even normal aging (Badaut and Bix, 2014; ElAli et al., 2014; Winkler et al., 2014; Muoio et al., 2014). Because the neurovascular unit is unique to the human body, the way cells die in these units is also unique.

The lack of support from any component of the vascular unit cells or matrix causes a particular apoptosis-like phenomenon known as anoikis (Frisch and Screaton, 2001). Currently, the entire therapeutic approach in brain lesions and restoration has been developed around the neurovascular unit.

### *1.2.2. Damage Mechanisms (DMs) and EDA*

Different pathophysiological mechanisms are triggered by various etiologic agents or biological events and produce a range of both acute and chronic neurological disorders.

There are a limited number of pathophysiological processes (Figure 1) that have many similarities to various CNS diseases. In stroke, excitotoxicity, oxidative stress, inflammation and apoptotic-like processes are predominant. In neurodegenerative disorders, protein misfolding plays an important role, in addition to the aforementioned processes. Excitotoxicity, inflammation and apoptosis-like processes represent the backbone common to most neuropathologies, and *modulation* of these processes is the key to efficient neuroprotection and neurorestoration in all neurological disorders.

The classic perception of the effects of brain lesions is that they are a linear sum of independent events (e.g., excitotoxicity, inflammation, apoptosis-like and oxidative stress) that generate the *pathways of pathological cascades*. This concept led to the development of the *subtractive suppressive strategy* for neuroprotection therapies. The rationale for this strategy is the presumption that if a certain pathophysiological process is pharmacologically suppressed, this will simply subtract the amount of damage created, below the death threshold.

Current basic and clinical data do not confirm this assumption. For this reason, the subtractive suppressive strategy for neuroprotection therapies has failed. This failure occurs because the interference between DM and EDA has not been properly considered, and not because the key cell death pathway is yet to be discovered. Even from empirical molecular pathway models, we know that it is impossible to interfere with the DMs without influencing EDA.

The historical concept that neuroprotection means the suppression of pathophysiological processes, the idea that a single mechanism/ molecule may be effective in clinical practice, is now obsolete and represents the root cause of failure of clinical neuroprotection. This indicates a failure of the reductionist approach to the problem. Therefore, when one acute pathophysiological process is pharmacologically suppressed (e.g., excitotoxicity and inflammation), the long-term endogenous drivers of restoration (e.g., plasticity and trophicity) are disturbed.

Neurotrophicity, neuroprotection, neuroplasticity (Kalivas and Volkow, 2005; Muresanu, 2003) and neurogenesis (detail definitions to see whole neurorestorative process and mechanisms in Chapter 3 of Section One) are the most important neurobiological processes for neurorestoration that act together under genetic control toward EDA, which attempts to counteract pathophysiological processes (i.e., DM).

When studying endogenous neuroprotection, we must distinguish between two different aspects: the so-called absolute and relative mechanisms. The absolute aspect refers to all of the mechanisms that determine the activation of DNA expression, followed by protein synthesis induction.

The relative aspect refers to all of the mechanisms that ultimately determine neuroprotective activities with preponderant expression in the membrane, cytosol and organelles.

*Pharmacological neuroprotection* involves the same patterns. Pharmacologically, the absolute mechanisms are predominantly controlled by neurotrophic factors and neurotrophic-like molecules, but the relative mechanisms mainly utilize ion channel blockers, agonists and antagonists of specific receptors, antioxidants, chelators of various metals and many other agents (Muresanu, 2007).

Therefore, all of these biological mechanisms can be naturally or pharmacologically activated. To successfully counteract pathophysiological mechanisms, the effect of EDA must be pharmacologically enhanced. *The key issue is that the neurobiological processes of EDAs share a common biological background with the pathophysiological mechanisms of DMs.* Pathophysiological mechanisms (PMs) have a dual character due to a common biological background with EDAs. For example, excitotoxicity (a pathophysiological mechanism), neurotrophicity and neuroplasticity (neuroreparatory processes) share N-methyl-D-aspartate receptors (NMDAR) activity as their common important driver. Further, inflammation is an important contributor to neuroregeneration because it stimulates neuroplasticity via trophic factors.

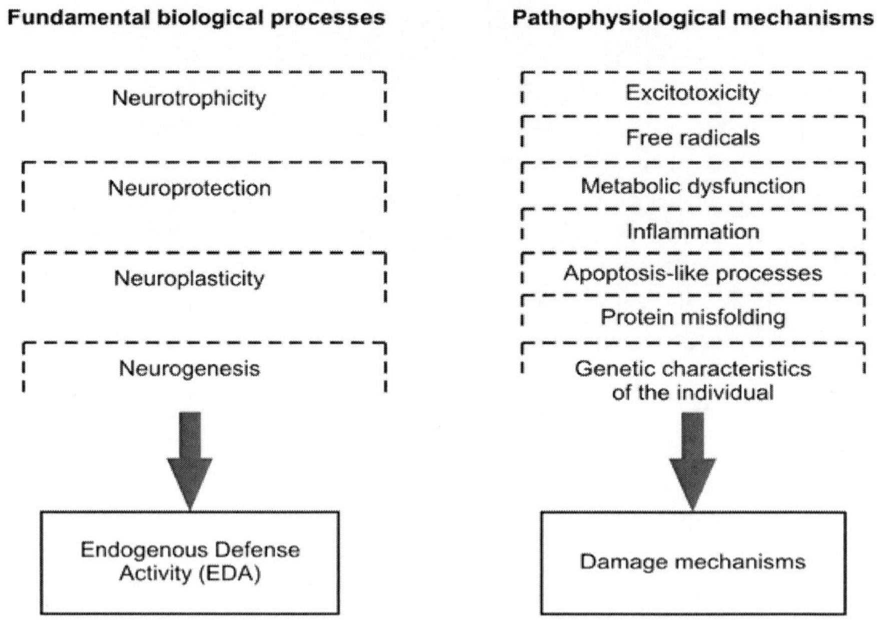


(Muresanu, 2011)

Figure 1. Pathophysiological processes.

Disturbances in the regulation of each of the four major players of EDA are themselves causes of some pathological conditions. For instance, a neurotrophicity deficit will always increase susceptibility to lesions. Thus far, no pathologies have been discovered that arise due in an excess of neurotrophicity or neuroprotection. For neuroplasticity, both up-regulation and down-regulation generate pathologies. Down-regulation generates a deficit of recovery, whereas up-regulation generates hundreds of neuropathological patterns of plasticity, including neuropathic pain, multiple sclerosis, movement disorders, tinnitus, impulse control disorders and obsessive-compulsive disorders. With regard to neurogenesis, both up-regulation and down-regulation generate pathological conditions, including down-regulation in Alzheimer's disease. Up-regulation of oligodendrogenesis and astrogenesis beyond normal regeneration is responsible for neuroproliferative disorders.

### *1.2.3. The Dual Character of DMs*

#### 1.2.3.1. Excitotoxicity

*Excitotoxicity* is the pathological process by which nerve cells are damaged by excess glutamate and other excitatory amino acid receptor ligands. NMDAR activation is one of the key features of excitotoxicity. The continuous activity of NMDARs is crucial for cell survival, and this is achieved through the regulation of neurotrophicity and neuroplasticity via calcium-controlled proteolytic systems (e.g., the calpain system) (Wu et al., 2005; Lai et al., 2014).

*Physiological patterns of synaptic NMDAR activity* actually promote neuronal cell survival by controlling the minimum calcium influx into the neuron. These very small quantities of calcium activate "high-affinity calcium-dependent molecules" (e.g., mu-calpain) and play the physiological role of conducting proteolytic activity, which is an important factor in neurotrophicity and neuroplasticity. This process is highly regulated by neurotrophic factors (Hutter et al., 1998). Key pro-survival pathways involving NMDARs are essential for neurotrophicity and neuroplasticity (Hetman and Kharebava, 2006; Lai et al., 2014).

The phosphoinositide 3-kinase (PI3K)–Akt cascade is strongly activated by NMDARs in many but not all neuronal types (Brunet et al., 2001). Synaptic NMDAR signaling also activates the Ras–extracellular signal-regulated kinase (1/2 ERK)1/2 cascade with pro-survival consequences, including cAMP-response element-binding protein (CREB) activation, BAD inactivation and antagonism of glycogen synthase kinase 3 (GSK3)β–induced apoptosis (Hardingham et al., 2001). Further, synaptic NMDAR-dependent calcium transients trigger a number of transcriptional changes that mediate long-lasting neuroplasticity via CRE-dependent gene expression (Hardingham et al., 2002; Hardingham and Bading, 2010).

*When NMDARs are over-activated by glutamate in pathological conditions*, such as stroke or trauma, large quantities of calcium enter the cells and activate "low-affinity calcium-dependent molecules", such as mu-calpain. The latter molecules have non-selective and uncontrolled proteolytic activities that lead to cell death. There are several fundamental mechanisms implicated in NMDAR-dependent cell death (Arundine et al., 2004; Bano et al., 2005; Stout et al., 1998; Zhou et al., 2013; Lai et al., 2014).

Cleavage of the plasma membrane $Na^+/Ca^{2+}$ exchanger by the $Ca^{2+}$-dependent protease, calpain, leads to necrosis. Mitochondrial dysfunction caused by excessive $Ca^{2+}$ uptake through the uniporter also leads to apoptosis-like processes. Finally, over-activation of the $Ca^{2+}$-dependent neuronal nitric oxide synthase (nNOS) by NMDAR activity has toxic downstream effects: p38 mitogen-activated protein kinase (MAPK) signaling, mitochondrial dysfunction and transient receptor potential melastatin channel (TRPM) activation leading to apoptosis-like processes.

Next, we examine NMDAR involvement in pro-survival (e.g., neurotrophicity and neuroplasticity) and pro-death signaling (excitotoxicity). (Figure 2)

*The first factor* that influences NMDAR receptor activation is the magnitude of stimulation (e.g., intensity or duration); low levels of activation are protective. $Ca^{2+}$ effectors of survival have considerably lower requirements for $Ca^{2+}$ than death effectors. Therefore, the ($Ca^{2+}$) threshold for the activation of pro-survival signaling by PI3K, ERK1/2 and calcium- and calmodulin-dependent kinase IV–CREB must be lower than the intracellular($Ca^{2+}$) that triggers toxic levels of calpain activation, mitochondrial uptake or nitric oxide production. Therefore, the pro-survival effector affinity for $Ca^{2+}$ is high. Certain potential death effectors, such as mu-calpain and the mitochondrial uniporter, have higher thresholds for $Ca^{2+}$ and intrinsically low $Ca^{2+}$ affinity (Soriano et al., 2007).

*The second important factor* is NMDAR location. *Extrasynaptic NMDAR activity* promotes the inactivation of CREB by dephosphorylation and early excitotoxic events (e.g., mitochondrial depolarization), concomitant with the inactivation of the ERK1/2 pathway, which causes necrosis and induces apoptosis-like processes. However, *synaptic NMDAR activity* promotes the activation of CREB and the ERK1/2 pathway.

Synaptic NMDAR activity does not disturb mitochondrial function, and it offers overall neuroprotective activity and promotes neurotrophicity and neuroplasticity (Hardingham and Bading, 2010; Parsons and Raymond, 2014).

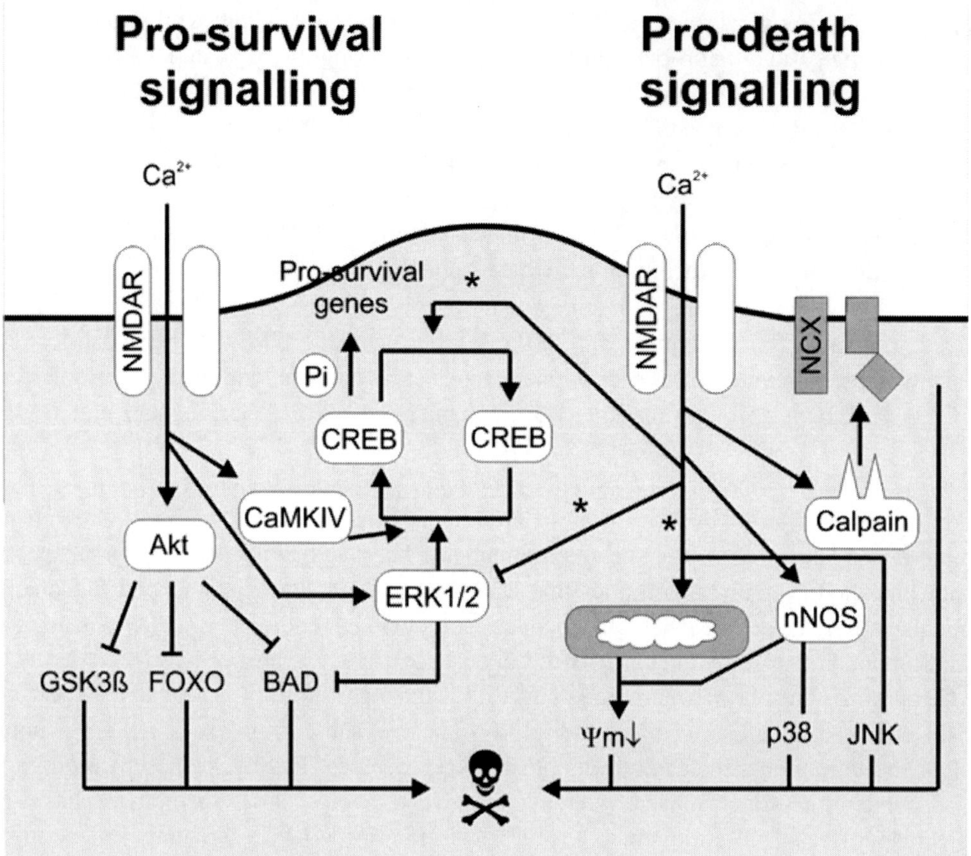


(Adapted after G.E. Hardingham, 2006; Biochemical Society 2006)

Figure 2. Pro-survival and pro-death signaling.

### 1.2.3.2. Inflammation

The pathological role of inflammation has been recognized in almost all neurological conditions. This well-orchestrated process, situated on the borderline between physiology and pathology, tends to become highly destructive when prolonged or deregulated. However, inflammatory cells and mediators may also have beneficial functions and contribute to tissue repair processes. There is evidence demonstrating that inflammation plays a positive role in neuroprotection and neuroplasticity (Iseda et al., 2004; Kotter et al., 2001). Neurotrophic factors are the major players in this process, and are produced by activated immune cells to participate in neuronal cell protection and neuroplasticity (Masson et al., 2000). Neurotrophic factors either bind directly to their receptors or act by modulating the local immune response. Even a very potent pro-inflammatory molecule such as tumor necrosis factor-α has neuroprotective and neurotrophic effects via trophic factors when activating R2 (Arnett et al., 2003; Marchetti et al., 2004; Bartsch et al., 2010; Sharma, 2010).

The very low permeability of the BBB extends to immune cells and molecules. Usually, resident cells in the CNS (particularly astrocytes and microglia) regulate immune reactivity within the CNS. Other alien immune entities enter the CNS only through highly regulated processes mediated by adhesion molecules, chemokines, cytokines and matrix metalloproteinases (Becher and Antel, 1996; Windhangen et al., 1995; Pachter et al., 2003).

### 1.2.3.3. Apoptosis and Apoptosis-Like Processes

Apoptosis is a positive process that maintains the number and quality of cells. If a cell has a DNA lesion, it activates the p53 gene. Then, the cell will halt in the G1 phase of the cell cycle by bcl-2 activation, repair its DNA and recommence division. Alternatively, altered DNA repair may cause the activation of "bax", which leads to apoptotic death. If apoptosis is not effective, then malignant clone formation will occur.

From the above highlights of the links between DM and EDA, we can draw the following conclusions:

1. NMDAR activity plays a positive role during physiological activation by generating neurotrophicity and neuroplasticity or a deleterious role by overactivation-induced excitotoxicity generating pathological processes (e.g., stroke, trauma and neurodegenerative disorders).
2. Inflammation generally has a negative impact, but it can positively influence neuroprotection and neuroplasticity via neurotrophic factors.
3. Apoptosis is a positive process, but apoptotic-like processes are always negative. Apoptotic-like processes must be endogenously and therapeutically controlled.

In this light, there is a compelling body of basic and clinical evidence indicating that even the *subtractive suppressive strategy* was an important achievement that generated beneficial results for neuroprotection in animal models, such as reducing the volume of ischemic lesions in experimental stroke. Yet, this strategy failed from the clinical neurorecovery perspective. It is becoming evident that pharmacological intervention should address *modulation* not *suppression*. The more pathophysiological processes are modulated, the better the chances are for therapeutic success. Therefore, drugs with pleiotropic mechanisms of action are the best candidates for acute neuroprotection.

The *concept of a pleiotropic effect* is only related to neuroprotection and represents the capacity of a pharmacological agent to interfere in more than one pathophysiological process (Figure 1).

The best approach for clinical neuroprotection is modulating (not suppressive) pleiotropic drugs that down-regulate extrasynaptic NMDAR excitotoxicity and, at the same time, decrease the negative effects of inflammation, increase the positive effects of inflammation and prevent apoptotic-like processes. In this way, the valuable processes that support recovery (e.g., neuroplasticity and neurotrophicity) are not hindered.

Important biological molecules such as neurotrophic factors may also have a concomitant supportive effect on the EDA side by stimulating neurotrophicity, neuroprotection, neuroplasticity and neurogenesis. This capacity of a molecular agent is described as a *multimodal effect* (Figure 1; Figure 3).

A unimodal agent influences only one neurobiological process of EDA whereas a pleiotropic multimodal agent will influence more neurobiological processes. *Pleiotropic neuroprotective and multimodal effects* are fundamentally different but highly complementary.

There are suppressive chemical agents that cause pleiotropic effects, but these agents are not very helpful in clinical practice because they lack the multimodal effect. Biological agents (e.g., neurotrophic factors and related molecules) with *modulating and neuroprotective pleiotropic effects* are better because they also usually have *multimodal* effects. These agents are capable of pharmacologically bridging acute neuroprotective processes with the long-term recovery processes. The pharmacological consequences of the evolution of "neuroprotection and neurorecovery" concepts are depicted in Figure 3.

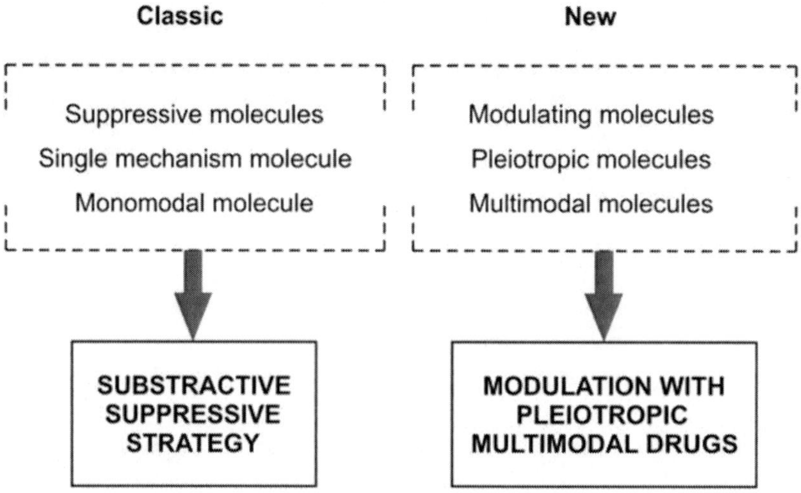


(Muresanu, 2011)

Figure 3. Pharmacological consequences of the evolution of neuroprotection and neurorecovery.

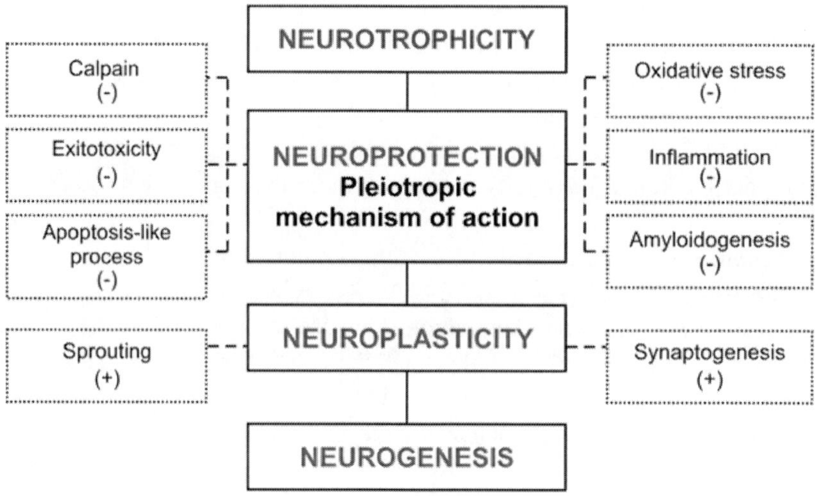


(Muresanu, 2011)

Figure 4. The mechanism of action of modulating, pleiotropic, neuroprotective and multimodal drugs.

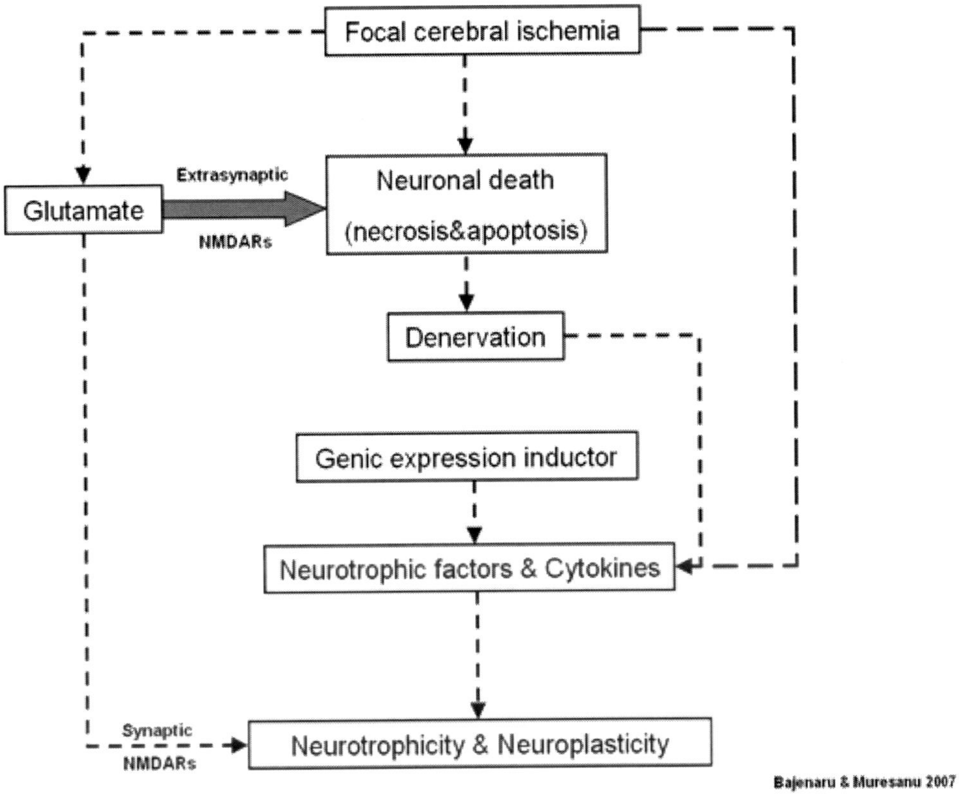


Figure 5. The dual roles performed by glutamate makes it a potent and indispensable factor for neurotrophicity and neuroplasticity processes.

The concept and mechanism of action of modulating pleiotropic multimodal drugs (e.g., neurotrophic factors) are presented in Figure 4. We can better understand the mechanism of action of pleiotropic multimodal drugs by following the example of how neuroprotection or neuroplasticity are endogenously integrated during an acute injury, such as stroke or trauma, where glutamate plays a dual role (Figure 5).

From this intuitive example, we learned that in the first hours after an acute injury, the large amount of glutamate (which acts predominantly on extrasynaptic NMDARs) is deleterious due to its final cell death effect. Beyond 48 to 72 h, glutamate becomes the key player in controlling neurorestoration via synaptic NMDARs that stimulate neuroplasticity and neurotrophicity. A multimodal pharmacological agent modulates both protection and plasticity within the continuous EDA process.

All of these concepts and data are supported by the results of RCTs in neuroprotection and neurorestoration. In one of the most accurate meta-analyses, "Clinical Trials for Cytoprotection in Stroke", Labiche and Grotta (2004) underscored the fact that all of the trials that have studied the effect of *unimodal suppressive single mechanism* drugs have negative or neutral results. Only two drugs, Cerebrolysin and citicoline, which are *non-suppressive, pleiotropic, multimodal drugs*, demonstrated positive trends (Table 1). Larger RCTs are necessary to ultimately confirm these positive results. We have similar situations in acute traumatic brain injury clinical trials for neuroprotection. In a systematic review written by

Maas et al., the only drug that showed significant results was progesterone, which is also a non-suppressive, pleiotropic, multimodal agent (Maas et al., 2010; Xiao et al., 2008).

## 1.3. Neuroplasticity and Neurorestoration in Acute and Chronic Neurological Disorders

EDA of the nervous system is a polychromic continuous process that simultaneously performs and integrates the neurobiological processes of neurotrophicity, neuroprotection, neuroplasticity and neurogenesis. *Neuroregeneration* is the morphological outcome of the interactions between these basic neurobiological processes that develop in a particular biological and individual context. *Neurorestoration* is the positive outcome that produces clinically relevant results with immediate functional and late structural effects. Immediate and late effects generate two types of changes: *restitution and substitution. Restitution* is an intrinsic process involving biochemically and genetically induced events, such as a reduction of edema, the absorption of heme and the restoration of axonal transport and ionic currents. *Substitution* depends on external stimuli, such as practice, which drives activity-dependent plasticity through learning. (Barnes et al., 2003).

## 1.4. Neurorestoration – Biological Background

All neurobiological processes can be endogenously or exogenously activated. The altered regulation of any of the four components of EDA may generate pathological conditions. Further, altered neuroplasticity, in the form of both up- and down-regulation, generates pathologies (Read et al., 2001).

Normally, these processes are regulated via key endogenous players, such as neurotrophic factors and neurotrophic-like molecules. To successfully compete with pathological processes and support neurorestoration, EDA should be exogenously enhanced by pharmacological intervention, physical means, electromagnetic stimulation, psychological support, environmental stimulation, cell transplantation or any demonstrated combinations of these factors capable of improving a patient's condition. From the pharmacological perspective, it is clear that focusing on molecules that are capable of mimicking the structure and function of endogenous molecules with non-suppressive pleiotropic neuroprotective and multimodal mechanisms is the best approach in neuroprotection and neuroplasticity (Muresanu et al., 2011; Sharma et al., 2014). Both processes occur in a particular sequence in the continuous process of EDA. Indeed, the brain uses the same molecules for both neuroprotection and neuroplasticity, although in different combinations. These molecules are activated during altered gene expression induced by lesion; brain ischemia regulates the expression of more genes than any other condition (Danton and Dietrich, 2003; Ginsberg 1997). However, many activated genes are not translated into proteins after injury. Endogenous neuroprotection is maximally effective approximately 72 h following an insult. Any further positive clinical outcome is driven by the processes of neuroplasticity and neurogenesis. A brief overview of post-lesion regulation is presented in Table 2.

**Table 1. Past and Current Cytoprotective Clinical Trials**

| Drugs | Phase | Latest Extent of Time Window | Adeq. Power | Adeq Dose | Dose-Limiting AEs | Homogen Patient Population | Linked to TPA | Biologic Imaging Marker | Results |
|---|---|---|---|---|---|---|---|---|---|
| Calcium Antagonists | | | | | | | | | |
| Nimodipine | 3 | 6-48 h | + | | Hypotension | | | | Neutral |
| Nicardipine | 2 | 12 h | | | Hypotension | | | | Neutral |
| Glutamate Antagonists | | | | | | | | | |
| Selfotel | 3 | 6-12 h | + | No | Neuropsych | | | | Negative |
| Dextrorphan | 2 | 48 h | | Yes | Neuropsych | | | | Neutral |
| Cerestat | 3 | 6-24 h | + | Yes | Hypertension | | | | Negative |
| AR-R15696 | 2 | 12 h | | Yes | Neuropsych | | | | Neutral |
| Magnesium | 3* | 2-12 h | + | Yes | No | + | | + | ? |
| AMPA Antagonists | | | | | | | | | |
| YM872 | 2b | 3-6 h | + | ? | ? | + | + | + | Neutral |
| ZK200775 | 2 | 24 h | | ? | Sedation | | | + | Negative |
| Indirect Glutamate Modulators | | | | | | | | | |
| Eliprodil | 3 | ? | ? | ? | ? | ? | ? | ? | Negative |
| Gavestinel | 3 | 6 h | +† | Yes | No | + | | | Neutral |
| Sipatrigine | 2 | 12 h | | ? | Neuropsych | + | | | Negative |
| Fosphenytoin | 2/3 | 4 h | + | ? | No | | | | Neutral |
| BMSS-204352 | 3 | 6 h | + | ? | No | + | | + | Neutral |
| Lifarizin | 2 | ? | | ? | Hypotension | | | | Neutral |
| Lubeluzole | 3 | 4-8 h | +† | No | Cardiac | + | + | | Neutral |

**Table 1. (Continued)**

| Drugs | Phase | Latest Extent of Time Window | Adeq. Power | Adeq Dose | Dose-Limiting AEs | Homogen Patient Population | Linked to TPA | Biologic Imaging Marker | Results |
|---|---|---|---|---|---|---|---|---|---|
| Other Neurotrans Modulators | | | | | | | | | |
| Trazadone | 2 | ? | ? | ? | ? | ? | ? | ? | Neutral |
| Repinotan | 3* | 6 h | +† | Yes | ? | + | | | ? |
| ONO-2506 | 2/3* | 6 h | + | ? | ? | + | | | ? |
| Opioid Antagonists | | | | | | | | | |
| Naloxone | 2 | 8-60 h | | ? | No | | | | Neutral |
| Nalmefene | 3 | 6 h | +† | ? | No | + | | | Neutral |
| GABA Agonist | | | | | | | | | |
| Clonethiazole | 3 | 12 h | +† | Yes | Sedation | + | | | Neutral |
| Diazepam | 3* | 12 h | + | ? | ? | | | | ? |
| Free Radical Scavengers | | | | | | | | | |
| Tirilazad | 3 | 6 h | + | ? | No | | | + | Negative |
| Ebselen | 3* | 48 h | + | ? | ? | + | | | ? |
| NXY-059 | 2b/3* | 6 h | +† | ? | ? | + | | | Negative |
| Anti-inflammatory Agents | | | | | | | | | |
| Enlimomab | 3 | 6 h | + | Yes | Fever | + | | | Negative |
| LeukArrest | 3 | 12 h | ? | ? | ? | | | | Neutral |
| FK-506 | 2* | 12 h | | ? | ? | + | | | ? |
| Steroids | 2 | 48 h | | ? | Infection | | | | Negative |

| Drugs | Phase | Latest Extent of Time Window | Adeq. Power | Adeq Dose | Dose-Limiting AEs | Homogen Patient Population | Linked to TPA | Biologic Imaging Marker | Results |
|---|---|---|---|---|---|---|---|---|---|
| Membrane Stabilizers/Trophic Factors | | | | | | | | | |
| GM1 | 3 | 72 h | + | ? | No | | | | Neutral |
| Cerebrolysin | 2 | 12-24 h | | ? | No | | | | Positive Trend |
| Citicoline | 3 | 24 h | +† | ? | No | + | | + | Positive Post hoc |
| EPO | 2a* | | | | | | | | |
| bFGF | 2/3 | 6 h | + | ? | Hypotension | + | | | Negative |
| Hypothermia | 2* | 5-24 h | | Yes | Pneumonia, arrhythmias, hypotension | + | | + | ? |
| Caffeinol Oxygen Delivery | 2* | 4-6 h | | Yes | No | + | | | ? |
| DCLHb | 2 | 18 h | | ? | HTN | | | | Negative |
| HBO | 2/3* | 24 h | | ? | ? | | | | Neutral |

Only relevant to phase 2b or 3 efficacy trials.
* Currently enrolling.
† Not adequately powered for TPA subgroup.
+ = positive; HTN = hypertension; AE = adverse effects; Neuropsych = Neuropsychiatric side effects.

The identification of when particular changes occur (early or late) and the interpretation of their influence is often difficult. *Early changes* reflect neuroprotective efforts induced by cell damage and have little relevance to recovery potential. *Late changes* generally suggest recovery processes, but simultaneous overlapping events add complexity to the identification of individual changes. With regard to gene expression, patterns of gene expression change and it is not simply individual genes that must be considered. It is important to acknowledge the remarkable flexibility of endogenous programs (Ginsberg 1997). For simplicity, 72 h is considered a distinguishing time point: the first 72 h after insult represents the early time window, and anything after 72 h represents the late time window.

## 1.5. Pharmacological Modulation in Neuroprotection and Restoration

Pharmacological modulation as a support for classical neurorehabilitation treatments, such as kinetotherapy, physiotherapy, speech therapy and occupational therapy, represents a promising approach for promoting restoration.

Below, we emphasize several pharmacological agents that are relevant for current or future clinical therapy.

### *1.5.1. D-Amphetamine (AMPH)*

D-amphetamine is a drug that increases the release of norepinephrine, dopamine and serotonin in the synaptic cleft. Allthought high doses induce the excessive release of dopamine resultin in neurotoxicity, moderate doses proved that can induce neuroprotection (Rau et al., 2011). By stimulating the presynaptic release of catecholaminergic terminals, AMPH disinhibits the inhibitory circuits, which results in the long-term facilitation of sensorimotor synapses. AMPH facilitates the development of long-term potentiation (LTP) in a dose-dependent manner and enhances memory retrieval (Gold et al., 1984).

**Table 2. Post-lesional regulation [J Neuropathol Exp Neurol, Vol 61, October, 2002]**

| - = no report; ↑ = upregulation; ↓ = downregulation | | | | | |
|---|---|---|---|---|---|
| Early regulation<br>≤ 3 days post-lesion | | | Late regulation<br>> 3 days post-lesion | | |
| Molecule | Ipsi-lesional | Contra-lesional | Ipsi-lesional | Contra-lesional | Involvement in experience – induced plasticity |
| Immediate early gene/transcription factor | | | | | |
| c-Fos | ↑ | – | ↑ | ↑ | Environmental enrichment |
| c-Jun | ↑ | – | ↑ | – | Learning |
| JunB | ↑ | – | – | – | Environmental enrichment |
| NGFI-A | ↑ | – | ↑ | – | Environmental enrichment |
| NGFI-B | ↑ | – | – | ↑ | Learning |

| | | | | | |
|---|---|---|---|---|---|
| - = no report; ↑ = upregulation; ↓ = downregulation | | | | | |
| NGFI-C | ↑ | – | – | – | Used-induced |
| Krox-20 | ↑ | – | – | – | – |
| Arc | ↑ | – | – | ↑ | Environmental enrichment |
| CREB (increased phosphorylation | ↑ | – | ↑ in c. callosum | ↑ | Used-induced |
| NF-kB | Controversial results | | | | Learning |
| Kinase network molecules | | | | | |
| MAP kinase | ↑ | – | – | ↑ | Learning |
| CaM kinase | ↓ | – | ↑ | – | Physical exercise |
| Neurotransmitter receptors | | | | | |
| GluR1 | ↓ | – | ↓ | – | Environmental enrichment |
| GluR2 | ↓ | – | ↓ | – | – |
| GluR3 | ↓ | – | ↓ | – | – |
| NMDAR (receptor binding) | – | ↑ | ↑ | ↑ | Environmental enrichment |
| mGluR3 | ↓ | – | – | – | Learning |
| mGluR2 | ↓ | – | ↓ | ↓ | Learning |
| GABAR (receptor binding) | ↓ | – | ↓ | ↓ | Learning |
| Growth factors/receptors | | | | | |
| NGF | ↑ | – | ↑ | ↑ | Environmental enrichment |
| BDNF | ↑ | ↑ | – | – | Environmental enrichment |
| NT3 | ↓ | – | ↓ | – | Environmental enrichment |
| bFGF | ↑ | – | ↑ | ↑ | Learning/physical exercise |
| GDNF | ↑ | – | – | – | Environmental enrichment |
| PDGF | ↑ | – | ↑ | – | – |
| IGF | – | – | ↑ | ↑ | – |
| TGF-β1 | ↑ | – | ↑ | – | – |
| Trk B | ↑ | ↑ | – | – | Learning |
| Neuropilin -1, -2 | ↑ | – | ↑ | – | – |
| TNF-α | ↑ | ↑ | – | – | – |
| APP | – | – | ↑ | – | Learning |
| Growth – associated/cytoskeletal molecules | | | | | |
| GAP – 43 | ↑ | – | ↑ | ↑ | Learning |
| SCG – 10 | – | ↑ | – | ↑ | – |
| α – tubulin | – | – | ↑ | – | Learning |

**Table 2. (Continued)**

| | | | | | |
|---|---|---|---|---|---|
| - = no report; ↑ = upregulation; ↓ = downregulation | | | | | |
| MAP – 2 | ↑ | – | ↑ | – | Learning |
| apoE | ↓ | – | ↑ | – | Learning |
| apoD | ↑ | – | ↑ | ↑ | – |
| Synapse-related molecules | | | | | |
| Synaptophysin | – | – | ↑ | ↑ | Environmental enrichment |
| synapsin-I | ↑ | – | ↑ | – | Learning |
| SNAP-25 | – | – | ↑ | – | – |
| Adhesion molecules | | | | | |
| PSA-NCAM | ↑ | – | ↑ | – | Learning |
| L1 | ↓ | – | ↑ | – | Learning |
| F3 | ↓ | – | ↓ up to 1 week then ↑ | ↑ | – |
| Tenascin-C | ↑ | – | ↑ | – | – |

Additionally, through catecholaminergic release, AMPH contributes to the alleviation of neuronal metabolic depression (Queen et al., 1997). Another mechanism that enhances neuroplasticity is the promotion of alternative circuit activation (Dietrich et al., 1990). AMPH enhances the expression of proteins, including neurotrophins, which may be involved in dendritic and axonal sprouting by the induction of the immediate early gene c-fos (Stroemer et al., 1998).

Some basic research with AMPH suggested that it facilitates motor recovery after brain lesions, such as TBI and stroke (Hovda et al., 1984). Mayfield et al. (1993) tested the effects of AMPH on reaction time in rats. The animals were trained to release a lever in response to an auditory or visual stimulus to avoid a mild foot shock. Successful avoidance was not affected by AMPH treatment, but response latencies were dose-dependently decreased (Mayfield et al., 1993). Hurwitz et al. (1991) demonstrated that AMPH, when administered in multiple injections following cerebrovascular insult, facilitates behavioral recovery from a sensorimotor deficit subsequent to thrombotic infarction of the primary somatosensory cortex in rats. In these experiments, rats received 2 or 4 mg/kg AMPH or saline 24 h prior to testing on days 4, 6, 9 and 11. The results demonstrated a dose-response effect (e.g., the 4 mg/kg amphetamine group recovered earlier than the 2 mg/kg amphetamine group), and both AMPH groups recovered more completely than the saline-injected group (Hurwitz et al., 1991). In another study, Stroemer et al. (1998) demonstrated that multiple intraperitoneal AMPH treatments, accompanied by behavioral training during the period of drug effect, enhance behavioral recovery of sensorimotor function of the contralateral forelimb after neocortical infarction. They also demonstrated that AMPH treatment improves behavioral recovery in both a sensorimotor and a spatial memory task. The authors proposed that AMPH treatment induces neural sprouting and synaptogenesis (Stroemer et al., 1998). However, in other studies on animal models of cervical contusion and stroke, the combined pharmacological intervention with amphetamine with motor training, did not prove any kinematic improvement or neuroprotection (Alaverdashvili M. et al., 2007; Krisa et al., 2012). In contrast, in a study on TBI animal models treatment with low-dose AMPH in the first 3 h after the injury restored learning and memory function to near normal ability (Rau et al., 2012). In a recent study the administration of AMPH 0.500mg/kg/h in the first 12 h after severe TBI, proved to be neuroprotective by reducing the expression of key pro-inflammmatory genes, and the administration in the first 8 h preserved axonal density (Rau, 2014).

AMPH was one of the first drugs investigated in rehabilitation clinical trials. Their results on motor functions, aphasia and cognitive rehabilitation were controversial, most probably because of the diversity of methodology: time post-stroke of study initialtion; drug ingestion interval before rehabilitation treatments; rehabilitation treatment type, intensity, duration; timing of final outcome measures; what the outcome measures actually assess amd adequate subject description (Walker-Batson, 2013). Indeed, some studies suggest a beneficial role of AMPH in the rehabilitation efforts in stroke patients (Bütefisch et al., 2002; Sawaki et al., 2002; Pleger et al., 2004; Loubinoux et al., 1999), but also there are several studies that could not evidentiate a difference between AMPH treatment and placebo (Platz, 2005; Gladstone et al., 2006). A review that analyzed 11 completed trials concluded that there was no evidence that AMPH decreased death rate or dependency after ischemic stroke, but AMPH use was associated with significant effects on hemodynamic measures (Sprigg et al., 2009). Two more recent reviews (Harbeck-Seu et al., 2011; Walker-Batson, 2013) concluded that the majority of studies could not demonstrate an efficacy of AMPH treatement upon rehabilitation. There were also concerns about the safety of this drug.

### *1.5.2. Rasagiline (N-Propargyl-1-(R)-Aminoindan)*

Rasagiline is a selective, irreversible, second-generation monoamine oxidase-B (MAO-B) inhibitor. It was approved by the U.S. Food and Drug Administration in 2006 for the treatment of idiopathic Parkinson's disease as an initial monotherapy or as an adjunct to levodopa. It is structurally similar to selegiline, but unlike selegiline, rasagiline is not derived from AMPH, is not metabolized to a neurotoxic l-methamphetamine derivative, and does not have sympathomimetic activity. Both rasagiline and selegiline demonstrate potent neuroprotective and anti-apoptotic effects under experimental conditions. Additionally, the neuroprotective activity of rasagiline is observable at concentrations below the MAO-B inhibition threshold and in cell systems that do not contain MAO-B (Maruyama et al., 2002). Rasagiline suppresses oxidative stress in dopaminergic neurons by increasing the expression of the antioxidative enzymes superoxide dismutase and catalase (Carrillo et al., 2000). Additionally, rasagiline has the capacity to down-regulate genes that are suspected to play a role in neurodegeneration, such as those encoding oxidative stress proteins, glutamate and AMPA receptors, inducible nitric oxide synthase (iNOS) and inflammatory transcription factors. Basic research has demonstrated that rasagiline also has a potent anti-apoptotic activity that is exerted by increasing the activity of the Bcl-2 and protein kinase C (PKC) genes and by down-regulating the pro-apoptotic FAS and Bax genes (Youdim et al., 2003).

In addition, rasagiline binds directly to methyl-4-phenyl-1,2,3,6-tetrahydropyridine (MPTP) and stabilizes the mitochondrial membrane potential to prevent the pro-apoptotic decline in mitochondrial membrane potential (DCm) due to a permeability transition and activation of apoptotic processes, including activation of caspase 3, nuclear translocation of glyceraldehyde-3-phosphate dehydrogenase and nucleosomal DNA fragmentation. Rasagiline also inactivates glyceraldehyde phosphodehydrogenase (GAPDH), which is over-expressed during apoptosis (Mandel et al., 2005).

The activation of GAPDH is another pathway of apoptosis-induced cell death that is associated with glucose, and the intermediate metabolism of GAPDH translocation is a downstream signal of mitochondria in Bcl-2 over-expressing cells (Maruyama et al., 2001). Other neuroprotective mechanisms of rasagiline occur via an increase in the protein and mRNA levels of GDNF (Maruyama et al., 2004) and by the prevention of N- MPTP-induced neurotoxicity (Kupsch et al., 2001).

Rasagiline also processes amyloid precursor protein (APP) into the neuroprotective-neurotrophic soluble APP alpha (sAPPα) using PKC and the MAP kinase-dependent activation of α-secretase. Laboratory studies have demonstrated that treatment with rasagiline decreases the level of APP, which prevents the increased generation of beta-amyloid peptides, which play a central role in the pathogenesis of Alzheimer's disease (Mandel et al., 2005).

Four pivotal clinical trials, TEMPO, LARGO, PRESTO and ADAGIO, have investigated rasagiline. All of these trials demonstrated that the drug is associated with improved outcomes in patients with early PD and reduces the off-time in patients with moderate to advanced PD with motor fluctuations (Chen et al., 2004).

The ADAGIO study, one of the largest studies concerning PD, included 1,176 patients with very early PD who were randomized to receive 1 or 2 mg rasagiline per day for 72 weeks (early start) or a placebo for 36 weeks followed by 1 or 2 mg rasagiline per day for 36 weeks (delayed start). The study was conducted to test whether rasagiline was a possible disease-modifying therapy. At either dose, rasagiline had to meet three pre-specified trial efficacy endpoints, which were a combination of slope and difference measures, to be considered a 'disease modifying' therapy. The authors reported that a daily dose of 1 mg of rasagiline provided neuroprotective benefits, but similar results were not found with the 2 mg dose. The authors theorized that perhaps the milder subjects at baseline benefited so much symptomatically from 2 mg rasagiline that it masked any possible disease-modifying effect, which could only be tested by examining slightly more severe subjects (Olanow et al., 2009).

### *1.5.3. Dopamine*

Dopamine (DA) is a catecholamine neuromodulator that activates five types of receptors and their variants: D1, D2, D3, D4 and D5. DA is produced in several areas of the brain, including the substantia nigra and the ventral tegmental area(VTA), and is a neurohormone released by the hypothalamus. Dopaminergic transmission is recognized as an important modulator of human cognition, motivation, behavioral adaptation, movement, addiction, pain and memory. Abnormal dopaminergic transmission plays a major role in PD and mental disorders, such as schizophrenia and other psychoses (Schnider et al., 2010; Arias-Carrión et al. 2007).

The effects of DA binding to its metabotropic receptors include modifications of synaptic plasticity, which is the substrate of learning and memory. The strength of synaptic transmission can be modified on a long-term basis by specific patterns of activation, such as high frequency trains that produce LTP. DA enhances LTP regarding motor memory in the hippocampus, striatum and cerebral cortex (Garris et al., 1994). Additionally, normal aging, which is characterized by a decreased ability to encode novel information and to express LTP, is associated with diminished brain DA activity (Jay, 2003).

To evaluate the efficacy of carbidopa/levodopa (carbidopa L-dopa) in reducing left spatial neglect after stroke, Mukand et al. (2001) treated four right-handed female patients (who suffered right brain stroke and left unilateral spatial neglect) with carbidopa L-dopa. Treatment led to a beneficial response in three of the patients, and the authors concluded that a larger randomized controlled study that can address the issues of dose, duration of treatment and a refined criteria for a carbidopa L-dopa trial was necessary.

To test the efficacy of carbidopa L-dopa in combination with physiotherapy, Scheidtmann et al. (2001) performed a prospective placebo-controlled, double-blinded study in which they tested 53 primary stroke patients. For the first 3 weeks, patients received single doses of levodopa (100 mg) or a placebo daily in combination with physiotherapy. For the second 3 weeks, patients received only physiotherapy. The results showed that a single dose of levodopa was well-tolerated and, when given in combination with physiotherapy, enhanced motor recovery in patients with hemiplegia (Scheidtmann et al., 2001).

Floel et al. (2005) conducted a study in which they assessed the effect of L-dopa premedication on the training-dependent encoding of an elementary motor memory in young and elderly healthy volunteers. The study demonstrated that the upregulation of dopaminergic activity resulted in beneficial effects on the formation of motor memories, particularly in elderly adults. In another clinical study, Floel et al. (2005) tested the effects of a single oral dose of levodopa on the formation of a motor memory using TMS to measure motor excitability. They demonstrated that patients receiving levodopa had enhanced motor training ability to encode an elementary motor memory relative to placebo. In another study using a different design, Restemeyer et al. (2007) used a double-blinded, placebo-controlled crossover trial to test if a single dose of levodopa could improve motor functions and change motor excitability. The authors applied the Nine Hole Peg Test as a measure of dexterity, a dynometer to measure grip strength and the Action Research Arm Test, which allows the evaluation of proximal and distal arm function. Additionally, the patients were tested for their motor excitability using TMS techniques. Compared to the placebo, levodopa neither improved motor functions nor changed motor excitability as tested by TMS. In two different studies, despite the two different methodologies (in one levodopa was administrated 100mgx2 in the first day and 100mg in the second day before one session of procedural motor learning, while in the other one 100mg/day for 5 weeks was administrated without motor learning), a significant improvement of motor function was found (Rosser et al., 2008; Acler et al., 2009).

In 2010, a multi-center prospective, randomized, double-blinded, placebo-controlled trial was initiated to test whether L-dopa and carbidopa drug treatment, in combination with occupational and physical therapy, improved functional recovery, including walking ability and arm function. In this study, 572 patients with stroke were randomized to receive L-dopa and carbidopa or a placebo within 7 to 14 days post-stroke. The patients were evaluated using the following scales: the Rivermead Mobility Index, Barthel Index, Northwick Park Nursing Dependency, Nottingham Extended Activities of Daily Living Scale, General Health Questionnaire, Caregiver Burden Index, EQ-5D, the ABILHAND questionnaire, Fatigue Assessment Scale and Musculoskeletal symptoms/signs and Pain Manikin. A Modified Rankin Scale was used such that results from this study can be related to other clinical trials. Additionally, a standardized questionnaire was developed to record the patients' and therapists' perspective of the use of L-dopa as part of the rehabilitation treatment. There is no published data yet (Bharkta et al).

Two more recent studies found an improvement in motor function, but only when levodopa was combined with physiotherapy (Lokk et al., 2011; Acler M and Mananotti P, 2013).

### 1.5.4. Reboxetine

Reboxetine is a new antidepressant that belongs to the category of selective norepinephrine reuptake inhibitors and has an affinity for the muscarinic, cholinergic, dopaminergic and alpha 1 adrenergic receptor families. A recent review of the treatment of major depression concluded that reboxetine is ineffective and potentially harmful (Eyding et al., 2010). In addition to being an antidepressant, reboxetine has been studied as a potential treatment that induces neuroplasticity in post-ischemic stroke. Animal experiments indicate that noradrenergic agents can improve recovery from stroke (Feeney et al., 2004). Linner et al. (2001) analyzed the effects of reboxetine on the somatodendritic and terminal regions of the mesolimbocortical DA system in rats using single cell recordings and microdialysis following the administration of reboxetine in doses that appear to yield clinically-relevant plasma concentrations. This study demonstrated that the systemic administration of reboxetine preferentially increases the burst firing of dopaminergic neurons in the VTA but does not produce a significant effect on the average firing frequency. Increased excitability in the VTA dopaminergic neurons consequently increases neuronal activity in reward-related learning.

Zittel et al. (2007) used a double-blinded, placebo-controlled, crossover study to analyze the effects of reboxetine administration in chronic hemiparetic patients. Ten patients were enrolled in this pilot study and were given a single dose of reboxetine. Three different motor assessments (i.e., tapping speed, grip strength and dexterity evaluation) were performed before drug intake, 1.5 h later and after the physiotherapy session. TMS was used to investigate motor excitability by measuring motor thresholds and the amplitudes of motor-evoked potentials; both hands were studied. The results demonstrated an improvement of motor functions, especially simple movements (including enhanced hand-tapping speed and grip strength of the affected hand), but it did not modify the performance of more complex motor tasks. Additionally, there was no improvement in motor performance after physiotherapy, and the TMS data did not indicate a relevant change of corticospinal excitability.

In a more recent study with placebo-controlled, double-blind and crossover design, 5 mg of reboxetine was administered in 11 stroke patients in the subacute and chronic stage. Behavioral performance was tested twice, about 2.5 h after drug administration on each testing day. Before the second behavioral testing, patients were scanned with fMRI. The results showed improvement in motor function that was related to a rearrangement of cortical interactions. Howerver, the reboxetine-improved motor performance represented a short-term effect (Wang et al., 2011).

Currently, there is an ongoing randomized, placebo-controlled, double-blinded, crossover study to analyze if the combination of reboxetine/transcranial direct current stimulation is more effective at enhancing the motor functions of daily life (assessed by the Jebsen Taylor test) compared to reboxetine or tDCS alone (Gerloff et al., STIMBOX, ongoing clinical study).

### 1.5.5. Serotonin

Serotonin is implicated in learning and memory formation due to its impact on neuroplasticity. Serotonin affects LTP and long-term depression (LTD) by enhancing or blocking each, depending on the sub-receptor specificity, the location of plasticity induction and the frequency of application (Nitsche et al., 2009). Due to its neuromodulatory function, serotonin has been proposed as a potential therapy for neurorehabilitation.

To test the capacity of paroxetine and selective serotonin reuptake inhibitors (SSRI) to modulate behavior and cortical motor activity, Loubinoux et al. (2005) conducted a double-blinded, placebo-controlled, fMRI study in healthy subjects. Paroxetine improved the efficiency of motor responses, which demonstrates a clear modulation of sensory and motor cerebral activation, and improved behavior efficiency. Laboratory studies have demonstrated that treatment with fluoxetine provides strong protection against delayed cerebral ischemic injury, and these neuroprotective effects may be associated with its anti-inflammatory effects (Lim et al. 2009).

In a prospective, double-blinded, crossover, placebo-controlled fMRI study, eight patients with pure motor hemiparesia were tested for motor deficit. The patients received a single dose of fluoxetine or a placebo. Patients who received fluoxetine displayed hyperactivation in the ipsilesional primary motor cortex. Moreover, fluoxetine significantly improved the motor skills of the affected side (Pariente et al., 2001). A similar result with fluoxetine was obtained in several clinical studies (Berends et al. 2009; van Genderen et al., 2008).

Nitsche et al. (2009) used a single-blinded, placebo-controlled, randomized crossover study to test whether the administration of citalopram in combination with tDCS enhances motor cortex excitability. They applied anodal excitability-enhancing or cathodal excitability-diminishing tDCS after a single dose of citalopram or a placebo. Their results demonstrated that citalopram modulated tDCS-induced plasticity by increasing the facilitatory plasticity induced by anodal tDCS and by converting the inhibitory plasticity induced by cathodal tDCS into facilitation. Robol et al. (2004) tested motor cortex excitability using single and paired TMS before and after the oral administration of citalopram. Their findings suggest that a single oral dose of citalopram induces a significant but transitory suppression of motor cortex excitability in normal subjects. A similar conclusion was reached after a prospective, randomized, double-blinded, placebo-controlled study. Twenty patients with unilateral stroke that received citalopram or a placebo in combination with physiotherapy were enrolled. Motor cortex excitability was studied using single and paired TMS. A significant decrease of motor cortex excitability in stroke patients with effects on both the affected and unaffected hemispheres, which was associated with a better motor recovery, was observed (Acler et al., 2009).

A meta-analysis from 2012 identified 56 completed trials of SSRI of which 52 trials (4059 participants) were elected. The results suggest that SSRIs can improve dependence, disability, neurological impairment, anxiety and depression after stroke. There was not a significant increase in seizures, gastro-intestinal side-affects or bleeding. There was a high risk of bias due to the heterogeneity between trials and methodological limitations in a substantial proportion of the trials (Mead et al., 2013).

### 1.5.6. Cannabis

Several clinical and laboratory studies suggest that cannabis may be an effective treatment for MS spasticity. A review published in 2009 analyzed trials published between 2002 and 2007. From these 38 studies, only six double-blinded, randomized, placebo-controlled trials were selected. These studies included a total of 481 patients with MS who were administered a combined extract of both $\Delta^9$-tetrahydrocannabinol (THC) and cannabidiol (CBD). The subjective experience of symptom reduction was generally found to be significant, but objective measures of spasticity failed to reveal significant changes. However, the authors concluded that there is evidence that the combined extracts of THC and CBD may reduce the symptoms of spasticity in patients with MS. Additionally, the combined extracts of THC and CBD may attenuate the side effects of THC alone (Lakhan et al., 2009).

Another review published in 2010 concluded that the therapeutic effects of cannabis-based medicine on spasticity that have been reported in clinical trials could best be described as moderate and occurred mainly in subjective scores rather than in objective measurements. Additionally, the therapeutic benefit from these drugs was considered quite small in return for any adverse side effects that were experienced (Smith et al., 2010).

Studies regarding the neuroprotective properties of cannabinoids in MS have demonstrated a reduction in inflammation, a modulation of the immune system, and protection against apoptosis. There are several studies that highlight the neuroprotective potential of cannabinoids, which can slow the progression of MS (Croxford et al., 2008; Loría et al., 2010). Cannabinoids have also been studied as potential neuroprotective treatments for PD (García-Arencibia et al., 2009), Huntington's disease (Lastres-Becker et al., 2003), Alzheimer's disease (Ramírez et al., 2005), stroke (Fernández-López et al., 2010) and head trauma (Mechoulam et al., 2002).

### 1.5.7. Bone Morphogenic Protein-7 (BMP7)

BMP7 (also known as osteogenic protein 1) is a member of the TGF-β superfamily. Several laboratory studies have indicated that the expression of TGF-β is enhanced after ischemic injury in the brain.

BMP7 given parenterally after a stroke can pass through the BBB on the ischemic side and induce a spontaneous improvement in locomotor function by interfering with apoptotic pathways to reduce cerebral infarction. Additionally, there is an upregulation of BMP7 mRNA in the contralateral hemisphere after stroke (Chang et al., 2003; Shen et al. 2008; Shen et al., 2009; Lin et al., 1999).

### 1.5.8. Cerebrolysin

Neurotrophic factors are polypeptides or proteins that play a role in regulation of key cellular processes and are part of the growth factors group. Neurotrophic factors regulate the proliferation, survival, migration and differentiation of cells underlying plasticity of the nervous system. Their gene expression is enhanced after brain injury, but in most cases, this endogenous over-expression is not able to compensate quickly enough for the consequences of disturbed homeostasis leading to secondary injuries. Neurotrophic stimulation of natural neuroprotection and neurorepair (Figure 1) is therefore a target for development of new therapies (Nieto-Sampedro et al., 1982; Truettner et al., 1999).

The only drug available for clinical use containing active fragments of various neurotrophic factors is Cerebrolysin, which is obtained using a standardized biological method of controlled breakdown of highly purified specific proteins.

Active neurotrophic factor fragments quickly pass the BBB and stimulate neurotrophic signaling pathways of the nervous system. Cerebrolysin neuropeptides were shown to modulate activity of the relevant protein kinases (like PI3K/AKT), which ultimately leads to the activation of transcription factors and the production of proteins involved in the stimulation of natural plasticity and repair processes (like various endogenous NTFs and sonic hedgehog (Shh) (Zhang, 2010; Zhang, 2013; Ubhi, 2013).

Cerebrolysin possesses a pleiotropic neuroprotective therapeutic effect (e.g., anti-excitotoxic, anti-inflammatory, anti-apoptotic and antioxidant) by simultaneously modulating several pathogenic links in the pathological cascade in stroke, traumatic brain injury and neurodegenerative diseases (Riley et al., 2006; Wronski et al., 2000).

Cerebrolysin inhibits APP phosphorylation and its transport from the cellular body to the synapse, thus decreasing the production of β42 amyloidal, which is involved in the molecular mechanisms of dementia (Masliah et al., 1999). This multimodal mechanism of action is summarized on Figure 4.

Multiple clinical studies have confirmed the efficacy of Cerebrolysin treatment and recommend it as a pivotal medication in all acute and neurorestoration therapeutic strategies.

To date, > 10,200 patients have enrolled in 139 completed clinical trials with Cerebrolysin; approximately a quarter of these patients were enrolled in clinical trials for stroke. Almost all of these trials have been designed as randomized, controlled, double-blinded trials, and Cerebrolysin has been given as an add-on treatment to anti-platelet medication. In most of these trials, the study endpoint was day 21 after stroke or approximately day 30, except for the trials performed by Herrschaft, Ladurner and Haffner with a study endpoint/follow-up visit performed on day 90. Correspondingly, the study duration was 21, 30 or 90 days. One trial (Skvortsova et al., 2004) was designed as a dose-response trial; trials with investigation on day 90 were considered for the evaluation of long-term efficacy (Ladurner et al., 2005; Muresanu, 1999; Haffner et al., 2001; Skvortsova et al., 2004).

The data suggests that Cerebrolysin is an effective adjuvant treatment for ischemic stroke. The results of these clinical trials demonstrate significant improvements in cognitive performance and clinical outcome in the rehabilitation phase of stroke. In the acute phase, Cerebrolysin induces an accelerated recovery pattern that overlaps with the therapeutic window and clinical effects of early mobilization and results in the significantly improved survival rate post-stroke.

Cognitive functions, motor functions and daily living activities were significantly better with Cerebrolysin, and early Cerebrolysin treatment was related to improved clinical outcome. Further, Cerebrolysin demonstrated a fast onset of action and a pharmacological support for rehabilitation (Labiche and Grotta, 2004). A large randomized, double-blind, placebo-controlled, multicenter phase II clinical trial, called Cerebrolysin and Recovery after Stroke, has recently completed the enrollment phase in 9 (nine) centers in Europe.

The clinical efficacy of Cerebrolysin in dementia has also been evaluated in a number of studies in patients with Alzheimer's disease and vascular dementia. Assessment of therapeutic efficacy was performed in the domains of cognition, activities of daily living, global assessment and behavior according to scientific standards and under consideration of the applicable guidance on dementia guidelines treatment (Alvarez et al., 2006; Muresanu et al., 2008; Ruether et al., 2002). The recently published Cochrane review of Cerebrolysin trials in vascular dementia confirmed clinical benefits in cognitive and global domains (Chen, 2013).

### 1.5.9. Deleterious Drugs in Clinical Practice of Neurorestoration

Brustein and Rossignol (1999) investigated the effects of noradrenergic and serotoninergic drugs on locomotion after spinal lesions of the ventral and ventrolateral quadrants in a *Felis catus* animal model. Norepinephrine and methoxamine, an α1-adrenergic agonist, caused locomotor improvement in contrast to clonidine, an α2-adrenergic agonist, which had a detrimental effect on walking. All serotoninergic drugs (5HT, the neurotransmitter itself; its precursor, 5HTP; and quipazine, a 5HT1, 2 and 3 agonist) improved locomotion, except the agonist 8-hydroxy-dipropylaminotetralin (DPAT). However, compared to clonidine, the detrimental effect of DPAT was short-lived and less intensive.

Other animal studies have reported similar results. The post-lesion systemic administration of adrenergic receptor antagonists (yohimbine, an α1 and α2 antagonist, idazoxan, an α2 adrenergic receptor antagonist and an inidazoline receptor antagonist) was beneficial, but the α2 adrenergic receptor agonist clonidine impaired motor recovery (Feeney et al., 1990; Sutton et al., 1992; Goldstein et al., 1995).

In addition to yohimbine and prazosin, α1 adrenergic receptor antagonists, Freeney et al. (1990) investigated phenoxybenzamine (α1 adrenergic receptor antagonist), haloperidol (dopaminergic receptor antagonist), prazosin (α1 adrenergic receptor antagonist), propranolol (β1 and 2 adrenergic receptor antagonist) and methoxamine (α1 adrenergic receptor antagonist). Their results indicate that drugs with adrenergic antagonist effects, but not propranolol, had a negative effect on motor rehabilitation. The same negative effect was found with haloperidol. Additionally, a single administration of clonidine transiently reinstated hemiplegic symptoms. In another study of recovery after traumatic brain injury in which haloperidol and risperidone (which also has a high affinity for D2 dopaminergic receptors) were tested, only risperidone delayed motor recovery, but both agents impaired cognitive functions (Wilson et al., 2003).

Systemic phenytoin administration in rats with induced-cortical lesions produces a significant increase in the severity of the resulting hemiplegic syndrome (Brailowsky et al., 1986).

In addition, both phenytoin and carbamazepine may have negative effects on cognitive performance in patients recovering from brain trauma, particularly on tasks with significant motor and speed components (Smith et al., 1994).

Benzodiazepines also have detrimental effects on neurorehabilitation. Diazepam, which acts as an indirect γ-Aminobutyric acid (GABA) agonist, delays motor recovery in rats following unilateral damage to the anterior-medial region of the neocortex, a delay that is more serious when diazepam is administrated in the acute phase of the brain damage (Schallert et al., 1986). Intracortical infusion of the inhibitory neurotransmitter GABA increases the hemiparesis produced by a small motor cortex lesion in rats (Brailowsky et al., 1986; Goldstein et al., 1995). Goldstein et al. (1990) tested the effect of detrimental drugs on neurorehabilitation. They conducted a retrospective study with two groups of patients that had a recent ischemic stroke: a "detrimental drug" group and the "neutral drug" group. The detrimental drug group included patients that received phenytoin, benzodiazepines (e.g., triazolam, chlordiazepoxide or alprazolam), neuroleptics (e.g., chlorpromazine, prochlorperazine or haloperidol) or antihypertensive drugs (i.e., clonidine or prazosin) during hospitalization.

The results indicate that the patients who received the detrimental drugs had a slower recovery; they had poorer sensorimotor function and were less independent in activities of daily living activities. In another retrospective study, Goldstein et al. (1995) tested the effect of detrimental drugs on patients enrolled in a multi-center study concerning the effects of GM1 ganglioside after ischemic stroke.

The detrimental group also included patients who were prescribed the anti-hypertensives clonidine or prazosin, the anticonvulsants phenobarbital or phenytoin, a benzodiazepine or a DA receptor antagonist. This study provided data regarding medications prescribed for patients over the first 28 days after a carotid-distribution ischemic stroke. The results demonstrated that the patients who received detrimental drugs had poorer recoveries compared to patients from the neutral group.

Additionally, the study highlighted that benzodiazepines were the most commonly prescribed of the potentially detrimental medications, and that triazolam was the one most commonly given. The authors concluded that the routine prescription of benzodiazepines should be avoided and that DA receptor antagonists, adrenergic receptor antagonists and α2 adrenergic receptor agonists, such as clonidine, should be used with caution and avoided if possible.

Aside from the beneficial effect of DA, excessive DA receptor stimulation is detrimental to prefrontal cortex cognitive function and leads to the impairment of working memory performance. Laboratory studies suggest that both D1 and D2 receptor families contribute to the detrimental actions of DA in the prefrontal cortex, and the two may synergize to take the prefrontal cortex "off-line" during stress (Zahrt et al., 1997).

Also SSRIs were associated with detrimental effects such as increased risk of hemorrhagic stroke with increased severity and mortality (Mortensen et al., 2014).

Nicotine profoundly decreases, in a dose-dependent manner, the expression of the polysialylated (PSA) forms of the neural cell adhesion molecule (PSA-NCAM) in the hippocampus (dentate gyrus) and induces long-term functional impairments due to SCI in rats (Abrous et al., 2002). These effects result from secondary apoptotic death that is regulated, in part, by SCI-induced decreases in the protein levels of the anti-apoptotic protein Bcl-xL. In an experiment examining motor rehabilitation after SCI in rats, Cittelly et al. (2008) showed that anti-apoptotic treatment targeting Bcl-xL (Tat-Bcl-xL and Tat-BH4) shifts neuronal apoptosis to necrosis, increases the inflammatory response and impairs locomotor recovery.

# 2. Herbal Medicines

*Yi-Lin Chen, Horng-Jyh Harn and Shinn-Zong Lin*

## 2.1. Introduction

One of the biggest challenges in using traditional medicinal plants in regenerative medicine is to define the relationship between Chinese herbal medicines and neuronal cell protection. Although genetic methods have been used successfully and significant progress has been made (Sato N. et al., 2003), we are still far from the goal of conveniently and easily controlling neuronal cell fate for use in regenerative medicine.

## 2.2. Traditional Chinese Medicines

Native cultures all over the world have traditionally used herbs to maintain health and treat disease. In China, more than 400 different formulas derived from more than 3,200 herbs and 300 extracts from minerals or animals are used as herbal medicines. Chinese herbal medicine is a major component of traditional Chinese medicines, which focuses on restoring a balance of energy, body, and spirit to maintain health, as opposed to treating a particular disease or medical condition. Herbs are used with the goal of restoring balance by nourishing the body. Chinese herbal medicine is not based on diagnosis and treatment like the conventional concepts of Western medicine, but instead treats the patient's main complaints and patterns of symptoms rather than the underlying causes. Practitioners of Chinese herbal medicine attempt to prevent and treat imbalances caused by cancer and other diseases with complex combinations of herbs, minerals, and plant extracts. One aspect of Chinese herbal medicine is to restore or strengthen immunity and resistance to disease. Treatments with this goal are named “Fu Zheng” and are used as complementary therapies intending to reduce the side-effects associated with conventional Western treatments.

*TCM and Neurodegenerative Diseases*

The herbs to be discussed in this chapter are listed by category of use in Table 3. Many Chinese herbs or herbal extracts prevent the degeneration of dopaminergic neurons and alleviate the symptoms caused by the neurotoxins 1-methyl-4-phenyl-1,2,3,6-tetrahydropyridine and 6-hydroxydopamine, both *in vitro* and *in vivo*. Herbs or herbal extracts that produce these effects include the following: the polyphenols or catechins found in green tea (Bournival J. et al. 2009; Chen, L. W. et al. 2007; Guo S. et al. 2005; Levites Y. et al. 2001,2002; Li R. et al. 2004; Pan T. et al. 2003); oil from *Ganoderma lucidum* spores ( Zhu WW et al., 2005); triptolide from *Tripterygium wilfordii* Hook (Li F. Q. et al. 2003,2004); the polysaccharides found in *Nerium indicum* flowers (Chen, L. W. et al. 2007); ginseng and ginsenoside found in *Panax* spp. (Chen X. C. et al. 2003; Radad, K. et al. 2004 a,b; Rudakewich M. et al. 2001; Watanabe H. et al. 1991); the *Ginkgo biloba* extract, EGb 761 (Cao F. et al. 2003; Ramassamy C. et al. 1990; Rojas P. et al. 2001; Sloley B. D. et al. 2000; Szasz B. K. 2008; Yang S. F. et al. 2001); tetrahydroxystilbene glucoside, one of the main active ingredients in heshouwu, which is derived from *Polygonum* roots (Li J. X. et al. 2005). Chinese herbs and herbal extracts have shown the potential to attenuate the progression of PD by rescuing nigral dopaminergic neurons from progressive cell death (Li L. et al. 1998; Zhang J. F. et al. 2005; Zhang Q. J. et al. 2004). Chinese herbs and herbal extracts may promote neuronal cell survival and neurite growth and may facilitate functional recovery from brain injuries by invoking distinct mechanisms that are related to their neuroprotective roles as antioxidants (Li L. et al. 1998; Rojas P. et al. 2008), dopamine transporter inhibitors (Zhao G et al., 2007, 2008), monoamine oxidase inhibitors (Sloley B. D. et al. 2000; Zhao H. W. et al. 2002), free radical scavengers (Guo S. et al. 2005, 2007), modulators of cell survival genes and cell signaling (Levites Y. et al. 2002; Mizumaki Y. et al. 2002), anti-apoptotic agents (Kim, E. H. et al. 2003; Yu M. S. et al. 2007; Zhao H. W. et al. 2002), and agents that improve blood circulation within the brain (Jingyi W. et al. 1997).

**Table 3. Herbs that are used by TCM practitioners to treat neurodegenerative diseases**

| Category of use | Latin name (source) | Chinese name (pinyin) |
|---|---|---|
| Blood circulation–promoting and stasis-removing drugs | *Paeoniae rubra* (root) | Chi Shao |
| | *Radix Achyranthis Bidentatae* | Niu Xi |
| | *Radix Salviae Miltiorrhizae* | Dan Shen |
| | *Corydalis sp.* (rhizome) | Yan Hu Suo |
| | *Radix Notoginseng* | San Qi |
| | *Rhizoma Chuanxiong* | Chuan Xiong |
| | *Crocus sp.* (stigma) | Xi Hong Hua |
| Qi-regulating drugs | *Toosendan sp.* | Chuan Lian Zi |
| | *Fructus Aurantii Immaturus* | Zhi Shi |
| | *Rhizoma Cyperi* | Xiang Fu |
| Expectorants, antitussives, and anti-asthmatics | *Pinelliae sp.* (unprocessed rhizome) | Sheng Ban Xia |
| | *Ginkgo sp.* (leaf) | Yin Xing Ye Pian |
| | *Unprocessed Rhizome Arisaematis* | Sheng Tian Nan Xing |
| | *Fructus Perillae* | Zi Su Zi |
| Heat-clearing drugs | *Cortex Moutan* | Mu Dan Pi |
| | *Radix Sophorae Flavescentis* | Ku Shen |
| | *Herba Patriniae* | Bai Jiang Cao |
| | *Herba Houttuyniae* | Yu Xing Cao |
| | *Fructus Gardeniae* | Zhi Zi |
| | *Spica Prunellae* | Xia Ku Cao |
| | *Rhizoma Coptidis* | Huang Lian |
| | *Radix Scutellariae* | Huang Qin |
| Awakening drugs | *Borneolum Syntheticum* | Bing Pian |
| | *Rhizoma Acori Tatarinowii* | Shi Chang Pu |
| Tranquilizers | *Radix Polygalae* | Yuan Zhi |
| | *Semen Ziziphi Spinosae* | Suan Zao Ren |
| | *Cortex Albiziae* | He Huan Pi |
| | *Succinum* | Hu Po |
| Tonics | *Radix Ginseng* | Ren Shen |
| | *Radix Paeniae Alba* | Bai Shao |
| | *Radix Codonopsis* | Dang Shen |
| | *Radix Glycyrrhizae* | Gan Cao |

Some lignan compounds (e.g., sesamin, sesamolin) act as neuroprotective agents against oxidative injury and excitotoxicity (Hou R. C. et al. 2003). Lignans can also inhibit lipopolysaccharide-induced cyclooxygenase-2 expression in macrophages (Yun K. J. et al. 2007). The natural compound isochaihulactone, which is purified by chloroform extraction from Nan-Chai-Hu (Chai Hu of the South), the root of *Bupleurum scorzonerifolium*, is an important component of this Chinese herb (Hou R. C. et al. 2003). The pretreatment of PC12 cells with isochaihulactone increased cell viability and decreased membrane damage, reactive oxygen species production, and poly (ADP-ribose) polymerase degradation in response to $H_2O_2$. Isochaihulactone also decreased the expression of cyclooxygenase-2, *via* downregulation of nuclear factor-κB, and the resulting peroxidation of lipids in $H_2O_2$-treated PC12 cells.

These results suggest that isochaihulactone is an antioxidant. The antioxidant activity of isochaihulactone was observed at concentrations of 5 μM and 10 μM, whereas 40 μM isochaihulactone did not show antioxidant effects. In primary astrocyte cultures, isochaihulactone decreased reactive oxygen species production in response to $H_2O_2$-induced oxidative stress at much higher concentrations of 30 μM and 60 μM (data not shown). The reason for the difference in the effective concentrations may be related to the different cell types that were used.

Chronic systemic exposure to d-galactose causes the acceleration of senescence in mice.

Administration of isochaihulactone (10 mg/kg/d, subcutaneously) for 6 weeks concomitant with d-galactose administration significantly increased the activity of superoxide dismutase and GPx and decreased plasma levels of malondialdehyde.

A health food product, 20070721-GX, contains a mixture of extracts from Chinese herbs, and we recently found that this compound is a potent stem cell growth factor. Administration of 20070721-GX for at least 2 months to eleven volunteers increased the number of circulating $CD34^+$ cells 4.9-fold when compared with the number of circulating $CD34^+$ cells after administration of placebo ($1.47 \pm 0.11\%$ for the experimental group vs. $0.3 \pm 0.1\%$ for the control group). This is another example of the many herbal medicines that may be applied in stem cell biology.

The differentiation of ESCs can be directed toward neurons with a Chinese herbal medicine, which may allow for clinical transplantation. This study also suggested a new approach for developing herbal medicines for inducing the differentiation of MSCs and ESCs. New pharmaceutical strategies for treating PD will hopefully be developed through an understanding of the biological effects of Chinese herbs and herbal extracts.

In conclusion, growing evidence indicates that Chinese herbs and herbal extracts may efficiently regulate the fate, proliferation, and differentiation of stem cells. Many reports focus on the effectiveness of Chinese herbal compounds on diseases, such as neurodegenerative diseases. Few reports, however, focus on the effects of Chinese herbal compounds on stem cell regulation. A greater understanding of the molecular mechanisms through which Chinese herbal compounds regulate stem cells is the next challenge that will aid in neurorestoration for neurodegenerative diseases.

# 3. Factors and Protein Transduction Domain Fusion Proteins as a Therapeutic for Neurological Disorders

*Stephen D. Skaper and Hongyun Huang*

## 3.1. Introduction

In mammals and other vertebrates, soluble peptide growth factors play essential roles in intercellular communication. They exert their effects by signaling through surface membrane receptors that interact with diverse types of intracellular second-messenger systems. Many growth factors, moreover, have been found to sub-serve a wide variety of functions by acting on many cell types at different stages of development or in adult life. One of the major advances of molecular neuroscience over the past several decades has been to recognize that much of the cellular damage resulting from such CNS insults as stroke, trauma, and neurodegenerative disease may be caused by a limited number of endogenously generated molecules with neurotoxic activities. Less well-developed is the idea that endogenous mechanisms exist to provide neuroprotection, and that endogenous molecules may be produced specifically to service neuroprotective, and even neurorestorative, signaling functions (Sofroniew et al., 2001).

Since their discovery in the 1950s, neurotrophic factors have raised expectations that their clinical application to neurodegenerative diseases might provide an effective therapy for what are now untreatable conditions. There is an impressive volume of evidence for neuroprotective effects of neurotrophic factors in animal models of neurodegenerative diseases. These applications include abolishing cell loss in the septum following fimbria-fornix transection, a cholinergic model for Alzheimer's disease (Hefti, 1986, Williams et al., 1986), recovery from chemically-induced parkinsonism (Grondin et al., 2003, Kordower et al., 2000), motor neuron disease (Ishii, 1999; Sendtner, 1999), and spinal cord injury (Kobayashi et al., 1997; Ramer et al., 2000; Schnell et al., 1994). While showing great promise for the treatment of such disorders, delivery of therapeutic proteins across the blood-brain barrier is severely limited by the size and biochemical properties of the proteins. Gene therapy is one promising method for circumventing this problem, but conditions for high-efficiency targeting and long-term protein expression have not yet been developed.

Cell-penetrating peptides are small, usually basic domains that have the ability to deliver other peptides across the plasma membrane and the blood-brain barrier. This technology has now been employed by a great many labs for the intracellular delivery of fluorophores, small compounds, nucleic acids, and liposomes. One approach of protein transduction, in particular, has made use of full-length proteins generated that contain an $NH_2$-terminal 11-amino acid protein transduction domain (PTD) from the human immunodeficiency virus-1 (HIV-1) transactivator protein (Tat) [first identified in 1988 (Frankel and Pabo, 1988; Green and Loewenstein, 1988). Here we provide a brief overview of the neurotrophins and neuropoietic cytokines ("neurokines"), followed by a discussion of the principles of protein transduction domain technology, and conclude with a recent application of this approach to a neurotrophic protein.

## 3.2. Factors: An Overview

### *3.2.1. Neurotrophins*

Neurotrophins are a family of proteins that play a fundamental role in the regulation of neural function, plasticity, development and survival (for reviews, see Korsching, 1987; Lewin and Barde, 1996; Segal and Greenberg, 1996; McAllister et al., 1999; Poo, 2001; Sofroniew et al., 2001; Numakawa et al., 2010); in regulating synaptic plasticity and in the guidance of axon growth cones (Bibel and Barde, 2000; Kaplan and Miller, 2000; Lu et al., 2005); and have their effects on the proliferation, differentiation, and survival of neurons both during development and in adulthood (Lewin and Barde, 1996). In mammals, they consist of four structurally related protein members: nerve growth factor (NGF), brain derived neurotrophic factor (BDNF) (Barde et al., 1982; Leibrock et al., 1989), neurotrophin-3 (NT-3) (Ernfors et al., 1990; Maisonpierre et al., 1990) and neurotrophin-4/5 (NT-4/5) (Hallböök et al., 1991; Ip et al., 1992) are derived from the same ancestral gene (Hallböök et al., 2006). Initially, neurotrophins are synthesized as precursor proteins (proneurotrophins), similar to other neuropeptides. They are then cleaved intracellularly by various enzymes that give rise to the mature protein that is released into the extracellular medium (Lee et al., 2001). Each of these proteins in their mature form (with an approximate molecular weight of 13 kDa) is a protein complex with a mate (dimer), thereby activating specific receptors (Chao, 2003). Also several excellent reviews describe the signaling pathways stimulated by the neurotrophins that affect the survival, differentiation and function of the cell within the nervous system (Chao, 2003; Lu et al., 2005; Reichardt, 2006).

Neurotrophins exert their function mediated by two types of transmembrane receptors: the family of tropomyosin-receptor-kinase receptors (Trk) (Huang and Reichardt, 2003) act in cell proliferation, survival or chemotaxis, and the pan neurotrophin receptor, p75NTR (p75 neurotrophin receptor) can mediate two responses. On the one hand, when coexpressed with Trks, p75NTR enhances the affinity and specificity of neurotrophin binding to Trks to promote survival signaling. On the other hand, the activation of p75NTR by proneurotrophins can initiate apoptosis when p75NTR is coexpressed with sortilin, a member of the VpS10p family of receptors (Nykjaer et al., 2004). All the neurotrophins bind with similar affinity to p75NTR, but each binds specifically with high affinity to a different Trk receptor (Kaplan and Miller, 2000).

In addition to the neurotrophins, a number of polypeptide factors have been shown to possess neurotrophic activities. These include vascular endothelial growth factor (VEGF) (Ferrara et al., 2003), GDNF (Lindsay and Yancopoulos, 1996), insulin-like growth factor (Doré et al., 1997), and basic fibroblast growth factor (Walicke et al., 1986). Transforming growth factor-β (Farkas et al., 2003) and Sonic hedgehog (Miao et al., 1997) are other proteins capable of promoting survival of specific CNS neuron populations and protect these cells from toxic insults. Here simply describe NGF and BDNF.

**NGF.** It is the founding and best characterized member of the neurotrophin family, and was discovered during a search for survival factors that could explain the deleterious effects of deletion of target tissues on the subsequent survival of motor and sensory neurons (Levi-Montalcini, 1987). During normal development, neurons die at the time that their processes enter the target. These studies were important because they identified the target as playing a key role in neuronal development (Levi-Montalcini and Hamburger, 1951; Levi-Montalcini et al., 1954). It may be important that the NGF family's expression and actions acquire target-derived factor, and present autocrine and non-target-derived paracrine modes of factor (Bothwell, 1995).

**BDNF.** It is a homodimer of 27 kDa, which was identified by Barde and cloned by Leibrock in the 80's, is produced primarily in the brain and spinal cord by glial cells (Barde et al., 1982; Leibrock et al., 1989). Its importance has been demonstrated in neural development and cell survival, including dorsal root ganglion cells (Acheson et al., 1995) or in cortical and hippocampal neurons (Huang and Reichardt, 2001). In addition, it promotes neuronal cell differentiation from endogenous progenitor cells in the ventricular wall of the adult forebrain (Kirschenbaum and Goldman, 1995) and it has an essential role in neuronal cell survival or neuroprotection in the CNS. In vivo, BDNF application can protect a variety of neurons from brain injury (Wu and Pardridge, 1999; Schäbitz et al., 2000), regulate vascular development (Donovan et al., 2000); and have a neuroprotective effect by intravenous delivery after the onset of focal cerebral ischemia (Schäbitz et al., 2000). It also participates in the regulation of synaptic plasticity arising from the activity associated with learning and memory processes (Pang et al., 2004; Lu et al., 2005). Chronic sublethal hypoxia can elicit persistent angiogenesis induced by increased VEGF and BDNF secretion by endothelial cells and astrocytes (Kim et al., 2004).

### *3.2.2. Vascular Endothelial Growth Factor (VEGF)*

VEGF is the major angiogenic factor in developmental (Ferrara et al., 2003), pathological angiogenesis (Plate et al., 1992; Lafuente et al., 1999; Marti et al., 2000; Bulnes and Lafuente, 2007) and also in pathological vascular permeability (Dvorak, 2006). However, VEGF has strong neuroprotective, neurotrophic and neurogenic properties (Jin et al., 2002; Rosenstein and Krum, 2004; Storkebaum et al., 2004) to exert a direct mitogenic action on neural precursors (Jin et al., 2002; Rosenstein et al., 2003; Greenberg and Jin, 2005) or promote the proliferation and differentiation of neuronal precursors, releasing neurotrophic factors (Louissaint et al., 2002). VEGF also can mediate vascular permeability, inducing the leakage of the BBB in some pathological situations (Schoch et al., 2002; Nordal and Wong, 2005) and affect other neural cell types except neurons such as, endothelial cells, astrocytes (Rabchevsky et al., 1998; Krum and Kraibullina, 2003), Schwann cells and microglia. Furthermore, exogenous infusion of this factor stimulates the production of other astroglial mitogenic factors like bFGF, thereby augmenting the proliferative action of VEGF alone (Krum et al., 2002). It should be remembered that VEGF plays a dual role in different neurodegenerative pathologies (MS, PD). In addition, neuronal and axonal loss might be a result of diminished grey matter perfusion. Intracerebral infusion reduces the severity of disease in the EAE model in rats, which indicates the extreme relevance of these two roles of VEGF.

### *3.2.3. Insulin-Like Growth Factor - I (IGF-I)*

It is a protein related to insulin (Rinderknecht and Humbel, 1978) and is one of the main mediators of growth hormone action (Daughaday and Rotwein, 1989). It is a single-stranded protein of 70 amino acids with three intramolecular disulphide bridges and a molecular weight of 7,649 KDa. It is not yet well known how IGF-I is transported into the CNS; the possible reason may be that neuronal activity drives localized BBB to transport IGF-I (Nishijima et al., 2010).

It is a well-known angiogenic factor (Dunn, 2000) to modulate vessel formation during brain development (Bar et al., 1988; Dunn, 2000) and it also modulates the basal angiogenic activity and repair in the gradual decline of vascular density that accompanies brain aging (Sonntag et al., 1997). It is a survival factor for sensory and motor neurons (Russo et al., 2005), acting as a neuroprotector against excitotoxicity and oxidative stress (Heck et al., 1999; Vincent et al., 2004) or for oligodendrocyte precursors against cytotoxicity (Ness et al., 2004) and for mature oligodendrocytes from death-inducing effects (Mason et al., 2000). It exerts effects on the proliferation of neural and oligodendrocyte progenitor, recovering cells from ischemic stroke through regeneration, and also enhances the proliferation of endogenous neural progenitors in rats (Dempsey et al., 2003). It promotes synaptogenesis and neurogenesis in the hippocampal dentate gyrus (O'Kusky et al., 2000) and modulates brain plasticity via neuritic outgrowth, synaptogenesis and neurotransmitter release (Torres-Aleman, 1999; Aberg et al., 2006).

### *3.2.4. Erythropoietin (EPO)*

It is a 34 KDa glycoprotein purified in 1977 by Goldwasser and Kung (Myake et al., 1977) and isolated by Lin et al. (1985). Initially it was described as the principal regulator of erythropoiesis, since it inhibited the programmed cell death of erythrocytes and in consequence, allowed their maturation (Jelkmann, 2007). However, more studies have shown that this cytokine acts in different tissues, including the nervous system (Nagai et al., 2001). Although it is mainly produced in the fetal liver and adult kidney (Jelkmann, 1992), EPO and its specific receptor (EPOR) have been described in several regions of the mammalian brain (Marti et al., 1996; Genc et al., 2004). Neurons, glia and brain capillary endothelial cells (Digicaylioglu et al., 1995; Juul et al., 1998; Nagai et al., 2001) were shown to express the cytokine and its receptor. Furthermore, expression of EPO and EPOR in the adult brain is enhanced by hypoxia (Marti et al. 1996), and other stimuli such as hypoglycemia, insulin and IGF-1 release. Reactive oxygen species lead to an increased expression of EPO, also by activating the hypoxia-inducible factor-l alpha (Masuda et al., 1997; Chandel et al., 1998).

EPO and EPOR are detected in the CNS during fetal development (Juul et al., 1998) and remain in the brain throughout adulthood (Marti et al., 1996). Expression of EPOR in the embryonic stage suggests a role for EPO in brain development and tissue maintenance (Noguchi et al., 2007). Konishi et al. (1993) first described the neurotrophic function of EPO both in vitro and in vivo. Moreover, EPO has been shown to induce a variety of cellular responses as it has been described as a neuroprotective, neurogenic, neurotrophic and angiogenic factor (Digicaylioglu and Lipton, 2001; Rabie and Marti, 2008; Sakanaka et al., 1998). Neurotrophic effects of EPO include the ability to stimulate axonal regrowth, neurite formation, dendritic sprouting and neurotransmitter synthesis, release (Yamamoto et al., 2000; Weber et al., 2002) and neurogenesis (Shingo et al., 2001). EPO also induces BDNF gene expression (Viviani et al., 2005), which is closely related to neurogenesis.

Besides its effects on neurons, EPO-induced neurorestoration may be attributed to an improvement in brain vascularization or angiogenic effect (Yasuda et al., 1998). In addition, EPO helps in the preservation of BBB integrity during injury, probably by restoring expression of tight junction proteins (Li et al., 2007), reducing vascular inflammation (Chen et al., 2007) and reacting free radical expression (Li et al., 2007). Finally, EPO attenuates inflammation by reducing reactive astrocytosis and microglia activation and by inhibiting immune cell recruitment into the injured area. Several studies have found that EPO reduced the production of inflammatory mediators leading to a smaller size of infarcts in cerebral ischemia (Brines and Cerami, 2005; Villa et al., 2003; Wang et al., 2007) and injury attenuation in multiple sclerosis (Agnello et al., 2002). EPO treatment can counteract degenerative processes in Parkinson's disease and ALS by the inhibition of apoptosis and the stimulation of axonal regeneration (Grunfeld et al., 2007). Administration of EPO in experimental models of traumatic brain and spinal cord injury leads to morphological, functional and cognitive recovery (Yatsiv et al., 2005), increased neurogenesis in the dentate gyrus (Lu et al., 2005) and reduced brain edema (Verdonck et al., 2007).

### *3.2.5. Neuropoietic Cytokines*

Although neurotrophic factors represent a group of ligands that were originally identified for their ability to support neuronal cell survival, several of these factors can also exert unique actions on cells outside the nervous system. As discussed above, the first family of neurotrophic factors is collectively known as the neurotrophins, and comprises several members that are related to NGF. The second family is represented by CNTF, a neuropoietic cytokine that is distantly related to a number of hematopoietic cytokines (Ip, 1998; Ip and Yancopoulos, 1996). Unlike the neurotrophins, which use a family of receptor tyrosine kinases, CNTF utilizes a multicomponent "cytokine receptor" system, which includes a specificity conferring α-receptor components acting in concert with signal-transducing β-receptor components, which are shared with its distant cytokine relatives.

CNTF is a 23 kDa cytoplasmic protein, which is expressed in both the peripheral nervous system and CNS beginning in the late embryonic period (Barbin et al., 1984; Stöckli et al., 1991). CNTF exhibits a variety of activities, affecting both the differentiation and survival of neuronal and glial cells (Ernsberger et al., 1989; Oppenheim et al., 1991; Louis et al., 1993), and also shares structural and functional properties with the cytokines interleukin-6, leukemia inhibitory factor, interleukin-11, and oncostatin M (Bazan, 1991). For this reason, CNTF is often referred to as a 'neurokine' (Taga and Kishimoto, 1992). CNTF promotes the survival of motor neurons in culture (Arakawa et al., 1990; Oppenheim et al., 1991), and prevents the degeneration of motor neurons after axotomy (Sendtner et al., 1990) and in mouse mutant progressive motor neuronopathy (Sendtner et al., 1992). These pre-clinical observations encouraged the potential for CNTF as a therapy for human motor neuron disease. However, these trials revealed adverse events, such as anorexia and weight loss, and increased deaths at the highest dose level (Miller et al. 1996a,b).

## 3.3. Neurotrophic Factors: Therapeutic Potential and Pitfalls

The power of neurotrophic factors to regulate neuronal cell survival in the developing nervous system and also to promote survival after injury or protect neurons in toxin-mediated disease models in animals has encouraged the idea that such proteins could be harnessed for the treatment of neurodegenerative disease. For example, the traditional perspective of applying neurotrophins in the context of Alzheimer's disease is based on the premise that neurotrophins are capable of up-regulating cholinergic function and of rendering neurons less vulnerable to certain processes causing degeneration (Hefti, 1986; Williams et al., 1986). Another example is that of GDNF, which acts on dopaminergic neurons. Administered intracerebrally, GNDF has neuroprotective and neurorestorative effects in toxin-induced rodent and non-human primate models of Parkinson's disease (Biju et al., 2010; Gash et al., 1996; Kordower et al., 2000). Dopaminergic neuroprotection by viral-mediated delivery or GDNF or the GDNF-related factor neurturin (Kotzbauer et al., 1996) has been demonstrated in animals (Choi-Lundberg et al., 1997; Kordower et al., 2000). Garcia and colleagues (2010), using recombinant cells secreting CNTF encapsulated in alginate polymers, showed that implantation of these bioreactors in the brain of amyloid β-peptide oligomer-infused mice led to a continuous secretion of recombinant CNTF, was associated with the robust improvement of cognitive performances, and led to full recovery of cognitive functions associated with the stabilization of synaptic protein levels in the Tg2576 Alzheimer disease mouse model. In the case of spinal cord injury, the transplantation of genetically modified cells (e.g. viral expression of neurotrophins either *in vivo* or *ex vivo* in stem cells) to lesion sites has been investigated as a means to augment axonal regeneration (Taylor et al., 2006; Zhou et al., 2003).

In spite of encouraging preclinical data, neurotrophic proteins have failed to show a beneficial effect in human trials of amytrophic lateral sclerosis (Lange et al., 1996; Ochs et al., 2000), and in some cases the side effects were severe (Turner et al., 2001). Randomized, controlled trials of GDNF in Parkinson's disease patients have proven negative, for the most part (Sherer et al., 2006; Yasuda and Mochizuki, 2010). Neurotrophic factor treatment of CNS diseases present an especially complex problem, since these polypeptides have poor pharmacokinetics and bioavailability and are not able to cross the blood-brain barrier. Intravenous administration of BDNF, conjugated to an anti-transferring antibody, is able to traverse the blood-brain barrier in rats and provide neuroprotection in focal transient brain ischemia (Wu and Pardridge, 1999). A cell-based approach for NGF delivery has shown promise in a phase I trial in Alzheimer's disease (Tuszynski et al., 2005).

## 3.4. Protein Transduction Domains as a Delivery Tool for Neuroregenerative Agents

In the past 15 years, many protein-based large molecule drugs and non-viral gene medicines have successfully been developed for therapeutic and/or diagnostic applications. In contrast to small (≤600 dalton) drugs, these large molecules have often limited pharmaceutical development or use as clinically-viable drugs. This limited access largely prohibits them from reaching appropriate sites (i.e. interior of cells and tissues) and from crossing epithelial and endothelial barriers. In the same period, many publications describing the use of peptide sequences that have been referred to as cell penetrating peptides, Trojan Horse peptides, protein transduction domains, or membrane-translocating sequences. The majority of cell penetrating peptides have been designed on the basis of known, naturally occurring protein domains, such as the *Drosophila* Antennapedia homeodomain-derivative penetratin (Derossi et al., 1998; Joliot et al., 1991; Perez et al., 1992), or the basic domain from HIV-1 Tat (Fawell et al., 1994; Nagahara et al., 1998; Schwarze et al., 1999), or the Herpes simplex virus-1 structural protein VP22 (Elliott and O'Hare, 1997). A number of cell penetrating peptides have been characterized as well, such as oligoarginines (Futaki et al., 2001; Wender et al., 2000) or transportan (Pooga et al., 1998). Extensive reviews of the various cell penetrating peptides, their mechanisms of transduction and applications, have been published (Dietz et al., 2004; Gump and Dowdy, 2007; Hervé et al., 2008). Here we will consider an overview of mechanism, followed by potential application to neurorestoration.

One of the most widely used protein transduction domains is that derived from HIV-1 Tat. The Tat protein is an 86 amino acid transcription factor involved in the replication cycle of the HIV-1 virus. It is rapidly taken up by cells and accumulates in the nucleus. Numerous truncated versions of Tat have been described, which penetrate different cell types (Vivès et al., 2003). Structure-activity studies of the fragment Tat (38-60) and additional truncated forms of this sequence revealed that the entire basic region of Tat ($Tat_{49-57}$, RKKRRQRRR) was a prerequisite for cellular peptide uptake (Vivès et al., 2003; Wender et al., 2000). One of the shortest peptides, Tat (48-60), which contains a nuclear translocation signal, was defined as the minimal translocating peptide. Analogs of the peptide corresponding to its retro-enantio form penetrated cells as efficiently as the parent peptide (Vivès et al., 2003; Wender et al., 2000). However, deletion of one or two arginine residues in the peptide sequence markedly reduced cell-penetrating ability, while the deletion of three non-basic residues within this sequence did not affect the translocation property.

The mechanism used by transducing peptides to permeate cell membranes has been the subject of considerable study in recent years. Early reports that Tat transduction occurred by a nonendocytic mechanism is now believed to have been artifactual, although other cell penetrating peptides might be taken up by way of direct membrane disruption (El-Andaloussi et al., 2005; Gupta et al., 2005). The current model for Tat-mediated protein transduction is a multistep process that involves binding of Tat to the cell surface, stimulation of macropinocytotic uptake of Tat and cargo into macropinosomes and endosomal escape into the cytoplasm (Gump and Dowdy, 2007). The first step, binding to the cell surface, is thought to be through ubiquitous glycan chains on the cell surface. As discussed above, the highly charged arginine residues present within Tat are necessary for transduction and the substitution of any of these residues dramatically reduces the efficiency of transduction (Wender et al., 2000). Tat and other polycationic transduction domains bind strongly to sulfated glycans like heparin sulphate, which can compete with the cell surface for binding to Tat and inhibit transduction (Rusnati et al., 1997). A role for cell-surface polyanionic glycan sugar chains in transduction of Tat, while generally assumed, is not universally accepted (see, for example: Silhol et al., 2002; Violini et al., 2002). Heparan and chondroitin sulfate glycans and sialic acids, with their negative charge that bind the highly basic Tat on the cell surface are thought to both serve as a binding pool for Tat but also to facilitate its interaction with the membrane. The role of heparan sulfate and other proteoglycans in Tat macropinocytosis has not been fully explored. It is possible that glycans serve not only to bind Tat but also to stimulate its endocytosis. Several proteoglycans that have been shown to interact with Tat peptide and full length HIV Tat protein, and these proteoglycans could serve as receptors for Tat and induce macropinocytosis (Argyris et al., 2004).

Stimulation of macropinocytosis by Tat occurs by an unknown mechanism that might include binding to a cell surface protein, or might also occur by way of proteoglycans or glycolipids. Uptake by way of macropinocytosis, a form of fluid phase endocytosis used by all cell types, is required for Tat and polyarginine transduction (Nakase et al., 2004; Wadia et al., 2004). The final step in Tat transduction is escape from macropinosomes into the cytoplasm; this process is likely to be dependent on the pH drop in endosomes that, along with other factors, facilitates a perturbation of the membrane by Tat and release of Tat and cargo (i.e. peptide, protein, drug, etc.) to the cytoplasm.

Full length Tat is neurotoxic, and partly responsible for acquired immunodeficiency syndrome-associated neurological disorders (e.g., Bruce-Keller et al., 2003; Haughey and Mattson, 2002; Song et al., 2003). Although intracerebral application of very high doses of a $Tat_{46-60}$ peptide, which includes the basic domain, is toxic in vivo (Sabatier et al., 1991), the basic domain $Tat4_{9-57}$ has been used in many applications in neuroscience without toxic effects. It has been particularly useful in the treatment of ischemic stroke and neurodegenerative disease. Tat conjugated protein kinase C delta (PKC-$\delta$) inhibitor peptides have shown promise in treatment of ischemia-reperfusion diseases in mouse and rat models. These Tat conjugated protein kinase C inhibitor peptides have strong activity in vitro; clinical trials are currently underway to assess the potential of their use to treat human disease (Bright et al., 2007; Inagaki et al., 2005). For example, the Bcl-2 family of proteins is a critical regulator of apoptosis (Becker and Bonni, 2004), and Tat-Bcl-2 family fusion proteins are obvious candidates to inhibit neurodegenerative processes. A Tat-Bcl-$x_L$ fusion protein quickly transduces cerebellar granule neurons in vitro, where it protects cerebellar granule cells against potassium and serum deprivation-induced apoptosis (Dietz et al., 2002). Tat-Bcl-$x_L$ also inhibits staurosporine-induced apoptosis in primary cortical neurons in vitro (Cao et al., 2002), is partly protective in a model for pneumococcal meningitis (Ebert et al., 2005), and protects against amyloid $\beta$-peptide toxicity (Pizzi et al., 2005). A Tat-Bcl-2 construct with a deleted loop domain also protected against apoptotic stimuli in primary cortical neurons and PC12 cells (Soane and Fiskum, 2005). Deletion of the loop domain removes several phosphorylation sites of the protein and enhances its anti-apoptotic activity. Another cell penetrating peptide fusion protein that provides protection against apoptotic stimuli, such as 6-hydroxydopamine, serum deprivation, and oxidative stress, is Tat-$\alpha$-synuclein, applied at low concentrations (Albani et al., 2004). At higher concentrations, intriguingly, the fusion protein is toxic (Recchia et al., 2008). Thus, $\alpha$-synuclein acts as a double-edged sword. The neuroprotective effect at low intracellular concentrations, while yet to be fully explained, could be mediated in part by heat shock protein-70 (Dietz, 2010). In contrast, in Parkinson's disease $\alpha$-synuclein appears to play an important role in disease pathogenesis (Recchia et al., 2004).

Multiple full length Tat fusion proteins, including Bcl-$X_L$, GDNF, a-synuclein and superoxide dismutase, have also been tested in vivo models of nerve injury, ischemia, and neurodegeneration (Choi et al., 2006a,b; Kilic et al., 2005, 2006). The majority of retinal ganglion cells undergo apoptotic death after optic nerve lesion (Weishaupt and Bähr, 2001), and many of these can be rescued by intraocular injection of Tat-Bcl-$X_L$ (Dietz et al., 2002). In the same model, a Tat-GDNF fusion protein enhanced the neuroprotective effect of GDNF alone (Kilic et al., 2004). Intravenously applied Tat-Bcl-$X_L$ reduced infarct size after 90 minutes of medial cerebral artery occlusion in mice, even when applied after the onset of reperfusion (Cao et al., 2002; Kilic et al., 2002); this was accompanied by an improved neurological score of the treated mice. A 30-minute episode of cerebral artery occlusion, which results in diffuse striatal neuron injury, was sensitive to the neuroprotective effects of Tat-Bcl-$X_L$ treatment – even after 2 hours of ischemia (Dietz et al., 2004). A mutant Tat-Bcl-$X_L$ (Tat-FNK) with a more flexible and mobile pore-forming domain displayed improved neuroprotection (Asoh et al., 2002). Tat-FNK has a higher cytoprotective activity than wild-type Bcl-xL (Asoh et al., 2000). Intraperitoneal injection of Tat-FNK in gerbils protected the hippocampal CA1 region against a 5-minute ischemic episode. The same protein did not protect against apoptosis induced by a fusion protein between the ligand-binding domain of the estrogen receptor and DeltaFosB (Tahara et al., 2003). An N-methyl-D-aspartic acid receptor/post-synaptic density protein 95 (PSD-95) interaction is important in mediating ischemic brain injury. Peptide sequences required for N-methyl-D-aspartic acid receptor/PSD-95 interaction, coupled to the Tat protein transduction domain alleviated ischemic brain damage in rats, even when applied 1 hour after occlusion (Aarts et al., 2002). In yet other example, GDNF linked to the Tat protein transduction domain efficiently penetrated the brain after intravenous application and reduced infarct size after middle cerebral artery occlusion through inhibition of apoptosis (Kilic et al., 2003). In similar models for transient and permanent ischemia, a fusion protein between the Tat cell penetrating peptide and the c-Jun N-terminal kinase(JNK) binding motif of JNK-interacting protein-1/isletbrain1was applied (Borsello et al., 2003). The protein significantly reduced infarct size after intracerebroventricular injection. Alzheimer's disease is characterized by the accumulation of amyloid β-peptide plaques and loss of cholinergic neurons in the basal forebrain. Tat-Bcl-$X_L$ protects neurons from Aβ-mediated apoptosis (Pizzi et al., 2005), and Tat-memapsin2 (β-secretase) inhibitor decreases Aβ levels in brain and plasma of transgenic Alzheimer mice (Chang et al., 2004). In addition, Tat-CNTF rescues learning and memory impairments in Aβ-treated mice. Following a different approach, Fu et al. (2004) delivered acetyltransferase (the enzyme required for acetylcholine synthesis) to the brain in an Alzheimer's disease transgenic mouse model by coupling the enzyme to the Tat cell penetrating peptide. In behavioral tests, these mice performed much better in long-term memory and spatial memory tasks. Table 4 summarizes the above studies.

**Table 4. Tat cell penetrating peptide-mediated applications for neuroregeneration**

| Tat-compound | Biological action | Reference |
|---|---|---|
| Tat-Bcl-$X_L$ | Rescue of cerebellar granule neurons after serum and $K^+$ deprivation;<br>Protection after optic nerve transection | Dietz et al., 2002 |
| Tat-Bcl-$X_L$ | Partial protection of neuroblastoma cells against pneumolysin | Ebert et al., 2005 |
| Tat-Bcl-$X_L$ | Protection in various models of brain infarct | Kilic et al., 2002 |
| Tat-Bcl-$X_L$ | Protection from cerebral infarct in vivo | Cao et al., 2002 |
| Tat-Bcl-$X_L$ | Protection from Aβ-induced neuron apoptosis | Pizzi et al., 2005 |
| Tat-Bcl-$X_L$ | Protection of retinal ganglion cells in experimental autoimmune optic neuritis | Diem et al., 2005 |
| Tat-FNK, a Bcl-$X_L$ derivative | Protection of primary cortical neurons and neuroblastoma cells against staurosporine or glutamate; reduction in cerebral ischemic damage | Asoh et al., 2002 |
| Tat-memapsin2 (β-secretase) inhibitor | Decreases Aβ levels in brain and plasma | Chang et al., 2004 |
| Tat-NR2B receptor-derived peptide (PSD-95/PDZ 1,2 domains) | Decreases ischemic brain damage by perturbing NMDAR-PSD-95 interaction | Aarts et al., 2002 |
| L-Tat-JNK inhibitor | Protection against malonate-induced striatal brain lesions | Asanuma et al., 2004 |

**Table 4. (Continued)**

| Tat-compound | Biological action | Reference |
|---|---|---|
| Tat-20 amino acid JNK-binding motif | Neuroprotection when applied intraventricularly or intraperitoneally following transient or permanent middle cerebral artery occlusion | Borsello et al., 2003 |
| PEP-1-SOD fusion protein | Protection against paraquat-induced dopaminergic neuron damage in a Parkinson's disease mouse model. | Choi et al., 2006a |
| Tat-α-synuclein | Protection from apoptotic or necrotic stimuli in PC12 cells, or toxicity | Albani et al., 2004 |
| Tat-α-synuclein | Protection against paraquat-induced dopaminergic cell death in vivo | Choi et al., 2006b |
| Tat-GDNF | Neuroprotection after systemic application in a brain infarct model | Kilic et al., 2003 |
| Tat-GDNF | Apoptosis inhibition in retinal ganglion cells after axotomy | Kilic et al., 2004 |
| Tat-CNTF | Rescues learning and memory impairments in Aβ-treated mice | Qu et al., 2008 |
| Tat-CNTF | Rescues motor neurons from death in neonatal rats subjected to sciatic nerve transection | Rezende et al., 2009 |

Aβ, amyloid β-peptide; JNK, c-Jun N-terminal kinase; NMDAR, N-methyl-D-aspartic acid receptor; NR2B, NMDAR subunit 2B; PSD-95, post-synaptic density protein 95; SOD, superoxide dismutase.

## 3.5. Application of a Protein Transduction Domain – CNTF Fusion Protein to Facilitate Neurorestoration

CNTF lacks a classical signal peptide sequence that serves to direct polypeptides out of the cell following synthesis. It is likely that CNTF resides within the cell, only to be released after injury. Strategies which facilitate intracellular entry of CNTF following administration would thus be of therapeutic interest. Indeed, as mentioned above, a fusion protein consisting of mature human CNTF and an 11-amino acid protein transduction domain rescued the learning and memory impairments induced by Aβ in mice (Qu et al., 2008).

In another study, Rezende et al. (2009) utilized a histidine-tragged Tat-CNTF fusion protein to examine the effect of this neurokine on recovery from sciatic nerve injury. CNTF is a member of a large cytokine family of proteins that display a four α-helix bundle topology (McDonald et al. 1995). The Tat domain and histidine tag fused to CNTF protein did not alter its secondary structure and, equally important, robust survival of chicken embryonic day 10 dorsal root ganglion neurons (Barbin et al., 1984) was observed in cultures supplemented with 1 nM recombinant human CNTF (rhCNTF), 1 nM Tat-CNTF, or 1 nM mouse NGF, but not Tat-green fluorescent protein (Figure 6), with $EC_{50}$ values of 0.037 nM, 0.042 nM, and 0.076 nM for rhCNTF, Tat-CNTF, and mouse NGF, respectively (Rezende et al., 2009).

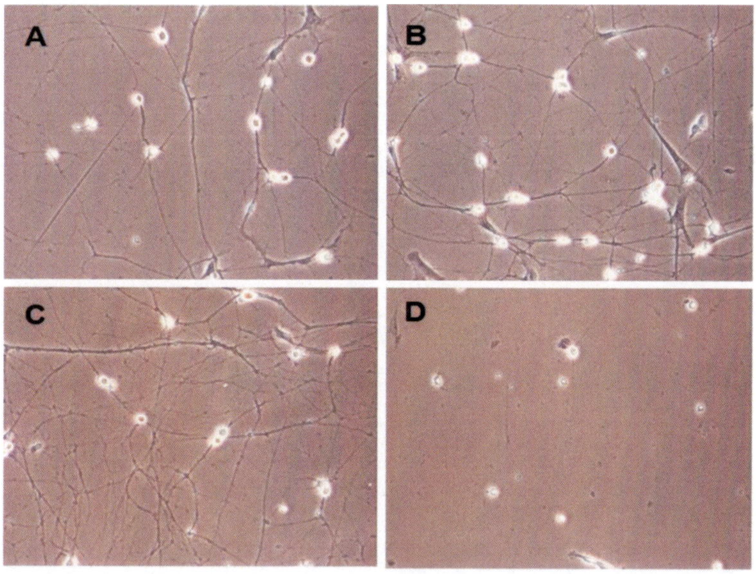


Figure 6. Tat-CNTF retains neurotrophic activity. Chicken embryonic day 10 dorsal root ganglion neurons were cultured for 48 hours with 50 ng/ml of rhCNTF (A), Tat-CNTF (B), mouse NGF(C), or medium only (D). Cultures were then fixed and photographed under phase contrast microscopy. Note that cultures supplemented with rhCNTF, Tat-CNTF, or NGF contain round, phase-bright cell bodies with neurites, while control cultures exhibit scattered debris and an occasional non-neuronal cell.

The neurotrophic activity of Tat-CNTF is thus likely attributable to the CNTF domain, with no interference from either the Tat domain or histidine tag. This is not unexpected, as the 14 amino acid N-terminus of CNTF is not required for neurotrophic activity (Negro et al., 1997).

CNTF and related cytokines induce the activation of receptor-associated just another kinase (JAK)/Tyk tyrosine kinases and subsequent recruitment and phosphorylation of signal transducers and activators of transcription (STAT) proteins, in particular STAT3 (Lelièvre et al., 2001). Phosphorylated STAT proteins dimerize and translocate to the nucleus where they activate target gene transcription (Heinrich et al., 1998; Levy and Darnell, 2002). Incubation of human neuroblastoma SH-SH5Y cells, which express an intact CNTF receptor complex (Kaur et al., 2002), to rhCNTF or Tat-CNTF caused a rapid and sustained increase in STAT3 phosphorylation (Figure 7). This indicates clearly that Tat-CNTF transduces cells and activates relevant signaling pathways.

The neuroprotective action of Tat-CNTF was evaluated using peripheral nerve lesion in neonatal rats. Rodent motor neurons are highly susceptible to injury when the peripheral nerve is transected during the first week of life (Schmalbruch, 1987; Pollin et al., 1991), perhaps because CNTF expression in peripheral nerve is very low during the period CNTF-responsive neurons undergo developmentally programmed cell death (Stöckli et al., 1991).

CNTF prevents the degeneration of these motor neurons after axotomy, and the effect is most evident between P2 and P7 (Sendtner et al., 1990).

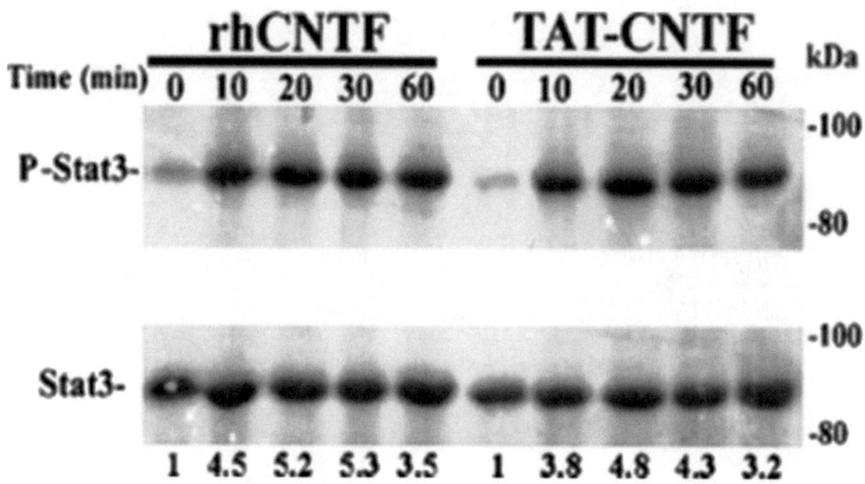


(Reprinted from Journal of Neurochemistry 109(6), A.C. Rezende, D. Peroni, A.S. Vieira, F. Rogerio, R.L. Talaisys, F.T.M. Costa, F. Langone, S.D. Skaper and A. Negro. Ciliary neurotrophic factor fused to a protein transduction domain retains full neuroprotective activity in the absence of cytokine-like side effects, 1680-1690 (Figure 2), Copyright (2009), with permission from Wiley-Blackwell Publishing Ltd.).

Figure 7. Tat-CNTF and rhCNTF induce STAT3 phosphorylation in human SH-5Y5Y neuroblastoma cells. Cells were incubated with 1 μM each of rhCNTF or Tat-CNTF. Cell lysates were subjected to Western blotting and probed with a phospho-STAT3 (P-Stat3) antibody, stripped, and reprobed for total STAT3. A representative blot is shown, with values for fold-increase given below each lane (normalized to total STAT3 amounts).

Subcutaneous or local injection of either rhCNTF or Tat-CNTF each reduced the morphological degenerative changes in spinal cord motor neurons following sciatic nerve axotomy (Figure 8), in keeping with earlier reports for CNTF (Sendtner et al., 1990). As Figure 8 shows, both rhCNTF and Tat-CNTF significantly reduce this motor neuron loss by comparable extents, demonstrating the biological efficacy of Tat-CNTF.

In conclusion, the power of neurotrophic factors to regulate neuronal cell survival in the developing nervous system and to promote also survival after injury or protect neurons in toxin-mediated disease models in animals has encouraged the idea that such proteins could be applied in the treatment of neurodegenerative diseases. However, the application of neurotrophic factors as therapeutic agents for these conditions faces limitations, including blood-brain barrier permeability. In this regard, protein transduction strategies are well suited for intracellular translocation of proteins. Tat and other protein transduction domains have enormous potential to solve age-old problems in the delivery of macromolecular therapeutics. The use of information rich macromolecules has great advantages in specificity and potency that most small molecule therapeutics cannot match. However, traditional gene therapy that uses viral delivery systems for the introduction of foreign nucleic acids as a means to treat disease is wrought with problems in delivery, serious toxicity and immunogenicity. The use of Tat as a delivery vehicle for therapeutic proteins, peptides, antisense and siRNAs avoids many of the drawbacks of gene therapy.

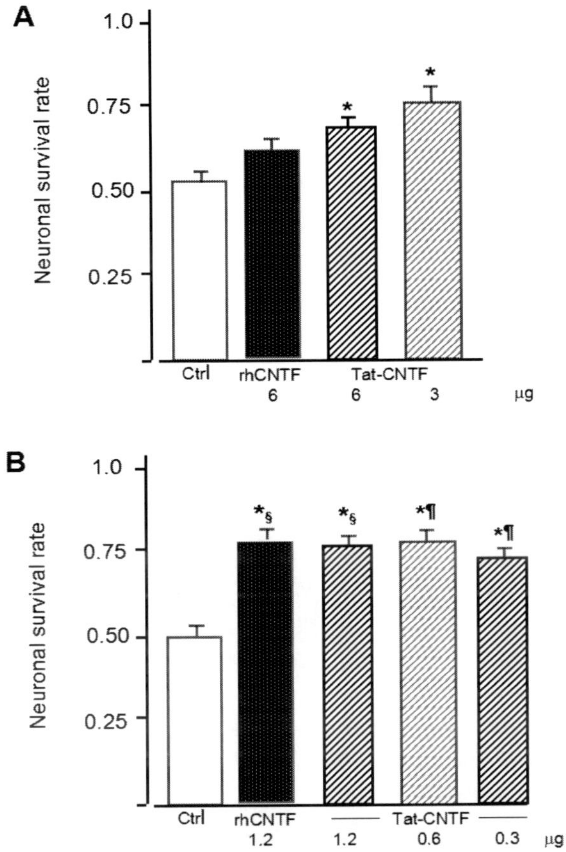


(Reprinted from Journal of Neurochemistry 109(6), A.C. Rezende, D. Peroni, A.S. Vieira, F. Rogerio, R.L. Talaisys, F.T.M. Costa, F. Langone, S.D. Skaper and A. Negro. Ciliary neurotrophic factor fused to a protein transduction domain retains full neuroprotective activity in the absence of cytokine-like side effects, 1680-1690 (Figure 6), Copyright (2009), with permission from Wiley-Blackwell Publishing Ltd).

Figure 8. Tat-CNTF rescues axotomized motor neurons from death. Following sciatic nerve transaction at postnatal day 2, one group of rats (panel A) received locally rhCNTF (6 µg, n=7) or Tat-CNTF (6 or 3 µg, n=6 and 7, respectively). A second group of lesioned rats (panel B) were dosed subcutaneously once daily with either rhCNTF (1.2 µg/g, n=7) or Tat-CNTF (1.2 µg/g, n=7; 0.6 µg/g, n=8; 0.3 µg/g, n=6, respectively). The ratio between the number of ventrolateral motor neurons counted in the lesioned and contralateral sides (neuron survival ratio) of lumbar enlargement at 5 days after sciatic nerve transection was determined. Neuronal survival ratio values are given as mean ± SD). Neuron survival ratio values for rats in all Tat-CNTF treatment groups differed significantly (*$p < 0.05$) from their respective phosphate-buffered saline (control) groups, but were not different ($p > 0.05$) from the corresponding rhCNTF group Moreover, daily subcutaneous dosing of rhCNTF or Tat-CNTF (1.2 µg/g) was more efficacious than the locally applied protein (6 µg/g) ($^{\S}p < 0.05$), while rats treated subcutaneously with 0.3-0.6 µg/g Tat-CNTF had neuron survival ratio values significantly greater ($^{\P}p <$ 0.05) than rats which received 6 µg rhCNTF locally.

The Tat sequence and protein transduction domain are capable, in principle, of crossing the plasma membrane in any cell type. For example, a TAT-β-galactosidase fusion protein injected in the rat-tail vein was found widely distributed in brain (Schwarze et al. 1999). The example of Tat-CNTF illustrates how a subcutaneously administered neurotrophic factor fusion protein can rescue axotomized motor neurons without producing the deleterious side effects of, in this case, CNTF (decrease in body weight together with fat mobilization in brown adipose tissue). The recent identification of fluid phase endocytosis as the mode of cellular entry for Tat and other protein transduction domains has enhanced our understanding of how transduction facilitates intracellular delivery. Many outstanding questions and contradictions still remain to be resolved in the field. Nevertheless, the current body of work regarding the mechanism of uptake gives a much clearer picture of how these macromolecules enter cells and how we might enhance the bioavailability to take advantage of them clinically.

## References

Aarts M., Liu Y., Liu L., Besshoh S., Arundine M., Gurd J. W., Wang Y. T., Salter M. W., Tymianski M. Treatment of ischemic brain damage by perturbing NMDA receptor-PSD-95 protein interactions. *Science,* 2002; 298: 846-50.

Aberg N. D., Brywe K. G., Isgaard J. Aspects of growth hormone and insulin-like growth factor-I related to neuroprotection, regeneration, and functional plasticity in the adult brain. *Scientific World Journal,* 2006; 6: 53-80.

Abrous D. N., Adriani W., Montaron M. F., Aurousseau C., Rougon G., Le Moal M., Piazza P. V., Nicotine Self-Administration Impairs Hippocampal Plasticity. *The Journal of Neuroscience,* 2002; 22(9):3656-3662.

Acheson A., Conover J. C., Fandl J. P., DeChiara T. M., Russell M., Thadani A., Squinto S. P., Yancopoulos G. D., Lindsay R. M. A BDNF autocrine loop in adult sensory neurons prevents cell death. *Nature,* 1995; 374:450-3.

Acler M., Manganotti P. Role, indications and controversies of levodopa administration in chronic stroke patients. *Eur. J. Phys. Rehabil. Med.,* 2013; 49:243-9.

Acler M., Robol E., Fiaschi A., Manganotti P. A double blind placebo RCT to investigate the effects of serotonergic modulation on brain excitability and motor recovery in stroke patients. *J. Neurol.,* 2009; 256(7):1152-8.

Agnello D., Bigini P., Villa P., Mennini T., Cerami A., Brines M. L., Ghezzi P. Erythropoietin exerts anti-inflammatory effect on the CNS in a model of experimental autoimmune encephalomyelitis. *Brain Res.,* 2002; 952:128-34.

Ahn A. C., Tewari M., Poon C.-S., Phillips R. S. The Limits of Reductionism in Medicine: Could Systems Biology Offer an Alternative? *PLoS Med.,* 2006; 3: 709-713.

Alaverdashvili M., Lim D. H., Whishaw I. Q. No improvement by amphetamine on learned non-use, attempts, success or movement in skilled reaching by the rat after motor cortex stroke. *Eur. J. Neurosci.,* 2007;25(11):3442-52.

Albani D., Peverelli E., Rametta R., Batelli S., Veschini L., Negro A., Forloni G. Protective effect of TAT-delivered α-synuclein: relevance of the C-terminal domain and involvement of HSP70. *FASEB J.,* 2004; 18: 1713-5.

Alvarez X. A., Cacabelos R., Laredo M., Couceiro V., Sampedro C., Figueroa J., Varela M., Corzo L., Gonzales A., Novoa-Fernandez L., Vargas M., Aleixandre M., Linares C., Granizo E., Muresanu D., Moessler H. A-24 week double-blind, placebo-controlled study of three dosage of cerebrolysin in patients with mild and Alzheimer´s disease. *European Journal of Neurology*, 2006, 13, 43-54.

Arakawa Y., Sendtner M., Thoenen H. Survival effect of ciliary neurotrophic factor (CNTF) on chick embryonic motoneurons in culture: comparison with other neurotrophic factors and cytokines. *J. Neurosci.*, 1990; 10: 3507-15.

Argyris E. G., Kulkosky J., Meyer M. E., Xu Y., Mukhtar M., Pomerantz R. J., Williams K. J. The perlecan heparan sulfate proteoglycan mediates cellular uptake of HIV-1 Tat through a pathway responsible for biological activity. *Virology,* 2004; 330: 481-6.

Arias-Carrión O., Pöppel E. DA, learning and reward-seeking behavior. *Act. Neurobiol. Exp.,* 2007;67 (4): 481–488.

Arnett H. A., Wang Y., Matsushima G. K., Suzuki K., Ting J. P. Y. Functional genomic analysis of remyelination reveals importance of inflammation in oligodendrocytes regeneration. *J. Neurosci.,* 2003; 23:9824–9832.

Arundine M., Tymianski M. Molecular mechanisms of glutamate-dependent neurodegeneration in ischemia and traumatic brain injury. *Cell. Mol. Life Sci.,* 2004; 61:657–668.

Asanuma T., Inanami O., Tabu K., Waki K., Kon Y., Kuwabara M. Protection against malonate-induced ischemic brain injury in rat by a cell-permeable peptidic c-Jun N-terminal kinase inhibitor, (L)-HIV-TAT48-57-PP-JBD20, observed by the apparent diffusion coefficient mapping magnetic resonance imaging method. *Neurosci. Lett.,* 2004; 359: 57-60.

Asoh S., Ohsawa I., Mori T., Katsura K., Hiraide T., Katayama Y., Kimura M., Ozaki D., Yamagata K., Ohta S. Protection against ischemic brain injury by protein therapeutics. *Proc. Natl. Acad. Sci. USA,* 2002; 99: 17107-12.

Asoh S., Ohtsu T., Ohta S. The super anti-apoptotic factor Bcl-xFNK constructed by disturbing intramolecular polar interactions in rat BclxL. *J. Biol. Chem.,* 2000; 275: 37240-5.

Badaut J., Bix G. J. Transl. Stroke Res. *Vascular neural network phenotypic transformation after traumatic injury: potential role in long-term sequelae*, 2014;5: 394-406.

Bano D., Young K. W., Guerin C. J., et al. Calpain cleavage of the plasma membrane Na+/$Ca^{2+}$ exchanger in excitotoxicity. *Cell,* 2005; 120:275–285.

Bar R. S., Boes M., Dake B. L., Booth B. A., Henley S. A., Sandra A. Insulin, insulin-like growth factors, and vascular endothelium. *Am. J. Med.,* 1988; 85:59-70.

Barbin G., Manthorpe M., Varon S. Purification of the chick eye ciliary neuronotrophic factor. *J. Neurochem*., 1984; 43: 1468-78.

Barde Y. A., Edgar D., Thoenen H. Purification of a new neurotrophic factor from mammalian brain. *EMBO J.,* 1982; 1:549-53.

Barnes M. P., Dobkin B. H., Bogousslavsky J. Recovery after Stroke. New York: Cambridge University Press; 2003.

Bartsch J. W., Wildeboer D., Koller G., Naus S., Rittger A., et al. Tumor necrosis factor-alpha (TNF-alpha) regulates shedding of TNF-alpha receptor 1 by the metalloprotease-disintegrin ADAM8: evidence for a protease-regulated feedback loop in neuroprotection. *J. Neurosci*., 2010; 30(36): 12210-8.

Bazan J. F. Neuropoietic cytokines in the hematopoietic fold. *Neuron,* 1991; 7: 197-208.

Becher B., Antel J. P. Comparison of phenotypic and functional properties of immediately ex vivo and cultured human adult microglia. *Glia,* 1996; 18:1–10.

Becker E. B., Bonni A. Cell cycle regulation of neuronal apoptosis in development and disease. *Prog. Neurobiol.*, 2004; 72: 1-25.

Berends H. I., Nijlant J., van Putten M., Movig K. L., IJzerman M. J. Single dose of fluoxetine increases muscle activation in chronic stroke patients. *Clin. Neuropharmacol.*, 2009;32(1):1-5.

Bezard E., Dovero S., Belin D., Duconger S., Jackson-Lewis V., Przedborski S., Piazza P. V., Gross C. E., Jaber M. Enriched environment confers resistance to 1-methyl-4-phenyl-1,2,3,6-tetrahydropyridine and cocaine: involvement of dopamine transporter and trophic factors. *J. Neurosci.*, 2003; 23:10999-1007.

Bharkta B., Cozens A., Farrin A., Ford G., Langan D., McCabe C., Newell O., Ruddock S., Sackley C., Skinner E., Walker M. DARS DA Augmented Rehabilitation in Stroke Does. Co-careldopa treatment in combination with routine NHS occupational and physical therapy, delivered early after stroke within a stroke service, improve functional recovery including walking and arm function? 2014 July 17th. Available from: http://www.controlled-trials.com/isrctn/pf/99643613.

Bibel M., Barde Y. A. Neurotrophins: key regulators of cell fate and cell shape in the vertebrate nervous system. *Genes Dev.*, 2000; 14:2919-37.

Biju K., Zhou Q., Li G., Imam S. Z., Roberts J. L., Morgan W. W., Clark R. A., Li S. Macrophage-mediated GDNF delivery protects against dopaminergic neurodegeneration: a therapeutic strategy for Parkinson's disease. *Mol. Ther.*, 2010; 18:1536-44.

Borsello T., Clarke P. G., Hirt L., Vercelli A., Repici M., Schorderet D. F., Bogousslavsky J., Bonny C. A peptide inhibitor of c-Jun N-terminal kinase protects against excitotoxicity and cerebral ischemia. *Nat. Med.*, 2003; 9: 1180-6.

Bothwell M. Functional interactions of neurotrophins and neurotrophin receptors. *Annu. Rev. Neurosci.*, 1995; 18: 223-53.

Bournival J., Quessy P., Martinoli M. G. Protective Effects of Resveratrol and Quercetin Against MPP(+) -Induced Oxidative Stress Act by Modulating Markers of Apoptotic Death in Dopaminergic Neurons. *Cell Mol. Neurobiol.*, 2009 Dec.; 29(8):1169-80.

Brailowsky S., Knight R. T., Blood K. y-aminobutyric acid induced potentiation of cortical hemiplegia. *Brain Res.*, 1986;362:322-30.

Brailowsky S., Knight R. T., Efron R. Phenytoin increases the severity of cortical hemiplegia in rats. *Brain Res.*, 1986;376(1):71-7.

Bright R., Steinberg G. K., Mochly-Rosen D. δPKC mediates microcerebrovascular dysfunction in acute ischemia and in chronic hypertensive stress in vivo. *Brain Res.*, 2007; 1144: 146-55.

Brines M., Cerami A. Emerging biological roles for erythropoietin in the nervous system. *Nat. Rev. Neurosci.*, 2005; 6:484-94.

Briones T. L., Rogozinska M., Woods J. Environmental experience modulates ischemia-induced amyloidogenesis and enhances functional recovery. *Journal Neurotrauma*, 2009; 26:613-25.

Bruce-Keller A. J., Chauhan A., Dimayuga F. O., Gee J., Keller J. N., Nath A. Synaptic transport of human immunodeficiency virus-Tat protein causes neurotoxicity and gliosis in rat brain. *J. Neurosci.*, 2003; 23: 8417-22.

Brunet A., Datta S. R., Greenberg M. E. Transcription-dependent and -independent control of neuronal survival by the PI3K-Akt signaling pathway. *Curr. Opin. Neurobiol.*, 2001; 11:297–305.

Brustein E., Rossignol S. Recovery of Locomotion After Ventral and Ventrolateral Spinal Lesions in the Cat. II. Effects of Noradrenergic and Serotoninergic Drugs. *The Journal of Neurophysiology,* 1999; 81:1513-1530.

Bulnes S., Lafuente J. V. VEGF immunopositivity related to malignancy degree, proliferative activity and angiogenesis in ENU-induced gliomas. *J. Mol. Neurosci.*, 2007; 33:163-72.

Bütefisch C. M., Davis B. C., Sawaki L., Waldvogel D., Classen J., Kopylev L., Cohen L. G. Modulation of use-dependent plasticity by d-amphetamine. *Ann. Neurol.*, 2002;51:59–68.

Cancedda L., Putignano E., Sale A., Viegi A., Berardi N., Maffei L. Acceleration of visual system development by environmental enrichment. *J. Neurosci.,* 2004; 24:4840-8.

Cao F., Sun S., Tong E. T. Experimental study on inhibition of neuronal toxical effect of levodopa by ginkgo biloba extract on Parkinson disease in rats. *J. Huazhong Univ. Sci. Technolog. Med. Sci.*, 2003; 23(2):151-153.

Cao G., Pei W., Ge H., Liang Q., Luo Y., Sharp F. R., Lu A., Ran R., Graham S. H., Chen J. In vivo delivery of a Bcl-xL fusion protein containing the TAT protein transduction domain protects against ischemic brain injury and neuronal apoptosis. *J. Neurosci.*, 2002; 22: 5423-31.

Carrillo M. C., Minami C., Kitani K. et al. Enhancing effect of rasagiline on super-oxide dismutase (SOD) and catalase (CAT) activities in the DArgic system in the rat. *Life Sci.,* 2000; 67:577-85.

Chandel N. S., Maltepe E., Goldwasser E., Mathieu C. E., Simon M. C., Schumacker P. T. Mitocondrial reactive oxygen species trigger hypoxia-induced transcription. *Proc. Natl. Acad. Sci. USA,* 1998; 95:11715-20.

Chang C. F., Lin S. Z., Chiang Y. H., Morales M., Chou J., Lein P., Chen H. L., Hoffer B. J., Wang Y. Intravenous administration of bone morphogenetic protein-7 after ischemia improves motor function in stroke rats. *Stroke,* 2003; 34(2):558-64.

Chang W. P., Koelsch G., Wong S., Downs D., Da H., Weerasena V., Gordon B., Devasamudram T., Bilcer G., Ghosh A. K., Tang J. In vivo inhibition of Aβ production by memapsin 2 (β-secretase) inhibitors. *J. Neurochem.*, 2004; 89: 1409-16.

Chao M. V. Neurotrophins and their receptors: a convergence point for many signalling pathways. *Nat. Rev. Neurosci.*, 2003; 4: 299-309.

Chen G., Shi J. X., Hang C. H., Xie W., Liu J., Liu X. Inhibitory effect on cerebral inflammatory agents that accompany traumatic brain injury in a rat model: a potential neuroprotective mechanism of recombinant human erythropoietin (rhEPO). *Neurosci. Lett.,* 2007; 425:177-82.

Chen J. J., Berchou R. C. Rasagiline, a selective, second-generation, irreversible inhibitor of monoamine oxidase type B, is effective in patients older and younger than 65 years of age with early-to-advanced Parkinson's disease (PD). *Pharmacotherapy,* 2004; 24:1448.

Chen L. W., Wang Y. Q., Wei L. C., Shi M., Chan Y. S. Chinese herbs and herbal extracts for neuroprotection of dopaminergic neurons and potential therapeutic treatment of Parkinson's disease. *CNS Neurol. Disord. Drug Targets*, 2007; 6(4):273-281.

Chen N., Yang M., Guo J., Zhou M., Zhu C., He L. Cerebrolysin for vascular dementia. *Cochrane Database Syst. Rev.,* 2013 Jan. 31; 1:CD008900.

Chen X. C., Zhu Y. G., Zhu L. A., Huang, C., Chen Y., Chen L. M., Fang F., Zhou Y. C., Zhao C. H. Ginsenoside Rg1 attenuates dopamine-induced apoptosis in PC12 cells by suppressing oxidative stress. *Eur. J. Pharmacol.*, 2003; 473(1):1-7.

Choi H. S., An J. J., Kim S. Y., Lee S. H., Kim D. W., Yoo K. Y., Won M. H., Kang T. C., Kwon H. J., Kang J. H., Cho S. W., Kwon O. S., Park J., Eum W. S., Choi S. Y. PEP-1-SOD fusion protein efficiently protects against paraquat-induced dopaminergic neuron damage in a Parkinson disease mouse model. *Free Radic. Biol. Med.*, 2006a; 41: 1058-68.

Choi H. S., Lee S. H., Kim S. Y., An J. J., Hwang S. I., Kim D. W., Yoo K. Y., Won M. H., Kang T. C., Kwon H. J., Kang J. H., Cho S. W., Kwon O. S., Choi J. H., Park J., Eum W. S., Choi S. Y. Transduced Tat-alpha-synuclein protects against oxidative stress in vitro and in vivo. *J. Biochem. Mol. Biol.*, 2006b; 39: 253-62.

Choi-Lundberg D. L., Lin Q., Chang Y. N., Chiang Y. L., Hay C. M., Mohajeri H., Davidson B. L., Bohn M. C. Dopaminergic neurons protected from degeneration by GDNF gene therapy. *Science,* 1997; 275: 838-41.

Cittelly D. M., Nesic O., Johnson K., Hulsebosch C., Perez-Polo J. R. Detrimental effects of antiapoptotic treatments in spinal cord injury. *Exp. Neurol.*, 2008;210(2):295-307.

Conforti L., Gilley J., Coleman M. P. Wallerian degeneration: an emerging axon death pathway linking injury and disease. *Nat. Rev. Neurosci.*, 2014; 15:394-409.

Croxford J. L., Pryce G., Jackson S. J., Ledent C., Giovannoni G., Pertwee R. G., Yamamura T., Baker D. Cannabinoid-mediated neuroprotection, not immunosuppression, may be more relevant to multiple sclerosis. *J. Neuroimmunol.*, 2008;193(1-2):120-9.

Danton G. H., Dietrich W. D. Inflammatory mechanisms after ischemia and stroke. *J. Neuropath. Exp. Neurol.,* 2003; 62:127–136.

Daughaday W. H., Rotwein P. Insulin-like growth factors I and II. Peptide, messenger ribonucleic acid and gene structures, serum, and tissue concentrations. *Endocr. Rev.,* 1989; 10:68-91.

Dempsey R. J., Sailor K. A., Bowen K. K., Tureyen K., Vemuganti R. Stroke induced progenitor cell proliferation in adult spontaneously hypertensive rat brain: effect of exogenous IGF-1 and GDNF. *J. Neurochem.*, 2003; 87:586-97.

Derossi D., Chassaing G., Prochiantz A. Trojan peptides: the penetration system for intracellular delivery, *Trends Cell Biol.,* 1998; 8: 84-7.

Diem R., Taheri N., Dietz G. P., Kuhnert A., Maier K., Sättler M. B., Gadjanski I., Merkler D., Bähr M. HIV-Tat-mediated Bcl-$X_L$ delivery protects retinal ganglion cells during experimental autoimmune optic neuritis. *Neurobiol. Dis.,* 2005; 20: 218-26.

Dietrich W. D., Alonso O., Busto R., Watson B. D., Loor Y., Ginsberg M. D. Influence of amphetamine treatment on somatosensory function of the normal and infarcted rat brain. *Stroke,* 1990; 21(11):147-50.

Dietz G. P. Cell-penetrating peptide technology to deliver chaperones and associated factors in diseases and basic research. *Curr. Pharm. Biotechnol.*, 2010; 11:167-74.

Dietz G. P. H., Kilic E., Bähr M. Delivery of bioactive molecules into the cell: the Trojan Horse approach. *Mol. Cell Neurosci.*, 2004; 27: 85-131.

Dietz G. P. H., Kilic E., Bähr M. Inhibition of neuronal apoptosis in vitro and in vivo using TAT-mediated protein transduction, *Mol. Cell Neurosci.*, 2002; 21: 29-37.

Digicaylioglu M., Bichet S., Marti H. H., Wenger R. H., Rivas L. A., Bauer C., Gassmann M. Localization of specific erythropoietin binding sites in defined area of the mouse brain. *Proc. Natl. Acad. Sci. USA*, 1995; 92:3717-20.

Digicaylioglu M., Lipton S. A. Erythropoietin-mediated neuroprotection involves cross-talk between Jak2 and NF-kappaB signalling cascades. *Nature*, 2001; 412:641-47.

Dingledine R., Varvel N. H., Dudek F. E. When and how do seizures kill neurons, and is cell death relevant to epileptogenesis? *Adv. Exp. Med. Biol.,* 2014; 813:109-22.

Donovan M. J., Lin M. I., Wiegn P., Ringstedt T., Kraemer R., Hahn R., Wang S., Ibañez C. F., Rafii S., Hempstead B. L. Brain-derived neurotrophic factor is an endothelial cell survival factor required for intramyocardial vessel stabilization. *Development,* 2000; 127:4531-40.

Doré S., Kar S., Quirion R. Rediscovering an old friend, IGF-I: potential use in the treatment of neurodegenerative diseases. *Trends Neurosci.,* 1997; 20: 326-31.

Dunn S. E. Insulin-like growth factor I stimulates angiogenesis and the production of vascular endothelial growth factor. *Growth Horm. IGF Res. Suppl.,* 2000; A:S41-2.

Dvorak H. F. Discovery of vascular permeability factor (VPF). *Exp. Cell Res.,* 2006; 312:522-6.

Ebert S., Dietz G. P. H., Mitchell T. J., Michel U., Bähr M., Nau R. Limited protection of Tat-Bcl-X(L) against pneumolysin-induced neuronal cell death. *Neurosci. Lett.*, 2005; 384: 349-53.

ElAli A., Thériault P., Rivest S. The role of pericytes in neurovascular unit remodeling in brain disorders. *Int. J. Mol. Sci.,* 2014; 16(15):6453-74.

El-Andaloussi S., Holm T., Langel U. Cell-penetrating peptides: mechanisms and applications. *Curr. Pharm. Des.,* 2005; 11: 3597-3611.

Elliott G., O'Hare P. Intercellular trafficking and protein delivery by a herpes virus structural protein. *Cell,* 1997; 88: 223-33.

Enhancers fluoxetine and fenozolone during hand sensorimotor tasks. *J. Cereb. Blood Flow Metab.*, 1999;19:1365–1375.

Ernfors P., Ibáñez C. F., Ebendal T., Olson L., Persson H. Molecular cloning and neurotrophic activities of a protein with structural similarities to nerve growth factor: developmental and topographical expression in the brain. *Proc. Natl. Acad. Sci. USA*, 1990; 87: 5454-8.

Ernsberger U., Sendtner M., Rohrer H. Proliferation and differentiation of embryonic chick sympathetic neurons: effects of ciliary neurotrophic factor. *Neuron*, 1989; 2: 1275-84.

Eyding D., Lelgemann M., Grouven U., Harter M., Kromp M., Kaiser T., Kerekes M. F., Gerken M., Wieseler B. Reboxetine for acute treatment of major depression: systematic review and meta-analysis of published and unpublished placebo and selective serotonin reuptake inhibitor controlled trials. *BMJ*, 2010; 341: c4737.

Farkas L. M., Dünker N., Roussa E. Unsicker K., Krieglstein K. Transforming growth factor-□s are essential for the development of midbrain dopaminergic neurons in vitro and in vivo. *J. Neurosci.*, 2003; 23: 5178-86.

Fawell S., Seery J., Daikh Y., Moore C., Chen L. L., Pepinsky B., Barsoum J. Tat-mediated delivery of heterologous proteins into cells. *Proc. Natl. Acad. Sci. USA,* 1994; 91: 664-8.

Feeney D. M., De Smet A. M., Rai S. Noradrenergic modulation of hemiplegia: facilitation and maintenance of recovery. *Restor. Neurol. Neurosci.*, 2004;22(3-5):175-90.

Feeney D. M., Westerberg V. S. Norepinephrine and brain damage: alpha noradrenergic pharmacology alters functional recovery after cortical trauma. *Can. J. Psychol.*, 1990; 44:233-52.

Fernández-López D., M. Pradillo J. M., García-Yébenes I., Martínez-Orgado J. A., Moro M. A., Lizasoain I. The Cannabinoid WIN55212-2 Promotes Neural Repair After Neonatal Hypoxia–Ischemia. *Stroke,* 2010;41:2956.

Ferrara N., Gerber H. P., LeCouter J. The biology of VEGF and its receptors. *Nat. Med.,* 2003; 9:669-76.

Floel A., Hummel C., Breitenstein C. Knecht C, Cohen LG. Effects on encoding of a motor memory in chronic stroke. *Neurology*, 2005; 65:472-474.

Floel A., Breitenstein C., Hummel F., Celnik P., Gigert C., Sawaki L., Knecht S., Cohen L. DArgic influences on formation of a motor memory. *Ann. Neurol.*, 2005;58:121-130.

Fong G. H., Zhang L., Bryce D. M., Peng J. Increased hemangioblast commitment, not vascular disorganization, is the primary defect in flt-1 knock-out mice. *Development,* 1999; 126:3015-25.

Frankel A. D., Pabo C. O. Cellular uptake of the tat protein from human immunodeficiency virus. *Cell,* 1988; 55: 1189-93.

Franklin T. B., Murphy J. A., Myers T. L., Clarke D. B., Currie R. W. Enriched environment during adolescence changes brain-derived neurotrophic factor and TrkB levels in the rat visual system but does not offer neuroprotection to retinal ganglion cells following axotomy. *Brain Res.,* 2006; 1095:1-11.

Friedman M., C. D. Furberg, and D. L. DeMets. Fundamentals of Clinical Trials. 3rd edition. New York :Springer-Verlag;1998.

Frisch S. M., Screaton R. A. Anoikis mechanisms. *Curr. Opin. Cell Biol.*, 2001; 13(5):555–562.

Fu A. L., Li Q., Dong Z. H., Huang S. J., Wang Y. X., Sun M. J. Alternative therapy of Alzheimer’s disease via supplementation with choline acetyltransferase. *Neurosci. Lett.,* 2004; 368: 258-62.

Futaki S., Suzuki T., Ohashi W., Yagami T., Tanaka S., Ueda K., Sugiura Y. Arginine-rich peptides. An abundant source of membrane-permeable peptides having potential as carriers for intracellular protein delivery, *J. Biol. Chem.,* 2001; 276: 5836-40.

Garcia P., Youssef I., Utvik J. K., Florent-Béchard S., Barthélémy V., Malaplate-Armand C., Kriem B., Stenger C., Koziel V., Olivier J. L., Escanye M. C., Hanse M., Allouche A., Desbène C., Yen F. T., Bjerkvig R., Oster T., Niclou S. P., Pillot T. Ciliary neurotrophic factor cell-based delivery prevents synaptic impairment and improves memory in mouse models of Alzheimer's disease. *J. Neurosci.*, 2010; 30: 7516-7527.

García-Arencibia M1, García C., Fernández-Ruiz J. Cannabinoids and Parkinson's disease. *CNS*, 2009 Dec.;8(6):432-9.

Garris P. A., Wightman R. M. Different kinetics govern DArgic transmission in the amygdala, prefrontal cortex and striatum: an in vivo volumetric study. *J. Neurosci.*, 1994;14:442-450.

Gash D. M., Zhang Z., Ovadia A., Cass W. A., Yi A., Simmerman L., Russell D., Martin D., Lapchak P. A., Collins F., Hoffer B. J., Gerhardt G. A. Functional recovery in parkinsonian monkeys treated with GDNF. *Nature,* 1996; 380: 252-5.

Genc S., Koroglu T. F., Genc K. Erythropoietin and the nervous system. *Brain Res.,* 2004; 1000:19-31.

Gerloff C., Liuzzi G., Hoope J., Hummel C. F., Heise F. K. Enhancement of Motor Function With Reboxetine and Transcranial Direct Current Stimulation (STIMBOX), ongoing clinical trial.

Ginsberg M. D. Injury mechanisms in the ischemic penumbra. Approaches to neuroprotection in acute ischemic stroke. *Cerebrovasc. Dis.*, 1997; 7(Suppl. 2):7–12.

Gladstone D. J., Danells C. J., Armesto A., McIlroy W. E., Staines W. R. Physiotherapy coupled with dextroamphetamine for rehabilitation after hemiparetic stroke: a randomized, double-blind, placebo-controlled trial. *Stroke*, 2006; 37:179-85.

Gold P. E., Delonay R. L., Merrin J. Modulation of long-term potentiation by peripherally administered amphetamine and epinephrine. *Brain Res.,* 1984;305:103–107.

Goldstein B. L. Common drugs may influence motor recovery after stroke. *J. of Neurology*, 1995;45:865-871.

Goldstein B. L. Prescribing of potentially harmful drugs to patients admitted to hospital after head injury. *J. of Neurology, Neurosurgery, and Psychiatry*, 1995;58:753-75.

Goldstein L. B., Matchar D. B., Morgenlander J. C., Davis. Influence of Drugs on the Recovery of Sensorimotor Function After Stroke. *JN. Neurorehabil. Neural Repair*, 1990; 3: 137-144.

Green M., Loewenstein P. M. Autonomous functional domains of chemically synthesized human immunodeficiency virus tat trans-activator protein. *Cell*, 1988; 55: 1179-88.

Greenberg D. A., Jin K. From angiogenesis to neuropathology. *Nature,* 2005; 438:954-9.

Grondin R., Zhang Z., Ai Y., Gash D. M., Gerhardt G. A. Intracranial delivery of proteins and peptides as a therapy for neurodegenerative diseases. *Prog. Drug Res*., 2003; 61: 101-23.

Grunfeld J. F., Barhum Y., Blondheim N., Rabey J. M., Melamed E.; Offen D. Erythropoietin delays disease onset in an amyothropic lateral sclerosis model. *Exp. Neurol*., 2007; 204:260-3.

Gump J. M., Dowdy S. F. TAT transduction: the molecular mechanism and therapeutic prospects. *Trends Mol. Med.,* 2007; 13: 443-8.

Guo S., Bezard E., Zhao B. Protective effect of green tea polyphenols on the SH-SY5Y cells against 6-OHDA induced apoptosis through ROS-NO pathway. *Free Radic. Biol. Med.,* 39(5):682-695; 2005.

Guo S., Yan J., Yang T., Yang X., Bezard E., Zhao B. Protective effects of green tea polyphenols in the 6-OHDA rat model of Parkinson's disease through inhibition of ROS-NO pathway. *Biol. Psychiatry*, 2007;62(12):1353-1362.

Gupta B., Levchenko T. S., Torchilin V. P. Intracellular delivery of large molecules and small particles by cell-penetrating proteins and peptides. *Adv. Drug Deliv. Rev.*, 2005; 57: 637-51.

Haffner Z., Gmeinbauer R., Moessler H. A randomized, double-blind, placebo-controlled trial with Cerebrolysin in acute ischaemic stroke. *Cerebrovasc. Dis*., 2001, 11/4: 76.

Hallböök F., Ibáñez C. F., Persson H. Evolutionary studies of the nerve growth factor family reveal a novel member abundantly expressed in Xenopus ovary. *Neuron,* 1991; 6: 845-58.

Hallböök F., Wilson K., Thorndyke M., Olinski R. P. Formation and evolution of the chordate neurotrophin and Trk receptor genes. *Brain Behav. Evol*., 2006; 68:133-44.

Hamm R. J., Temple M. D., O'Dell D. M., Pike B. R., Lyeth B. G. Exposure to environmental complexity promotes recovery of cognitive function after traumatic brain injury. *J. Neurotrauma,* 1996; 13:41-7.

Harbeck-Seu A., Brunk I., Platz T., Vajkoczy P., Endres M., Spies C. A speedy recovery *Curr. Opin. Anaesthesiol*., 2011 Apr;24(2):144-53.

Hardingham G. E. and Bading H. Synaptic versus extra synaptic NMDA receptor signalling: implications for neurodegenerative disorders. *Nat. Rev. Neurosci*., 2010; 11:682-96.

Hardingham G. E., Arnold F. J., Bading H. A calcium microdomain near NMDA receptors: on switch for ERK-dependent synapse-to-nucleus communication. *Nat. Neurosci.*, 2001; 4:565–566.

Hardingham G. E., Fukunaga Y., Bading H. Extrasynaptic NMDARs oppose synaptic NMDARs by triggering CREB shut-off and cell death pathways. *Nat. Neurosci.*, 2002; 5:405–414.

Hardingham G. E. Pro-survival signalling from the NMDA receptor. *Biochemical Society Transactions,* 2006; 34:936–938.

Haughey N. J., Mattson M. P. Calcium dysregulation and neuronal apoptosis by the HIV-1 proteins Tat and gp120. *J. Acquir. Immune Defic. Syndr.,* 2002; 31: S55-S61.

Hawkins B. T., Davis T. P. The blood-brain barrier/neurovascular unit in health and disease. *Pharmacol. Rev.*, 2005; 57:173–185.

Heck S., Lezoualc'h F., Engert S., Behl C. Insulin-like growth factor-1-mediated neuroprotection against oxidative stress is associated with activation of nuclear factor kappaB. *J. Biol. Chem.*, 1999; 274:9828 –35.

Hefti F. Nerve growth factor promotes survival of septal cholinergic neurons after fimbrial transactions. *J. Neurosci.*, 1986; 6: 2155-62.

Heinrich P. C., Behrmann I., Müller-Newen G., Schaper F., Graeve L. Interleukin-6-type cytokine signalling through the gp130/Jak/STAT pathway. *Biochem. J.,* 1998; 334: 297-314.

Hervé F., Ghinea N., Scherrmann J.-M. CNS delivery via adsorptive transcytosis. *The AAPS Journal,* 2008; 10: 455-72.

Hetman M., Kharebava G. Survival signaling pathways activated by NMDA receptors. *Curr. Top Med. Chem.*, 2006; 6:787–799.

Hoffman A. N., Malena R. R., Westergom B. P., Luthra P., Cheng J. P., Aslam H. A., Zafonte R. D., Kline A. E. Environmental enrichment-mediated functional improvement after experimental traumatic brain injury is contingent on task-specific neurobehavioral experience. *Neurosci. Lett.*, 2008; 431:226-30.

Hou, R. C.; Huang, H. M.; Tzen, J. T.; Jeng, K. C. Protective effects of sesamin and sesamolin on hypoxic neuronal and PC12 cells. *J. Neurosci. Res.,* 74(1):123-133; 2003.

Hovda D. A., Feeney D. M. Amphetamine with experience promotes recovery of locomotor function after unilateral frontal cortex injury in the cat. *Brain Res.,* 1984;298:358-61.

Huang E. J., Reichardt L. F. Neurotrophins: roles in neuronal development and function. *Annu. Rev. Neurosci.*, 2001; 24:677-736.

Huang E. J., Reichardt L. F. Trk receptors: roles in neuronal signal transduction. *Annu. Rev. Biochem.,* 2003; 72:609-42.

Hurwitz B. E., Dietrich W. D., McCabe P. M., Alonso O., Watson B. D., Ginsberg M. D., Schneiderman N. Amphetamine promotes recovery from sensory-motor integration deficit after thrombotic infarction of the primary somatosensory rat cortex. *Stroke,* 1991;22:648-54.

Hutter-Paier B., Grygar E., Fruhwirth M., Temmel I., Windisch M. Further evidence that Cerebrolysin protects cortical neurons from neurodegeneration in vitro. *J. Neural Transm. Suppl.*, 1998; 53:363–372.

Ickes B. R., Pham T. M., Sanders L. A., Albeck D. S., Mohammed A. H., Granholm A. C. Long-term environmental enrichment leads to regional increases in neurotrophin levels in rat brain. *Exp. Neurol.,* 2000; 164:45-52.

Inagaki K., Begley R., Ikeno F., Mochly-Rosen D. Cardioprotection by ε-protein kinase C activation from ischemia: continuous delivery and antiarrhythmic effect of an ε-protein kinase C-activating peptide. *Circulation,* 2005; 111: 44-50.

Ip N. Y., Ibáñez C. F., Nye S. H., McClain J., Jones P. F., Gies D. R., Belluscio L., Le Beau M. M., Espinosa R. III, Squinto S. P., Persson H., Yancopoulos G. D. Mammalian neurotrophin-4: structure, chromosomal localization, tissue distribution, and receptor specificity. *Proc. Natl. Acad. Sci. USA*, 1992; 89: 3060-4.

Ip N. Y., Yancopoulos G. D. The neurotrophins and CNTF: two families of collaborative neurotrophic factors. *Annu. Rev. Neurosci*., 1996; 19: 491-515.

Ip, N. Y. The neurotrophins and neuropoietic cytokines: two families of growth factors acting on neural and hematopoietic cells. *Ann. NY Acad. Sci*., 1998; 840: 97-106.

Iseda T., Nishio T., Kawaguchi S., et al. Spontaneous regeneration of the corticospinal tract after transection in young rats: a key role of reactive astrocytes in making favourable and unfavourable conditions for regeneration. *Neuroscience*, 2004; 126:365–374.

Ishii D. N., Pu S. F. In: Hefti F. Ed, Neurotrophic Factors. Berlin: Springer; 1999.

Jankowsky J. L., Melnikova T., Fadale D. J., Xu G. M., Slunt H. H., Gonzales V., Youkin S. G., Borchelt D. R., Savonenko A. V. Environmental enrichment mitigates cognitive deficits in a mouse model of Alzheimer´s disease. *J. Neurosci*., 2005; 25:5217-24.

Jay T. M. DA: a potential substrate for synaptic plasticity and memory mechanisms. *Progress in Neurobiology,* 2003; 69: 375–390.

Jelkmann W. Eryhtropoietin: structure, control of production, and function. *Physiol. Rev.,* 1992; 72:449-89.

Jelkmann W. Erythropoietin after a century of research: younger than ever. *Eur. J. Haematol*., 2007; 78:183-205.

Jin K., Zhu Y., Sun Y., Mao X. O., Xie L., Greenberg D. A. Vascular endothelial growth factor (VEGF) stimulates neurogenesis in vitro and in vivo. *Proc. Natl. Acad. Sci. USA*, 2002; 99:11946-50.

Jingyi W., Yasuhiro M., Naoya H., Seok R. C., Yoshiharu Y., Nagara T. Fumiko T., Shigeru M., Junji K. Observation on the effects of Chinese medicine zhenxuanyin for improving cerebral blood flow in rats with cerebral ischemia. *J. Tradit. Chin. Med.,* 1997;17(4):299-303.

Joliot A. H., Triller A., Volovitch M., Pernelle C., Prochiantz A. Alpha-2,8-polysialic acid is the neuronal surface receptor of antennapedia homeobox peptide, *New Biol*., 1991; 3: 1121-34.

Juul S. E., Anderson D. K., Li Y., Christensen R. D. Erythropoietin and erythropoietin receptor in the developing human central nervous system. *Pediatr. Res.,* 1998; 43:40-9.

Kalivas P. W., Volkow N. D. The neural basis of addiction: pathology of motivation and choice. *Am. J. Psychiatry*, 2005; 162:1403–1413.

Kaplan D. R., Miller F. D. Neurotrophin signal transduction in the nervous system. *Curr. Opin. Neurobiol.,* 2000; 10:381-91.

Kaur N., Wohlhueter A. L., Halvorsens W. Activation and inactivation of signal transactivator and activators of transcription by ciliary neutrotrophic factor in neuroblastoma cells. *Cell Signal,* 2002; 14: 419-29.

Kilic E., Dietz G. P. H., Hermann D. M., Bähr M. Intravenous Tat-Bcl-$X_L$ is protective after middle cerebral artery occlusion in mice, *Ann. Neurol*., 2002; 52: 617-22.

Kilic E., Kilic U., Hermann D. M. TAT fusion proteins against ischemic stroke: current status and future perspectives. *Front Biosci.*, 2006; 11: 1716-21.

Kilic E., Kilic U., Hermann D. M. TAT-GDNF in neurodegeneration and ischemic stroke. *CNS Drug Rev.,* 2005; 11: 369-78.

Kilic Ü., Kilic E., Dietz G. P. H., Bähr M. Intravenous TAT-GDNF is protective after focal cerebral ischemia in mice. *Stroke,* 2003; 34: 1304-10.

Kilic Ü., Kilic E., Dietz G. P. H., Bähr M. The TAT protein transduction domain enhances the neuroprotective effect of GDNF after optic nerve transaction. *Neurodegenerative Dis.,* 2004; 1: 44-9.

Kim H., Li Q., Hempstead B. L., Madri J. A. Paracrine and autocrine functions of brain-derived neurotrophic factor (BDNF) and nerve growth factor (NGF) in brain-derived endothelial cells. *J. Biol. Chem.,* 2004; 279:33538-46.

Kim, E. H.; Jang, M. H.; Shin, M. C.; Shin, M. S.; Kim, C. J. Protective effect of aqueous extract of Ginseng radix against 1-methyl-4-phenylpyridinium-induced apoptosis in PC12 cells. *Biol. Pharm. Bull.*, 2003; 26(12):1668-1673.

Kirschenbaum B., Goldman S. A. Brain-derived neurotrophic factor promotes the survival of neurons arising from the adult rat forebrain subependymal zone. *Proc. Natl. Acad. Sci. U S A,* 1995; 92:210-4.

Kobayashi N. R., Fan D. P., Giehl K. M., Bedard A. M., Wiegand S. J., Tetzlaff W. BDNF and NT-4/5 prevent atrophy of rat rubrospinal neurons after cervical axotomy, stimulate GAP-43 and Tα1-tubulin mRNA expression, and promote axonal regeneration. *J. Neurosci.,* 1997; 17: 9583-95.

Konishi Y., Chui D. H., Hirose H., Kunishita T., Tabira T. Trophic effect of erythropoietin and other haematopoietic factors on central cholinergic neurons in vitro and in vivo. *Brain Res.*, 1993; 609:29-35.

Kordower J. H., Emborg M. E., Bloch J., Ma S. Y., Chu Y., Leventhal L., McBride J., Chen E. Y., Palfi S., Roitberg B. Z., Brown W. D., Holden J. E., Pyzalski R., Taylor M. D., Carvey P., Ling Z., Trono D., Hantraye P., Déglon N., Aebischer P. Neurodegeneration prevented by lentiviral vector delivery of GDNF in primate models of Parkinson's disease. *Science,* 2000; 290: 767-73.

Korsching S., Thoenen H. Two-site enzyme immunoassay for nerve growth factor. *Methods Enzymology,* 1987; 147:167-85.

Kotter M. R., Setzu A., Sim F. J., et al. Macrophage depletion impairs oligodendrocyte remyelination following lysolecithin-induced demyelination. *Glia,* 2001; 35:204–212.

Kotzbauer P. T., Lampe P. A., Heuckeroth R. O., Golden J. P., Creedon D. J., Johnson Jr. E. M., Milbrandt J. Neurturin, a relative of glial-cell-line-derived neurotrophic factor. *Nature,* 1996; 384: 467-70.

Krisa L1., Frederick K. L., Canver J. C., Stackhouse S. K., Shumsky J. S., Murray M. Amphetamine-enhanced motor training after cervical contusion injury. J. Neurotrauma, 2012 Mar 20;29(5):971-89.

Krum J. M., Khaibullina A. Inhibition of endogenous VEGF impedes revascularization and astroglial proliferation: roles for VEGF in brain repair. *Exp. Neurol.*, 2003; 181:241-57.

Krum J. M., Mani N., Rosenstein J. M. Angiogenic and astroglial responses to vascular endothelial growth factor administration in adult rat brain. *Neuroscience,* 2002; 110:589-604.

Kupsch A., Sautter J., Götz M. E., Breithaupt W., Schwarz J., Youdim M. B., Riederer P., Gerlach M., Oertel W. H. Monoamine oxidase-inhibition and MPTP-induced neurotoxicity in the non-human primate: comparison of rasagiline (TVP 1012) with selegiline. *J. Neural Transm.*, 2001;108(8-9):985-1009.

Labiche L. A., Grotta J. C. Clinical trials for cytoprotection in Stroke. *NeuroRx.*, 2004; 1: 46–70.

Ladurner G., Kalvach P., Moessler H., Cerebrolysin Study Group. Neuroprotective treatment with cerebrolysin in patients with acute stroke: a randomised controlled trial. *J. Neural Transm.,* 2005, 112:415-428.

Lafuente J. V., Adan B., Alkiza K., Garibi J., Rossi M. and Cruz-Sánchez F. F. Expression of vascular endothelial growth factor (VEGF) and platelet-derived growth factor receptor-b (PDGFR-b) in human gliomas. *J. Mol. Neurosci.*, 1999; 13 (1-2): 177-185.

Lai T. W., Zhang S., Wang Y. T. Excitotoxicity and stroke: identifying novel targets for neuroprotection. *Prog. Neurobiol.*, 2014; 115:157-88.

Lakhan S. E., Rowland M. Whole plant cannabis extracts in the treatment of spasticity in multiple sclerosis: a systematic review. *BMC Neurol.*, 2009; 9:59.

Lange D. J., Felice K. J., Festoff B. W., Gawel M. J., Gelinas D. F., Kratz R., Lai E. C., Murphy M. F., Natter H. M., Norris F. H., Rudnicki S. Recombinant human insulin-like growth factor-1 in ALS: description of a double-blind, placebo-controlled study. North American ALS/IGF-1 Study Group. *Neurology,* 1996; 47: 93-4.

Lastres-Becker I., Bizat N., Boyer F., Hantraye P., Brouillet E., Fernández-Ruiz J. Effects of cannabinoids in the rat model of Huntington's disease generated by an intrastriatal injection of malonate. *Neuroreport.*, 2003; 14(6):813-6.

Laviola G., Hannan A. J., Macrì S., Solinas M., Jaber M. Effects of enriched environment on animal models of neurodegenerative diseased and psychiatric disorders. *Neurobiol. Dis.,* 2008; 31:159-68.

Lee R., Kermani P., Teng K. K., Hempstead B. L. Regulation of cell survival by secreted proneurotrophins. Science, 2001; 294:1945-8.

Leibrock J., Lottspeich F., Hohn A., Hofer M., Hengerer B., Masiakowski P., Thoenen H., Barde Y. A. Molecular cloning and expression of brain-derived neurotrophic factor. *Nature,* 1989; 341: 149-52.

Lelièvre E., Plun-Favreau H., Chevalier S., Froger J., Guillet C., Elson G. C. A., Gauchat J. F., Gascan H. Signaling pathways recruited by the cardiotrophin-like cytokine/cytokine-like.

Levi-Montalcini R., Hamburger V. Selective growth stimulating effects of mouse sarcoma on the sensory and sympathetic nervous system of the chick embryo. *J. Exp. Zool.*, 1951; 116: 321-61.

Levi-Montalcini R., Meyer H., Hamburger V. In vitro experiments on the effects of mouse sarcomas 180 and 37 on the spinal and sympathetic ganglia of the chick embryo. *Cancer Res.,* 1954; 14: 49-57.

Levi-Montalcini R. The nerve growth factor 35 years later. *Science,* 1987; 237: 1154-62.

Levites Y., Weinreb O., Maor G., Youdim M. B., Mandel S. Green tea polyphenol (-)-epigallocatechin-3-gallate prevents N-methyl-4-phenyl-1,2,3,6-tetrahydropyridine-induced dopaminergic neurodegeneration. *J. Neurochem.*, 2001; 78(5):1073-1082.

Levites Y., Youdim M. B., Maor G., Mandel S. Attenuation of 6-hydroxydopamine (6-OHDA)-induced nuclear factor-kappaB (NF-kappaB) activation and cell death by tea extracts in neuronal cultures. *Biochem. Pharmacol.*, 2002;63(1):21-29.

Levy D. E., Darnell J. E. Jr. STATs: transcriptional control and biological impact. *Nat. Rev. Mol. Cell Biol.*, 2002; 3: 651-62.

Lewin G. R., Barde Y. A. Physiology of the neurotrophins. *Annu. Rev. Neurosci.*, 1996; 19:289-317.

Li F. Q., Cheng X. X., Liang X. B., Wang X. H., Xue B., He Q. H., Wang X. M., Han J. S. Neurotrophic and neuroprotective effects of tripchlorolide, an extract of Chinese herb Tripterygium wilfordii Hook F, on dopaminergic neurons. *Exp. Neurol.,* 2003;179(1): 28-37.

Li J. X., Wang Z. B., Zhu L. Q., Zhu F., Cui W. Cell proliferation inhibitive and apoptosis promoting effects of sanchi extract on GES-1 cell after being transformed by MNNG. *Zhongguo Zhong Xi Yi Jie He Za Zhi*, 2005;25(8):719-722.

Li L. Protective effects of schisanhenol, salvianolic acid A and SY-L on oxidative stress induced injuries of cerebral cells and their mechanisms. *Sheng Li Ke Xue Jin Zhan*, 1998;29(1):35-38.

Li R., Huang Y. G., Fang D., Le W. D.(-)-Epigallocatechin gallate inhibits lipopolysaccharide-induced microglial activation and protects against inflammation-mediated dopaminergic neuronal injury. *J. Neurosci. Res.*, 2004;78(5):723-731.

Li Y., Lu Z. Y., Ogle M., Wei L. Erythropoietin prevents blood-brain barrier damage induce by focal cerebral ischemia in mice. *Neurochem. Res.,* 2007; 32:2132-41.

Li, F. Q.; Lu, X. Z.; Liang, X. B.; Zhou, H. F.; Xue, B.; Liu, X. Y.; Niu, D. B.; Han, J. S.; Wang, X. M. Triptolide, a Chinese herbal extract, protects dopaminergic neurons from inflammation-mediated damage through inhibition of microglial activation. *J. Neuroimmunol.*, 2004; 148(1-2):24-31.

Lim C. M., Kim S. W., Park J. Y., Kim C., Yoon S. H., Lee J. K. Fluoxetine affords robust neuroprotection in the postischemic brain via its anti-inflammatory effect. *J. Neurosci. Res.*, 2009 ;87(4):1037-45.

Lin F. K., Suggs S., Lin C. H., Browne J. K., Smalling R., Egrie J. C., Chen K. K., Fox G. M., Martin F., Stabinsky Z. Cloning and expression of the human erythropoietin gene. *Proc. Natl. Acad. Sci. USA,* 1985; 82:7580-4.

Lin S. Z., Hoffer B. J., Kaplan P., Wang Y. Osteogenic protein-1 protects against cerebral infarction induced by MCA ligation in adult rats. *Stroke*, 1999 ;30(1):126-33.

Lindsay R. M., Yancopoulos G. D. GDNF in a bind with known orphan: accessory implicated in new twist. *Neuron*, 1996; 17: 571-4.

Linner L. Reboxetine modulates the firing pattern of DA cells in the ventral tegmental area and selectively increases DA availability in the prefrontal cortex. *J. Pharmacol. Exp. Ther.*, 2001;297(2):540-6.

Lokk J1., Salman Roghani R., Delbari A. Effect of methylphenidate and/or levodopa coupled with physiotherapy on functional and motor recovery after stroke--a randomized, double-blind, placebo-controlled trial. *Acta. Neurol. Scand.*, 2011 Apr.;123(4):266-73.

Loría F., Petrosino S., Hernangómez M., Mestre L., Spagnolo A., Correa F., Di Marzo V., Docagne F., Guaza C. An endocannabinoid tone limits excitotoxicity in vitro and in a model of multiple sclerosis. *Neurobiol. Dis.,* 2010;37(1):166-76.

Loubinoux I., Boulanouar K., Ranjeva J. P., Carel C., Berry I., Rascol O., Celsis P., Chollet F. Cerebral functional magnetic resonance imaging activation modulated by a single dose of the monoamine neurotransmission enhances fluoxetine and fenozolone during hand sensorimotor tasks. *J. Cereb. Blood Flow Metabol.*, 1999;19:1365.

Loubinoux I., Tombari D., Pariente J., Gerdelat-Mas A., Franceries X., Cassol E., Rascol O., Pastor J., Chollet F. Modulation of behavior and cortical motor activity in healthy subjects by a chronic administration of a serotonin enhancer. *Neuroimage,* 2005; 27(2): 299-313.

Louis J. C., Magal E., Takayama S., Varon S. CNTF protection of oligodendrocytes again natural and tumor necrosis factor-induced death. *Science,* 1993; 259: 689-92.

Louissaint A. Jr., Raos S., Leventhal C., Goldman S. A. Coordinated interaction of neurogenesis and angiogenesis in the adult songbird brain. *Nature,* 2002; 13:945-60.

Lu B., Pang P. T., Woo N. H. The yin and yang of neurotrophin action. *Nat. Rev. Neurosci.*, 2005; 6:603-14.

Lu D., Mahmood A., Qu C., Goussev A., Schallert T., Choop P. Erythropoietin enhances neurogenesis and restores spatial memory in rats after traumatic brain injury. *J. Neurotrauma,* 2005; 22:1011-17.

Maas A. I., Roozenbeek B., Manley G. T. Clinical trials in traumatic brain injury: past experience and current developments. *Neurotherapeutics,* 2010 ; 7(1):115-26.

Maisonpierre P. C., Belluscio L., Squinto S., Ip N. Y., Furth M. E., Lindsay R. M., Yancopoulos G. D. Neurotrophin-3: a neurotrophic factor related to NGF and BDNF. *Science,* 1990; 247: 1446-51.

Mandel S., Weinreb O., Amit T. et al. Mechanism of neuroprotective action of the anti-Parkinson drug rasagiline and its derivatives. *Brain Res. Brain Res. Rev.,* 2005; 48: 379-87.

Marchetti L., Klein M., Schlett K., Pfizenmaier K., Eisel U. L. M. Tumor necrosis factor (TNF)-mediated neuroprotection against glutamate-induced excitotoxicity is enhanced by N-methyld-aspartate receptor activation. *J. Biol. Chem.,* 2004; 279(31):32869–32881.

Marti H. H., Wenger R. H., Rivas L. A., Straumann U., Digicaylioglu M., Henn V., Yonekawa Y., Bauer C., Gassmann M. Erythropoiein gene expresión in human, monkey and murine brain. *Eur. J. Neurosci.*, 1996; 8:666-76.

Marti H. J., Bernaudin M., Bellail A., Schoch H., Euler M., Petit E., Risau W. Hypoxia-induced vascular endothelial growth factor expression precedes neovascularisation after cerebral ischemia. *Am. J. Pathol.*, 2000; 156:965-76.

Maruyama W., Naoi M., Akao Y., Isobe K. The mechanism of neuroprotection by rasagiline. *Biomedical Gerontology*, 2001;25(1):10.

Maruyama W., Nitta A., Shamoto-Nagai M. et al. N-Propargyl-1 (R)-aminoindan, rasagiline, increases glial cell line-derived neurotrophic factor (GDNF) in neuroblastoma SH-SY5Y cells through activation of NF-kappaB transcription factor. *Neurochem. Int.,* 2004; 44:393-400.

Maruyama W., Takahashi T., Youdim M. B. et al. The anti-Parkinson drug, rasagiline, prevents apoptotic DNA damage induced by peroxynitrite in human DArgic neuroblastoma SH-SY5Y cells. *J. Neural. Transm.*, 2002; 109:467-81.

Masliah E., Armasolo F., Veinbergs I., Mallory M., Samuel W. Cerebrolysin ameliorates performance deficits, and neuronal damage in apolipoprotein E-deficient mice. *Pharmacol. Biochem. Behav.*, 1999 Feb;62(2):239-45.

Mason J. L., Jones J. J., Taniike M., Morell P., Suzuki K., Matsushima G. K. Mature oligodendrocyte apoptosis precedes IGF-1 production and oligodendrocyte progenitor accumulation and differentiation during demyelination/remyelination. *J. Neurosci. Res.*, 2000; 61:251-262.

Masson J. L., Jones J. J., Taniike M., Morelll P., Suzuki K., Matsushima G. K. Mature oligodendrocytes apoptosis precedes IGF-I production: an oligodendrocyte progenitor accumulation and differentiation during demyelination/remyelination. *J. Neurosci. Res.*, 2000; 61:251–262.

Masuda S., Chikuma M., Sasaki R. Insulin-like growth factors and insulin stimulates erythropoietin production in primary cultures astrocytes. *Brain Res.*, 1997; 746:63-70.

Mayfield R. D., Randall P. K., Spirduso W. W., Wilcox R. E. Apomorphine and amphetamine produce differential effects on the speed and success of reaction time responding in the rat. *Pharmacology, Biochemistry and Behavior*, 1993;46(4): 769-775.

McAllister A. K., Katz L. C., Lo D. C. Neurotrophins and synaptic plasticity. *Annu. Rev. Neurosci.*, 1999; 22:295-318.

McDonald N. Q., Panayotatos N., Hendrickson W. A. Crystal structure of dimeric human ciliary neurotrophic factor determined by MAD phasing. *EMBO J.*, 1995; 14: 2689-99.

Mead G. E., Hsieh C. F., Lee R., Kutlubaev M., Claxton A. et al. Selective serotonin reuptake inhibitors for stroke recovery: a systematic review and meta-analysis. *Stroke,* 2013; 44:844-50.

Mechoulam R., Panikashvili D., Shohami E. Cannabinoids and brain injury: therapeutic implications. *Trends in Molecular Medicine*, 2002; 8 (2): 58-61.

Miao N. Wang M., Ott J. A., D'Alessandro J. S., Woolf T. M., Bumcrot D. A., et al. Sonic hedgehog promotes the survival of specific CNS neuron populations and protects these cells from toxic insult In vitro. *J. Neurosci.*, 1997; 17: 5891-9.

Miller R. G., Bryan W. W., Dietz M. A., Munsat T. L., Petajan J. H., Smith S. A., Goodpasture J. C. Toxicity and tolerability of recombinant human ciliary neurotrophic factor in patients with amyotrophic lateral sclerosis. *Neurology,* 1996b; 47: 1329-31.

Miller R. G., Petajan J. H., Btyan W. W., Armon C., Barohn R. J., Goodpasture J. C., Hoagland R. J., Parry G. J., Ross M. A., Stromatt S. C. A placebo-controlled trial of recombinant human ciliary neurotrophic (rhCNTF) factor in amyotrophic lateral sclerosis. rhCNTF ALS Study Group. *Ann. Neurol.*, 1996a; 39: 256-60.

Mizumaki Y., Kurimoto M., Hirashima Y., Nishijima M., Kamiyama H., Nagai S., Takaku A., Sugihara K., Shimizu M., Endo S. Lipophilic fraction of Panax ginseng induces neuronal differentiation of PC12 cells and promotes neuronal survival of rat cortical neurons by protein kinase C dependent manner. *Brain Res.,* 2002;950(1-2):254-260.

Mortensen J. K., Larsson H., Johnsen S. P., Andersen G. Impact of prestroke selective serotonin reuptake inhibitor treatment on stroke severity and mortality. *Stroke,* 2014; 45:2121-3.

Moser K. V. and Humpel C. Vascular endothelial growth factor counteracts NMDA-induced cell death of adult cholinergic neurons in rat basal nucleus of Meynert. *Brain Res. Bull.,* 2005; 65:125-31.

Mukand J. A., Guilmette T. J., Allen D. G., Brown L. K., Brown S. L.,Tober K. L., VanDyck W. R. DArgic therapy with carbidopa L-dopa for left neglect after stroke: A case series. *Archives of Physical Medicine and Rehabilitation*, 2001;82(9):1279-82.

Muoio V., Persson P. B., Sendeski M. M. The neurovascular unit - concept review. *Acta. Physiol. (Oxf.)*, 2014; 210:790-8.

Muresanu D. F., Alvarez X. A., Moessler H., Buia M., Stan A., Pintea D., Moldovan F., Popescu B. O. A pilot study to evaluate the effects of Cerebrolysin on cognition and qeEEG in vascular dementia: cognitive improvement correlates with qEEG acceleration. *Journal of the Neurological Sciences*, 2008;267:112–119.

Muresanu D. F., Doppler E., Novak P. Neurotrophic factor treatment of neurological disorders: the benefits of a pleiotropic treatment approach. Commentary. *CNS Neurol. Disord. Drug Targets*, 2011 Jun.; 10:415-6.

Muresanu D. F. Cerebrolysin treatment efficacy study in middle cerebral artery ischemic stroke patients. Report, 1999.

Muresanu D. F. Neurotrophic factors. Bucuresti: Libripress; 2003.

Muresanu F. D. Neuroprotection and neuroplasticity – a holistic approach and future perspectives. *J. Neurol. Sci.*, 2007; 257:38–43.

Myake T., Kung C. K., Goldwasser E. Purification of human erythropoietin. *J. Biol. Chem.*, 1977; 252:5558-64.

Nagahara H., Vocero-Akbani A. M., Snyder E. L., Ho A., Latham D. G., Lissy N. A., Becker-Hapak M., Ezhevsky S. A., Dowdy S. F. Transduction of full-length TAT fusion proteins into mammalian cells: TATp27Kip1 induces cell migration, *Nat. Med.*, 1998; 4: 1449-52.

Nagai A., Nakagawa E., Choi H. B., Hatori K., Kobayashi S., Kim S. U. Erythropoietin and erythropoietin receptors in human CNS neurons, astrocytes, microglia, and oligodendrocytes grown in culture. *J. Neuropathol. Exp. Neurol.*, 2001; 60:386-92.

Nakase I., Niwa M., Takeuchi T., Sonomura K., Kawabata N., Koike Y., Takehashi M., Tanaka S., Ueda K., Simpson J. C., Jones A. T., Sugiura Y., Futaki S. Cellular uptake of arginine-rich peptides: roles for macropinocytosis and actin rearrangement. *Mol. Ther.*, 2004; 10: 1011-22.

Negro A., Grassato L., Polverino De Laureto P., Skaper S. D. Genetic construction, properties and application of a green fluorescent protein tagged ciliary neurotrophic factor. *Protein Eng.*, 1997; 10:1077-83.

Ness J. K., Scaduto R. C. Jr., Wood T. L. IGF-I prevents glutamate-mediated bax translocation and cytochrome C release in O4 oligodendrocyte progenitors. *Glia*, 2004; 46:183–94.

Neufeld G., Cohen T., Shraga N., Lange T., Kessler O., Herzog Y. The neuropilins: multifunctional semaphoring and VEGF receptors that modulate axon guidance and angiogenesis. *Trend Cardiovas. Med.*, 2002; 12:13-9.

Nieto-Sampedro M., Lewis E. R., Cotman C. W., Manthorpe M., Skaper S. D., Barbin G., Longo F. M., Varon S. Brain injury causes a time-dependent increase in neuronotrophic activity at the lesion site. *Science*,1982 ;217(4562):860-1.

Nishijima T., Piriz J., Duflot S., Fernandez A. M., Gaitan G., Gomez-Pinedo U., Verdugo J. M., Leroy F., Soya H., Nuñez A., Torres-Aleman I. Neuronal activity drives localized blood-brain barrier transport of serum insulin-like growth factor-I into the CNS. *Neuron*, 2010; 67:834-46.

Nithianantharajah J., Barkus C., Murphy M., Hannan A. J. Gene-environment interactions modulating cognitive function and molecular correlates of synaptic plasticity in Huntington's disease transgenic mice. *Neurobiol. Dis.*, 2008; 29:490-504.

Nithianantharajah J., Hannan A. J. Enriched environments, experience-dependent plasticity and disorders of the nervous system. *Nature Rev. Neurosci.*, 2006; 7:697-709.

Nithianantharajah J., Hannan A. J. The neurobiology of brain and cognitive reserve: mental and physical activity as modulators of brain disorders. *Prog. Neurobiol.*, 2009; 89: 369-82.

Nitsche M. A., Kuo M. F., Karrasch R., Wächter B., Liebetanz D., Paulus W. Serotonin affects transcranial direct current-induced neuroplasticity in humans. *Biol. Psychiatry,* 2009; 66(5): 503-8.

Noguchi C. T., Asavaritikrai P., Teng R., Jia Y. Role of erythropoietin in the brain. *Crit. Rev. Oncol. Hematol.*, 2007; 64:159-71.

Nordal R. A., Wong C. S. Molecular targets in radiation-induced blood-brain barrier disruption. *Int. J. Radiat. Oncol. Biol. Phys.,* 2005; 62:279-87.

Numakawa T., Suzuki S., Kumamaru E., Adachi N., Richards M., Kunugi H. BDNF function and intracellular signaling in neurons. *Histol. Histopathol.*, 2010; 25:237-58.

Nykjaer A., Lee R., Teng K. K., Jansen P., Madsen P., Nielsen M. S., Jacobsen C., Kliemannel M., Schwarz E., Willnow T. E., Hempstead B. L., Petersen C. M. Sortilin is essential for proNGF-induced neuronal cell death. *Nature*, 2004; 427:843-8.

Ochs G., Penn R. D., York M., Tonn J., Haigh J., Malta E., Traub M., Sendtner M., Toyka K. V. A phase I/II trial of recombinant methionyl human brain derived neurotrophic factor administered by intrathecal infusion to patients with amyotrophic lateral sclerosis. *Amyotroph. Lateral Scler. Other Motor Neuron Disord.*, 2000; 1: 201-6.

Ogunshola O. O., Stewart W. B., Mihalcik V., Solli T., Madri J. A., Ment L. R. Neuronal VEGF expression correlates with angiogenesis in postnatal developing rat brain. *Dev. Brain Res.,* 2000; 119:139-53.

O'Kusky J. R., Ye P., D'Ercole A. J. Insulin-like growth factor-I promotes neurogenesis and synaptogenesis in the hippocampal dentate gyrus during postnatal development. *J. Neurosci.*, 2000; 20:8435–42.

Olanow C. W1., Rascol O., Hauser R., Feigin P. D., Jankovic J., Lang A., Langston W., Melamed E., Poewe W., Stocchi F., Tolosa E.; ADAGIO Study Investigators. A double-blind, delayed-start trial of rasagiline in Parkinson's disease. *N. Engl. J. Med.*, 2009 Sep. 24;361(13):1268-78.

Oppenheim R. W., Prevette D., Yin Q. W., Collins F., MacDonald J. Control of embryonic motoneuron survival in vivo by ciliary neurotrophic factor. *Science*, 1991; 251: 1616-8.

Oppenheim R. W. Cell death during development of the nervous system. *Annu. Rev. Neurosci.,* 1991; 14: 453-501.

Ortuzar N., Argandoña E. G., Bengoetxea H., Lafuente J. V. Combination of intracortically administered VEGF and environmental enrichment enhances brain protection in developing rats. *J. Neural Transm.*, 2011 Jan.; 118(1):135-44.

Ortuzar N., Argandoña E. G., Bengoetxea H., Leis O., Bulnes S., Lafuente J. V. Effects of VEGF administration or neutralization on the BBB of developing rat brain. *Acta. Neurochir. Suppl.*, 2010; 106:55-9.

Pachter J. S., de Vries H. E., Fabry Z. The blood–brain barrier and its role in immune privilege in the central nervous system. *J. Neuropathol. Exp. Neurol.*, 2003; 62:593–604.

Pan, T.; Fei, J.; Zhou, X.; Jankovic, J.; Le, W. Effects of green tea polyphenols on dopamine uptake and on MPP+ -induced dopamine neuron injury. *Life Sci.*, 2003; 72(9):1073-1083.

Pang P. T., Teng H. K., Zaitsev E., Woo N. T., Sakata K., Zhen S., Teng K. K., Yung W. H., Hempstead B. L., Lu B. Cleavage of proBDNF by tPA/plasmin is essential for long-term hippocampal plasticity. *Science,* 2004; 306:487-91.

Pariente J., Loubinoux I., Carel C., Albucher J. F., Leger A., Manelfe C., Rascol O., Chollet F. Fluoxetine modulates motor performance and cerebral activation of patients recovering from stroke. *Ann. Neurol*., 2001;50(6):718-29.

Parsons M. P., Raymond L. A. Extrasynaptic NMDA receptor involvement in central nervous system disorders. *Neuron,* 2014; 82:279-93.

Perez F., Joliot A., Bloch-Gallego E., Zahraoui A., Triller A., Prochiantz A. Antennapedia homeobox as a signal for the cellular internalization and nuclear addressing of a small exogenous peptide, *J. Cell Sci*., 1992; 102: 717-22.

Pham T. M., Winblad B., Granholm A. C., Mohammed A. H. Environmental influences on brain neurotrophins in rats. *Pharmacol. Biochem. Behav*., 2002; 73:167-75.

Pizzi M., Sarnico I., Boroni F., Benarese M., Steimberg N., Mazzoleni G., Dietz G. P., Bähr M., Liou H. C., Spano P. F. NF-κB factor c-Rel mediates neuroprotection elicited by mGlu5 receptor agonists against amyloid β-peptide toxicity, *Cell Death Differ*., 2005; 12: 761-72.

Plate K. H., Breier G., Weich H. A., Risau W. Vascular endothelial growth factor is a potential tumor angiogenesis factor in human gliomas in vivo. *Nature,* 1992; 359:845-8.

Platz T., Kim I. H., Engel U., Pinkowski C., Eickhof C., Kutzner M. Amphetamine fails to facilitate motor performance and to enhance motor recovery among stroke patients with mild arm paresis: interim analysis and termination of a double blind, randomised, placebo-controlled trial. *Restor. Neurol. Neurosci*., 2005; 23:271-80.

Pleger B., Schwenkreis P., Grunberg C., Malin J. P., Tegenthoff M. Fluoxetine facilitates use-dependent excitability of human primary motor cortex. *Clin. Neurophysiol*., 2004;115: 2157–2163.

Pocock, S. J. Clinical Trials — a practical approach. Chichester — New York — Brisbane — Toronto — Singapore: John Wiley & Sons; 1983.

Pollin M. M., McHanwell S., Slater C. R. The effect of age on motor neuron death following axotomy in the mouse. *Development,* 1991; 112: 83-9.

Poo M. M. Neurotrophins as synaptic modulators. *Nat. Rev. Neurosci*., 2001; 2:24-32.

Pooga M., Hallbrink M., Zorko M., Langel U. Cell penetration by transportan, *FASEB J.,* 1998; 12: 67-77.

Qu H. Y., Zhang T., Li X. L., Zhou J. P., Zhao B. Q., Li Q., Sun M. J. Transducible P11-CNTF rescues the learning and memory impairments induced by amyloid-beta peptide in mice. *Eur. J. Pharmacol*., 2008; 594: 93-100.

Queen S. A., Chen M. J., Feeney D. M. d-Amphetamine attenuates decreased cerebral glucose utilization after unilateral sensorimotor cortex contusion in rats. *Brain Res.,* 1997;777(1-2):42-50.

Rabchevsky A. G., Weinitz J. M., Coulpier M., Fages C., Tinel M., Junier M. P. A role for transforming growth factor alpha as an inducer of astrogliosis. *J. Neurosci*., 1998; 18: 10541-52.

Rabie T., Marti H. H. Brain protection by erythropoietin: a manifold task. *Physiol.,* 2008; 23:263-74.

Radad K., Gille G., Moldzio R., Saito H., Rausch W. D. Ginsenosides Rb1 and Rg1 effects on mesencephalic dopaminergic cells stressed with glutamate. *Brain Res.*, 2004 b; 1021(1): 41-53.

Radad, K.; Gille, G.; Moldzio, R.; Saito, H.; Ishige, K.; Rausch, W. D. Ginsenosides Rb1 and Rg1 effects on survival and neurite growth of MPP+-affected mesencephalic dopaminergic cells. *J. Neural Transm.,* 2004 a; 111(1):37-45.

Ramassamy, C.; Clostre, F.; Christen, Y.; Costentin, J. Prevention by a Ginkgo biloba extract (GBE 761) of the dopaminergic neurotoxicity of MPTP. *J. Pharm. Pharmacol.,* 1990; 42(11): 785-789.

Ramer M. S., Priestley J. V., McMahon S. B. Functional regeneration of sensory axons into the adult spinal cord. *Nature*, 2000; 403: 312-6.

Ramírez B. G., Blázquez C., Gómez del Pulgar T., Guzmán M., de Ceballos M. L. Prevention of Alzheimer's Disease Pathology by Cannabinoids: Neuroprotection Mediated by Blockade of Microglial Activation. *The Journal of Neuroscience*, 2005; 25(8):1904-1913.

Rau T. F., Kothiwal A., Zhang L., Ulatowski S., Jacobson S. et al. Low dose methamphetamine mediates neuroprotection through a PI3K-AKT pathway. *Neuropharmacology*, 2011; 61(4):677-86.

Rau T. F., Kothiwal A. S., Rova A. R., Brooks D. M., Poulsen D. J. Treatment with low-dose methamphetamine improves behavioral and cognitive function after severe traumatic brain injury. *J. Trauma Acute Care Surg.*, 2012; 73:S165-72.

Rau T. F., Kothiwal A. S., Rova A. R., Brooks D. M., Rhoderick J. F. et al. Administration of low dose methamphetamine 12 h after a severe traumatic brain injury prevents neurological dysfunction and cognitive impairment in rats. *Exp. Neurol.*, 2014; 253: 31-40.

Read S. J., Parsons A. A., Harrison D. C., Philpott K., Kabnick K., O'Brien S. Stroke genomics:approaches to identify, validate, and understand ischemic stroke gene expression. *J. Cereb. Blood Flow Metab.*, 2001; 21:755–778.

Recchia A., Debetto P., Negro A., Guidolin D., Skaper S. D., Giusti P. α-Synuclein and Parkinson's disease. *The FASEB J.,* 2004; 18: 617-26.

Recchia A., Rota D., Debetto P., Peroni D., Guidolin D., Negro A., Skaper S. D., Giusti P. Generation of a α-synuclein-based rat model of Parkinson's disease. *Neurobiol. Dis.*, 2008; 30: 8-18.

Reichardt L. F. Neurotrophin-regulated signalling pathways. *Phil. Trans. Royal Soc. B.,* 2006; 361: 1545-64.

Restemeyer C., Weiller C., Liepert J. No effect of a levodopa single dose on motor performance and motor excitability in chronic stroke. A double-blind placebo-controlled cross-over pilot study. *Restor. Neurol Neurosci.*, 2007;25(2):143-50.

Rezende A. C., Peroni D., Vieira A. S., Rogerio F., Talaisys R. L., Costa F. T. M., Langone F., Skaper S. D., Negro A. Ciliary neurotrophic factor fused to a protein transduction domain retains full neuroprotective activity in the absence of cytokine-like side effects. *J. Neurochem.,* 2009; 109: 1680-90.

Riley C., Hutter-Paier B., U., Windisch M., E. Doppler, H. Moessler, R. Wronski. A peptide preparation protects cells in organotypic brain slices against death after glutamate intoxication. *J. Neural Transm.*, 2006;113:103-110.

Rinderknecht E., Humbel R. E.. The amino acid sequence of human insulin-like growth factor I and its structural homology with proinsulin. *J. Biol. Chem.*, 1978; 253:2769–76.

Robol E., Fiaschi A., Manganotti P. Effects of citalopram on the excitability of the human motor cortex: a paired magnetic stimulation study. *J. Neurol. Sci.*, 2004 ;221(1-2):41-6.

Rojas P., Garduno B., Rojas C., Vigueras R. M., Rojas-Castaneda J., Rios C., Serrano-Garcia N. EGb761 blocks MPP+-induced lipid peroxidation in mouse corpus striatum. *Neurochem. Res.*, 2001;26(11):1245-1251.

Rojas P.; Serrano-Garcia N.; Mares-Samano, J. J.; Medina-Campos O. N.; Pedraza-Chaverri J.; Ogren S. O. EGb761 protects against nigrostriatal dopaminergic neurotoxicity in 1-methyl-4-phenyl-1,2,3,6-tetrahydropyridine -induced Parkinsonism in mice: role of oxidative stress. *Eur. J. Neurosci.*, 2008;28(1):41-50.

Rosenstein J. M., Krum J. M. New roles for VEGF in nervous tissue-beyond blood vessels. *Exp. Neurol.*, 2004; 187:246-53.

Rosenstein J. M., Mani N., Khaibullina A., Krum J. M. Neurotrophic effects of vascular endothelial growth factor on organotypic cortical explants and primary cortical neurons. *J. Neurosci.*, 2003; 23:11036-44.

Rosenzweig M. R., Bennett E. L., Hebert M., Morimoto H. Social grouping cannot account for cerebral effects of enriched environments. *Brain Res.*, 1978; 153:563-76.

Rosenzweig M. R., Bennett E. L. Psychobiology of plasticity: effects of training and experience on brain and behaviour. *Behav. Brain Res.*, 1996; 78:57-65.

Rosser N., Heuschhmann P., Werching H., Breitenstein C., Knecht S., Floel A. Levodopa improves procedural motor learning in chronic stroke patients. *Ach. Phys. Med. Rehabil.*, 2008; 89:1633-41.

Rothwell P. Treating Individuals - From randomised trials to personalised medicine. London: Elsevier Health Sciences; 2007.

Rudakewich, M.; Ba, F.; Benishin, C. G. Neurotrophic and neuroprotective actions of ginsenosides Rb(1) and Rg(1). *Planta Med.*, 2001;67(6):533-537.

Ruether E,, Álvarez X, A,, Rainer M,, Moessler H. Sustained improvement of cognition and global function in patients with moderately severe Alzheimer's disease: a double-blind, placebo- controlled study with the neurotrophic agent Cerebrolysin. J. Neural Transm. Suppl., 2002;62:265–75.

Rusnati M., Coltrini D., Oreste P., Zoppetti G., Albini A., Noonan D., d'Adda di Fagagna F., Giacca M., Presta M. Interaction of HIV-1 Tat protein with heparin. Role of the backbone structure, sulfation, and size. *J. Biol. Chem.*, 1997; 272: 11313-20.

Russo V. C., Gluckman P., Feldman E. L., Werther G. A. The insulin-like growth factor system and its pleiotropic functions in the brain. *Endocr. Rev.*, 2005; 26:916 -43.

Sabatier J. M., Vives E., Mabrouk K., Benjouad A., Rochat H., Duval A., Hue B., Bahraoui E. Evidence for neurotoxic activity of tat from human immunodeficiency virus type 1, *J. Virol.,* 1991; 65: 961-7.

Sakanaka M., Wen T. C., Matsuda S., Masuda S., Morishita E., Nagao M., Sasaki R. In vivo evidence that erythropoietin protects neurons from ischemic damage. *Proc. Natl. Acas. Sci. USA,* 1998; 95:4635-40.

Sale A., Putignano E., Cancedda L., Landi S., Cirulli F., Berardi N., et al. Enriched environment and acceleration of visual system development. *Neuropharmacology,* 2004; 47: 649-60.

Sathasivam S. VEGF and ALS. *Neurosci. Res.*, 2008; 62:71-7.

Sato, N.; Sanjuan, I. M.; Heke, M.; Uchida, M.; Naef, F.; Brivanlou, A. H. Molecular signature of human embryonic stem cells and its comparison with the mouse. *Dev. Biol.*, 2003;260(2):404-413.

Saver J. L., Starkman S., Eckstein M., Stratton S., Pratt F. et al. Methodology of the Field Administration of Stroke Therapy - Magnesium (FAST-MAG) phase 3 trial: Part 1 - rationale and general methods. *Int. J. Stroke*, 2014;9:215-9.

Sawaki L., Cohen L. G., Classen J., Davis B. C., Bütefisch C. M. Enhancement of use-dependent plasticity by d-amphetamine. *Neurology,* 2002;59:1262–1264.

Schäbitz W. R., Sommer C., Zoder W., Kiessling M., Schwaninger M., Schwab S. Intravenous brain-derived neurotrophic factor reduces infarct size and counterregulates Bax and Bcl-2 expression after temporary focal cerebral ischemia. *Stroke*, 2000; 31:2212-7.

Schallert T., Hernandez T. D., BarthT. M. Recovery of function after brain damage: severe and chronic disruption by diazepam. *Brain Research,*1986;379:104–11.

Scheidtmann K., Fries W., Muller F., Koening E. Effect of levodopa in combination with physiotherapy on functional motor recovery after stroke: a prospective, randomised, double-blind study. *Lancet,* 2001; 82: 1279-82.

Schmalbruch H. Loss of sensory neurons after sciatic nerve section in the rat. *Anat. Rec.,* 1987; 219: 323-9.

Schnell L., Schneider R., Kolbeck R., Barde Y. A. Neurotrophin-3 enhances sprouting of corticospinal tract during development and after spinal cord lesion. *Nature,* 1994; 367: 170-3.

Schnider A., Guggisberg A., Nahum L., Gabriel D., Morand S. DArgic modulation of rapid reality adaptation in thinking. *Neuroscience,* 2010 ;167(3):583-7.

Schoch H. J., Fisher S., Marti H. H. Hypoxia-induced vascular endothelial growth factor expression causes vascular leakage in the brain. *Brain*, 2002; 125:2549-57.

Schwarze S. R., Ho A., Vocero-Akbani A., Dowdy S. F. In vivo protein transduction: delivery of a biologically active protein into the mouse. *Science,* 1999; 285: 1569-72.

Segal R. A., Greenberg M. E. Intracellular signaling pathways activated by neurotrophic factors. *Annu. Rev. Neurosci.*, 1996; 19:463-69.

Sendtner M., Kreutzberg G. W., Thoenen H. Ciliary neurotrophic factor prevents the degeneration of motor neurons after axotomy. *Nature,* 1990; 345: 440-1.

Sendtner M., Schmalbruch H., Stöckli K. A., Carroll P., Kreutzberg G. W., Thoenen H. Ciliary neurotrophic factor prevents degeneration of motor neurons in mouse mutant progressive motor neuronopathy. *Nature*, 1992; 358: 502-4.

Sendtner M. In: Hefti F. Ed., *Neurotrophic Factors.* Berlin, Springer. 1999; 81-117.

Senger D. R., Galli S. J., Dvorak A. M., Perruzzi C. A., Harvey V. S., Dvorak H. F. Tumor cell secrete a vascular permeability factor that promotes accumulation of ascites fluid. *Science,* 1983; 219:983-5.

Shalaby F., Rossant J., Yamaguchi T. P., Gertsenstein M., Wu X. F., Breitman M. L., Schuh A. C. Failure of blood-island formation and vasculogenesis in Flk-1-deficient mice. *Nature,* 1995; 376:62-6.

Sharma H. S., Menon P. K., Lafuente J. V., Aguilar Z. P., Wang Y. A., et al. The role of functionalized magnetic iron oxide nanoparticles in the central nervous system injury and repair: new potentials for neuroprotection with Cerebrolysin therapy. *J. Nanosci. Nanotechnol.,* 2014 Jan.;14(1):577-95.

Sharma H. S. A combination of tumor necrosis factor-alpha and neuronal nitric oxide synthase antibodies applied topically over the traumatized spinal cord enhances neuroprotection and functional recovery in the rat. *Ann. N Y Acad. Sci.,* 2010; 1199: 175-85.

Shen H., Luo Y., Kuo C. C., Deng X., Chang C. F., Harvey B. K., Hoffer B. J., Wang Y. 9-Cis-retinoic acid reduces ischemic brain injury in rodents via bone morphogenetic protein. *J. Neurosci. Res.*, 2009 ;87(2):545-55.

Shen H., Luo Y., Kuo C. C., Wang Y. BMP7 reduces synergistic injury induced by methamphetamine and ischemia in mouse brain. *Neurosci. Lett.,* 2008 ;442(1):15-8.

Sherer T. B., Fiske B. K., Svendsen C. N., Lang A. E., Langston J. W. Crossroads in GDNF therapy for Parkinson's disease. *Mov. Disord.*, 2006; 21: 136-41.

Shin J. A., Kang J. L., Lee K. E., Park E. M. Different temporal patterns in the expressions of bone morphogenetic proteins and noggin during astroglial scar formation after ischemic stroke. *Cell Mol. Neurobiol.*, 2012;32:587-97.

Shingo T., Sorokan S. T., Shimazaki T., Weiss S. Erythropoietin regulates in vitro and in vivo production of neuronal progenitors by mammalian forebrain neural stem cells. *J. Neurosci.*, 2001; 9733-43.

Silhol M., Tyagi M., Giacca M., Lebleu B., Vivès E. Different mechanisms for cellular internalization of the HIV-1 Tat-derived cell penetrating peptide and recombinant proteins fused to Tat. *Eur. J. Biochem.*, 2002; 269: 494-501.

Skvortsova V. I., Stakhovskaya L. V., Gubsky L. V., Shamalov N. A., Tikhonova I. V., Smychkov A. S., Randomized, Double-Blind, Placebo-Controlled Study of Cerebrolysin Safety and Efficacy in Treatment of Acute Ischemic Stroke. *Korsakov's Journal of Neurology and Psychiatry,* 2004, vol 11.

Sloley B. D., Urichuk L. J., Morley P., Durkin J., Shan J. J., Pang P. K., Coutts R. T. Identification of kaempferol as a monoamine oxidase inhibitor and potential Neuroprotectant in extracts of Ginkgo biloba leaves. *J. Pharm. Pharmacol.,* 2000;52(4): 451-459.

Sloviter R. Apoptosis: a guide for perplexed. *Trends Pharmacol. Sci.,* 2002; 23(1):19–24.

Smith K. R. Jr., Goulding P. M., Wilderman D., Goldfader P. R., Holterman-Hommes P., Wei F. Neurobehavioral effects of phenytoin and carbamazepine in patients recovering from brain trauma: a comparative study. *Arch. Neurol.*, 1994;51:653-60.

Smith P. F. New approaches in the management of spasticity in multiple sclerosis patients: role of cannabinoids. *Ther. Clin. Risk Manag.*, 2010;6:59-63.

Soane L., Fiskum G. TAT-mediated endocytotic delivery of the loop deletion Bcl-2 protein protects neurons against cell death. *J. Neurochem.*, 2005; 95: 230-43.

Sofroniew M. V., Howe C. L., Mobley W. C. Nerve growth factor signaling, neuroprotection, and neural repair. *Annu. Rev. Neurosci.*, 2001; 24:1217-81.

Soker S., Takashima S., Miao H. Q., Neufeld G., Klagsbrun M. Neuropilin-1 is expressed by endothelial and tumor cells as an isoform-specific receptor for vascular endothelial growth factor. *Cell,* 1998; 92:735-45.

Song L., Nath A., Geiger J., Moore A., Hochman S. Human immunodeficiency virus type 1 Tat protein directly activates neuronal N-methyl-D-aspartate receptors at an allosteric zinc-sensitive site. *J. Neurovirol.*, 2003; 9: 399-403.

Sonntag W. E., Lynch C. D., Cooney P. T., Hutchins P. M. Decreases in cerebral microvasculature with age are associated with the decline in growth hormone and insulin-like growth factor I. *Endocrinology*, 1997; 138:3515-20.

Soriano F. X1., Hardingham G. E. Compartmentalized NMDA receptor signalling to survival and death. *J. Physiol.*, 2007 Oct. 15;584(Pt 2):381-7.

Sprigg N., Bath P. M. Speeding stroke recovery? A systematic review of amphetamine after stroke. *J. Neurol. Sci.*, 2009;285(1-2):3-9.

Stöckli K. A., Lillien L. E., Näher-Noé M., Breitfeld G., Hughes R. A., Raff M. C., Thoenen H., Sendtner M. Regional distribution, developmental changes, and cellular localization of CNTF-mRNA and protein in the rat brain. *J. Cell Biol.*, 1991; 115: 447-59.

Storkebaum E., Lambrechts D., Carmeliet P. VEGF: once regarded as a specific angiogenic factor, now implicated in neuroprotection. *Bioessays,* 2004; 26:943-54.

Stout A. K., Raphael H. M., Kanterewicz B. I., Klann E., Reynolds I. J. Glutamate-induced neuron death requires mitochondrial calcium uptake. *Nat. Neurosci.*, 1998; 1:366–373.

Stroemer R. P., Kent T. A., Hulsebosch C. E. Enhanced Neocortical Neural Sprouting, Synaptogenesis, and Behavioral Recovery With D-Amphetamine Therapy After Neocortical Infarction in Rats. *Stroke,*1998;29:2381-2395.

Sutton R. L., Feeney D. M. a-Noradrenergic agonists and antagonists affect recovery and maintenance of beamwalking ability after sensorimotor cortex ablation in the rat. *Restorative Neurology and Neuroscience*, 1992;4: 1-11.

Szasz, B. K.; Lenkey, N.; Barth, A. M.; Mike, A.; Somogyvari, Z.; Farkas, O.; Lendvai, B. Converging effects of Ginkgo biloba extract at the level of transmitter release, NMDA and sodium currents and dendritic spikes. *Planta Med.,* 2008;74(10):1235-1239.

Taga T., Kishimoto T. Cytokine receptors and signal transduction. *FASEB J.,* 1992; 6: 3387-96.

Tahara K., Tsuchimoto D., Tominaga Y., Asoh S., Ohta S., Kitagawa M., Horie H., Kadoya T., Nakabeppu Y. DeltaFosB, but not FosB, induces delayed apoptosis independent of cell proliferation in the Rat1a embryo cell line. *Cell Death Differ.*, 2003; 10: 496-507.

Taylor L., Jones L., Tuszynski M. H., Blesch A. Neurotrophin-3 gradients established by lentiviral gene delivery promote short-distance axonal bridging beyond cellular grafts in the injured spinal cord. *J. Neurosci.*, 2006; 26: 9713-21.

Torres-Aleman I. Insulin-like growth factors as mediators of functional plasticity in the adult brain. *Horm. Metab. Res.*, 1999; 31:114-19.

Truettner J., Schmidt-Kastner R., Busto R., Alonso O. F., Loor J. Y., Dietrich W. D., Ginsberg M. D. Expression of brain-derived neurotrophic factor, nerve growth factor, and heat shock protein HSP70 following fluid percussion brain injury in rats. *J. Neurotrauma,* 1999;16(6):471-86.

Turner M. R., Parton M. J., Leigh P. N. Clinical trials in ALS: an overview. *Seminars in Neurology,* 2001; 21: 167-75.

Tuszynski M. H., Thal L., Pay M., Salmon D. P., U. H. S., Bakay R., Patel P., Blesch A., Vahlsing H. L., Ho G., Tong G., Potkin S. G., Fallon J., Hansen L., Mufson E. J., Kordower J. H., Gall C., Conner J. A phase 1 clinical trial of nerve growth factor gene therapy for Alzheimer disease. *Nat. Med.*, 2005; 11: 551-5.

Ubhi K., Rockenstein E., Vazquez-Roque R., Mante M., Inglis C., Patrick C., Adame A., Fahnestock M., Doppler E., Novak P., Moessler H., Masliah E. Cerebrolysin modulates pronerve growth factor/nerve growth factor ratio and ameliorates the cholinergic deficit in a transgenic model of Alzheimer's disease. *J. Neurosci. Res.*, 2013 Feb;91(2):167-77.

van Genderen H. I., Nijlant J. M., van Putten M. J., Movig K. L., Ijzerman M. J. Single Dose of Fluoxetine Increases Muscle Activation in Chronic Stroke Patients. *Clin. Neuropharmacol.*, 2008; 32(1):1-5.

van Praag H., Kempermann G., Gage F. H. Neural consequences of environmental enrichment. *Nature Rev. Neurosci.*, 2000; 1:191-8.

Verdonck O., Lahrech H., Francony G., Carle O., Farion R., Van de L. Y., Remy C., Segebarth C., Payen J. F. Erythropoietin protects from post-traumatic edema in the rat brain. *J. Cereb. Blood Flow Metab.*, 2007; 27:1369-76.

Villa P., Bigini P., Mennini T., Agnello D., Laragione T., Cagnotto A., Viviani B., Marinovich M., Cerami A., Coleman T. R., Brines M.; Ghezzi P. Erythropoietin selectively attenuates cytokine production and inflammation in cerebral ischemia by targeting neuronal apoptosis. *J. Exp. Med.*, 2003; 198:971-5.

Vincent A. M., Mobley B. C., Hiller A., Feldman E. L. IGF-I prevents glutamate-induced motor neuron programmed cell death. *Neurobiol. Dis.*, 2004; 16:407– 16.

Violini S., Sharma V., Prior J. L., Dyszlewski M., Piwnica-Worms D. Evidence for a plasma membrane-mediated permeability barrier to Tat basic domain in well-differentiated epithelial cells: lack of correlation with heparan sulfate. *Biochemistry,* 2002; 41: 12652-61.

Vivès E., Richard J. P., Rispal C., Lebleu B. TAT peptide internalization: seeking the mechanism of entry. *Curr. Protein Pept. Sci.*, 2003; 4: 125-32.

Viviani B., Bartesaghi S., Corsini E., Villa P., Ghezzi P., Garau A., Galli C. L., Marinovich M. Erythropoietin protects primary hippocampal neurons increasing the expression of brain-derived neurotrophic factor. *J. Neurochem.*, 2005; 93:412-43.

Wadia J. S., Stan R. V., Dowdy S. F. Transducible TAT-HA fusogenic peptide enhances escape of TAT-fusion proteins after lipid raft macropinocytosis. *Nat. Med.*, 2004; 10: 310-5.

Walicke P., Cowan W. M., Ueno N., Baird A., Guillemin R. Fibroblast growth factor promotes survival of dissociated hippocampal neurons and enhances neurite extension. *Proc. Natl. Acad. Sci. USA,* 1986; 83: 3012-6.

Walker-Batson D. Amphetamine and post-stroke *Eur. J. Phys. Rehabil. Med.,* 2013 Apr;49(2):251-60.

Wang L. E., Fink G. R., Diekhoff S., Rehme A. K., Eickhoff S. B., Grefkes C. Noradrenergic enhancement improves motor network connectivity in stroke patients. *Ann. Neurol.,* 2011;69:375-88.

Wang Y., Zhang Z. G., Rhodes K., Renzi M., Zhang R. L., Kapke A., Lu M., Pool C., Heavner G., Choop M. Post-ischemic treatment with erythropoietin or carbamylated erythropoietin reduces infarction and improves neurological outcome in a rat model of focal cerebral ischemia. *Br. J. Pharmacol.*, 2007; 151:1377-84.

Watanabe H., Ohta H., Imamura L., Asakura W., Matoba Y., Matsumoto K. Effect of Panax ginseng on age-related changes in the spontaneous motor activity and dopaminergic nervous system in the rat. *Jpn. J. Pharmacol.*, 1991;55(1):51-56.

Weber A., Maier R. F., Hoffmann U., Grips M., Hoppenz M., Aktas A. G., Heinemann U., Obiaden M., Schuchmann S. Erythropoietin improves synaptic transmission during and following ischemia in rat hippocampal slice cultures. *Brain Res.*, 2002; 958:305-11.

Weishaupt J. H., Bähr M. Degeneration of axotomized retinal ganglion cells as a model for neuronal apoptosis in the central nervous systemmolecular death and survival pathways, *Restor. Neurol. Neurosci.*, 2001; 19: 19-27.

Wender P. A., Mitchell D. J., Pattabiraman K., Pelkey E. T., Steinman L., Rothbard J. B. The design, synthesis, and evaluation of molecules that enable or enhance cellular uptake: peptoid molecular transporters. *Proc. Natl. Acad. Sci. USA,* 2000; 97: 13003-8.

Wick A., Wick W., Waltenberger J., Weller M., Dichgans J., Schulz J. B. Neuroprotection by hypoxic preconditioning requires sequential activation of vascular endothelial growth factor receptor and Akt. *J. Neurosci.*, 2002; 22:6401-7.

Will B., Galani R., Kelche C., Rosenzweig M. R. Recovery from brain injury in animals: relative efficacy of environmental enrichment, physical exercise or formal training (1990-2002). *Prog. Neurobiol.,* 2004; 72:167-82.

Williams L. R., Varon S., Peterson G. M., Wictorin K., Fischer W., Bjorklund A., Gage F. H. Continuous infusion of nerve growth factor prevents basal forebrain neuronal death after fimbria fornix transaction. *Proc. Natl. Acad. Sci. USA,* 1986; 83: 9231-35.

Wilson M. S., Gibson C. L., Hamm R. J. Haloperidol, but not olanzapine, impairs cognitive performance after traumatic brain injury in rats. *Am. J. Phys. Med. Rehabil.,* 2003;82: 871–9.

Windhangen A., Newcombe J., Dan-gond F., Strand C., Woodroofe M. N. B., Cuzner M. L. et al. Expression of co-stimulatory molecules B7–1 (CD80), B7–2 (CD86), and interleukin 12 cytokine in multiple sclerosis lesions. *J. Exp. Med.*, 1995; 182:1985–1996.

Winkler E. A., Sagare A. P., Zlokovic B. V. *Brain Pathol. The pericyte: a forgotten cell type with important implications for Alzheimer's disease?* 2014;24:371-86.

Wronski R., Tompa P., Hutter-Paier B., Crailsheim K., Friedrich P., Windisch M. Inhibitory effect of a brain derived peptide preparation on the Ca++-dependent protease, calpain. *J. Neural. Transm.,* 2000;107(2):145-57.

Wu D., Pardridge W. M. Neuroprotection with noninvasive neurotrophin delivery to the brain. *Proc. Natl. Acad. Sci. U S A,* 1999; 96:254-9.

Wu H. Y., Yuen E. Y., Lu Y. F., et al. Regulation of N-Methyl-D-aspartate receptors by calpain in cortical neurons. *J. Biol. Chem*., 2005; 280:21588–21593.

Xiao G., Wei J., Yan W., Wang W., Lu Z. Improved outcomes from the administration of progesterone for patients with acute severe traumatic brain injury: a randomized controlled trial. *Crit. Care*, 2008;12(2):R61.

Xie K., Wei D., Shi Q., Huang S. Constitutive and inducible expression and regulation of vascular endothelial growth factor. *Cytokine Growth Factor Rev*., 2004; 15:297-324.

Yamamoto M., Koshimura K., Kawaguchi M., Sohmiya M., Murakami Y., Kato Y. Stimulating effect of erythropoietin on the release of dopamine and acetylcholine from the rat brain slice. *Neurosci. Lett.,* 2000; 292:131-33.

Yan T., Feng Y., Zhai Q. Axon degeneration: Mechanisms and implications of a distinct program from cell death. *Neurochem. Int.,* 2010;56:529-34.

Yang S. F., Wu Q., Sun A. S., Huang X. N., Shi J. S. Protective effect and mechanism of Ginkgo biloba leaf extracts for Parkinson disease induced by 1-methyl-4-phenyl-1,2,3,6-tetrahydropyridine. *Acta. Pharmacol. Sin*., 2001;22(12):1089-1093.

Yasuda T., Mochizuki H. Use of growth factors for the treatment of Parkinson's disease. *Expert Rev. Neurother*., 2010; 10: 915-24.

Yasuda Y., Masuda S., Chikuma M., Inoue K., Nagao M., Sasaki R. Estrogen-dependent production of erythropoietin in uterus and its implication in uterine angiogenesis. *J. Biol. Chem.*, 1998: 273:25381-87.

Yatsiv I., Grigoriadis N., Simeonidou C., Stahel P. F., Schmidt O. I., Alexandrovitch A. G., Tsenter J., Shohami E. Erythropoietin is neuroprotective, improves functional recovery, and reduces neuronal apoptosis and inflammation in a rodent model of experimental closed head injury. *FASEB J.,* 2005; 19:1701-03.

Youdim M. B., Amit T., Falach-Yogev M. et al. The essentiality of Bcl-2, PKC and proteasome-ubiquitin complex activation in the neuroprotective-antiapoptotic action of the anti-Parkinson drug, rasagiline. *Biochem. Pharmacol.*, 2003; 66: 1635-41.

Yu M. S., Wong A. Y., So K. F., Fang J. N., Yuen W. H., Chang R. C. New polysaccharide from Nerium indicum protects neurons via stress kinase signaling pathway. *Brain Res.,* 2007;1153:221-230.

Yun K. J., Min B. S., Kim J. Y., Lee K. T. Styraxoside A isolated from the stem bark of Styrax japonica inhibits lipopolysaccharide-induced expression of inducible nitric oxide synthase and cyclooxygenase-2 in RAW 264.7 cells by suppressing nuclear factor-kappa B activation. *Biol. Pharm. Bull.*, 2007;30(1):139-144.

Zahrt J., Taylor J. R., Mathew R. G., Arnsten A. F. T. Supranormal Stimulation of D1 DA Receptors in the Rodent Prefrontal Cortex Impairs Spatial Working Memory Performance. *The Journal of Neuroscience*, 1997;17(21):8528–8535.

Zhang C., Chopp M., Cui Y., Wang L., Zhang R., Zhang L., Lu M., Szalad A., Doppler E., Hitzl M., Zhang Z. G. Cerebrolysin enhances neurogenesis in the ischemic brain and improves functional outcome after stroke. *J. Neurosci. Res.*, 2010 Nov. 15;88(15): 3275-81.

Zhang J. F., Sun G. S., Zhao G. H. Observation on therapeutic effect of herbs-partitioned moxibustion on Parkinson disease of 54 cases. *Zhongguo Zhen Jiu*, 2005;25(9):610-612.

Zhang L., Chopp M., Meier D. H., Winter S., Wang L., Szalad A., Lu M., Wei M., Cui Y., Zhang Z. G. Sonic hedgehog signaling pathway mediates cerebrolysin-improved neurological function after stroke. *Stroke*, 2013 Jul.; 44(7):1965-72.

Zhang Q. J., Zhang Y. Y., Huang W. Y. Traditional Chinese medicine in treatment of Parkinson's disease. *Zhong Xi Yi Jie He Xue Bao*, 2004;2(1):75-77.

Zhao G., Jiang Z. H., Zheng X. W., Zang S. Y., Guo L. H. Dopamine transporter inhibitory and anti-parkinsonian effect of common flowering quince extract. *Pharmacol. Biochem. Behav.*, 2008;90(3):363-371.

Zhao G., Li S., Qin G. W., Fei J., Guo L. H. Inhibitive effects of Fructus Psoraleae extract on dopamine transporter and noradrenaline transporter. *J. Ethnopharmacol.,* 2007;112(3): 498-506.

Zhao H. W., Li X. Y., Ginkgolide A. B., and huperzine A inhibit nitric oxide-induced neurotoxicity. *Int. Immunopharmacol.*, 2002; 2(11):1551-1556.

Zhou L., Baumgartner B. J., Hill-Felberg S. J., McGowen L. R., Shine H. D. Neurotrophin-3 expressed in situ induces axonal plasticity in the adult injured spinal cord. *J. Neurosci.*, 2003; 23: 1424-31.

Zhou S. and Zhou J. Neuritin, a neurotrophic factor in nervous system physiology. *Curr. Med. Chem.,* 2014; 21:1212-9.

Zhou X., Ding Q., Chen Z., Yun H., Wang H. *J. Biol. Chem. Involvement of the GluN2A and GluN2B subunits in synaptic and extrasynaptic N-methyl-D-aspartate receptor function and neuronal excitotoxicity*, 2013;16(288):24151-9.

Zhu S. W., Yee B. K., Nyffeler M., Winblad B., Feldon J., Mohammed A. H. Influence of differential housing on emotional behaviour and neurotrophin levels in mice. *Behav. Brain Res.*, 2006; 169:10-20.

Zhu, W. W.; Liu, Z. L.; Xu, H. W.; Chu, W. Z.; Ye, Q. Y.; Xie, A. M.; Chen, L.; Li, J. R. Effect of the oil from ganoderma lucidum spores on pathological changes in the substantia nigra and behaviors of MPTP-treated mice. *Di Yi Jun Yi Da Xue Xue Bao*, 2005;25(6):667-671.

Zittel S., Weiller C., Liepert J. Reboxetine improves motor function in chronic stroke. A pilot study. *J. Neurol.*, 2007; 254(2):197-201.

In: Neurorestoratology, volume 1
Editors: H. Huang, G. Raisman, P. R. Sanberg et al.
ISBN: 978-1-63463-599-8


Chapter 8

# Tissue Engineering and Bioengineering

*Anna Sarnowska*[1]*, *Marzena Zychowicz*[1], *Lenora Buzanska*[1], *Ying Li*[2], *Hongyun Huang*[2] *and Osamu Kano*[3,4]

[1] NeuroRepair Department, Medical Research Institute, Polish Academy of Sciences, Warsaw, Poland

[2] Centre of Neurorestoratology, Beijing Rehabilitation Hospital of Capital Medical University, Beijing, China

[3] Department of Neurology, Toho University Omori Medical Center, Otaku, Tokyo, Japan

[4] Department of Neurology, Methodist Neurological Institute, Houston, TX, US

## 1. Tissue Engineering – Biomaterials

*Anna Sarnowska, Marzena Zychowicz and Lenora Buzanska*

### 1.1. Introduction

Biomaterials are generally defined as natural or synthetic materials used in medical devices or implants for introduction into biological systems. They were first described as "a nonviable material used in a medical device, intended to interact with biological systems" [Williams DF, 1987]. As biocompatibility is their most important feature, the definition is often complimented with, "the ability of a material to perform with an appropriate host response in a specific application". Biocompatibility is defined in terms of performance or success for a specific medical treatment and may vary for different applications. More recent applications of biomaterials may not be intended for implantation; instead they are used

*Corresponding author: Anna SarnowskaE-mail:a_sarnowska@o2.pl; Hongyun Huang E-mail:hongyunh@gmail.com

extensively in cell and tissue culturing, the processing of biomolecules and the fabrication of bio-chips and biosensors for research and regenerative medicine.

The novel understanding of biomaterials and their biocompatibility is based on their ability to influence the fate: growth, differentiation and migration of cells in tissue regeneration. For this purpose, polymeric biomaterials are manufactured as three dimensional scaffold structures to provide both physical and chemical cues for living cells [Sun W et al., 2006; Weigel T et al., 2006; Ayres C et al., 2010]. For tissue engineering, polymeric biomaterials are of special interest for neurorestorative methods and are discussed in detail in this chapter.

Biodegradable polymeric materials used in regenerative medicine are classified into naturally derived or synthetic polymers and have shown promising results. Natural polymer agents include: collagen, alginate, chitosan, fibrin, and HA derivatives, whereas synthetic polymers approved by the Food and Drug Administration (FDA) for therapeutic application include: poly(glycolic acid), poly(lactic acid), poly(ε -caprolactone) and poly(lactic-co-glycolic acid) (PLGA) [Rezwan K et al., 2006;Zhang Z et al., 2013].

To perform their role as a successful cellular niche both *in vitro* and *in vivo*, biomaterials must provide a three dimensional structure to support transplanted cells [Teo EY et al., 2011] and micro-environmental cues resembling those of mammalian extracellular matrix (ECM) [Lutolf MP et al., 2005, 2009; Stabenfeldt SE, 2010; Phadke A et al., 2010; Zhang Z et al., 2013]. However, a significant challenge in developing artificial cell niches is to characterize the relevant chemical and physical features of native niches, which are unique for each tissue. The manufacture of an ideal scaffold is the focus of many research groups involved in neuro-regenerative medicine [Walker PA et al., 2009]. To achieve this goal, the artificial scaffolds require multi-component, fibrous and the nano-scale morphology, accompanied by chemical, surface electrical and mechanical properties that match the ECM of neural tissue [Leach JB et al., 2010]. The artificial matrices based on the natural and synthetic polymers and their combinations is a crucial area of research for tissue engineering and regenerative medicine [Lutolf MP et al., 2005, 2009; Zhang Z et al., 2013]. In this chapter we focus on the methods of scaffold fabrication for use in neurorestorative applications.

## 1.2. Scaffold Fabrication

*Conventional Scaffold Fabrication Methods: Phase Separation*

Phase separation is a technique that employs liquid-liquid or liquid-solid physical states to manufacture micro- and nano- skeletons [Sun W et al., 2006; Weigel T et al., 2006; Ayres CE et al., 2010]. Using this method, one material is used to construct the main body of scaffold, and the other acts as a porogen to determine the pore size. The materials most often used in this method are biocompatible and biodegradable aliphatic polyesters such as polylactide(PLA) and polyglycolide (PGA).

### 1.2.1. Solid-liquid

Solid-liquid phase separation is also called freeze drying or lyophilisation. Although the technique has a lot of limitations, the scaffolds created with this method and seeded with the appropriate cells have been used with success in bone tissue engineering [Fromstein JD et al.,

2008; Huang YX et al., 2008]. To enable the biological function of these scaffold surfaces, different molecular coatings such as collagen type I and III, matrigel, or elastin are added. These agents have been tested in preparations for CNS transplants and peripheral nerve conduits. [Barnes CP et al., 2007a; Cao Y et al., 2008].

### 1.2.2. Liquid-Liquid

Liquid-Liquid phase separation uses two different kinds of polymers with two different points of nucleation.

Thermally induced phase separationis a valuable and a somewhat robust method of producing scaffolds in the clinic [Wei G;Ma PX, 2004]. Phase separation occurs through cooling the solution to within a narrow temperature range. After phase separation, the solvent is removed by washing the scaffold in a substance that doesn't react with the scaffold material. When separation occurs spontaneously rather than at nucleation sites, this technique is known as spinodal decomposition. Nano-fibres created with spinodal decomposition produce nano-scale and porosities greater than 80% and are therefore suited for use in CNS applications.

### 1.2.3. Foaming process

This process is employed for the fabrication of porous materials and is achieved by passing through the polymer foaming agent under high pressure or high temperature. In this process, gases and liquids, such as nitrogen or water respectively are passed through the solid polymer or molten polymer mixture (combination of polymers) at high pressure and high temperature, for example for PLGA - 35-40 °C and 10-20 MPa [Singh L et al., 2004] PCL - 70-90 °C and 7-32 MPa. This allows the gases or water to form pores.

The foaming process could be initiated by the 'physical' action of the reacting agents that change their physical state as influenced by pressure or the temperature during the process. These include shape, size of particles or the chemical reaction that occurs during the passage of the substances through the material. The structure of the scaffold may also be manufactured by implementing a process of heterogeneous or homogeneous nucleation. For this process, different kinds of solid or cystic structures with sizes ranging from 30 to 700 μm are passed. Using the same method, the scaffold could be seeded with encapsulated cells [Jacobs MA, 2004], although, this suggests a low level of interconnectivity, their application in tissue engineering may be limited. Thus, the foaming processes are modified with leaching methods to increase the porosity of the scaffold [Yoon JJ;Park TG, 2001]. The preparation of scaffolds by a foaming process also allows the incorporation of pharmaceuticals or other bioactive substances.

### 1.2.4. Microsphere sintering

This technique is employed to form microspheres with the NIPS method or by ultrasound emulsification. To produce spheres, the polymer is sprayed on the surface of different non-solvent porogens and then the water is emulsified through the use of ultrasound in a polymer solution [Newman KD et al., 2004]. The water droplets in water-in-oil-in-water emulsion can then be loaded to carry substances, for example DNA. Following loading, the emulsion of water-in-polymer solution is moved into an aqueous polyvinyl alcohol (PVA) solution to complete the NIPS by stirring for 3 h. by vortex [Ruhe PQ et al., 2005]. The other method requires the pouring of the organic polymer solution into the aqueous PVA solution and to stir for a few hours. Both methods produce excellent spheres but the latter method is easier and less time consuming [Borden M et al., 2004].

### 1.2.5. Self Assembly

In this process the molecules undergo self-association to form the hierarchical structures without any external manipulations. The materials used in this technique range from simple peptides, lipids and proteins, to DNA [Ren K et al., 2005]. The system most often described uses peptide amphiphiles that are composed of a hydrophilic peptide head group (a N-alpha amino group) developed from collagen fragments attached to a hydrophobic tail group (a dialkyl chain moiety) [Ma PX et al., 2005; Vasita R et al., 2006]. The skeleton created with this method, has poor mechanical strength due to weak non-covalent interactions but can be used as a 'molecular carpet' [Harrington DA et al., 2006] e.g. for constructing peptide amphiphiles with bioactive heparin for binding and delivering different growth factors [Stendahl JC et al., 2008]. Scaffolds created from self-assembling peptides were used in nerve tissue engineering [Holmes TC et al., 2000] or cartilage repair [Kisiday J et al., 2002]. Cells seeded into these scaffolds have been reported to improve proliferation and differentiation, influencing the functional behaviours of certain cell [Hosseinkhani H et al., 2006; Zhang S, 2003].

### 1.2.6. Electrospinning (ELSP)

Unlike the mechanical processing method, the technique method employs a high-voltage electrostatic field (10–20 kV) to fabricate ultrafine (from micrometer to nanometer scale) fibres from both synthetic polymers and natural proteins [Boland ED et al., 2004; Matthews JA et al., 2002]. The electrostatic field generated between a metallic nozzle of a syringe and a metallic collector is used to create a sufficient surface charge to disrupt the surface tension in a pendent drop of the polymer fluid. The solvent evaporates from metallic nozzle and under the influence of the surface charge allows the formation of nanofibers [Pham QP et al., 2006]. Different processing parameters (e.g. viscosity, polymer/solution type, applied voltage, surface tension, needle size, spacing between needle and plate, and solution humidity, concentration, air velocity and temperature,) control the ELSP process and allow to modify the diameter [Ayres CE et al., 2007; Boland ED et al., 2004; Matthews JA et al., 2002] and morphology of the fibres [Nair LS et al., 2004]. This technique allows the formation of skeletons with different configurations, shapes and dimensions e.g. mats, cylinders, strands, stacked layers or coaxial tubes. The biological properties of scaffolds can be modulated through compositional settings; mixture of natural protein such as elastin, collagen types I–IV, gelatine, fibrinogen [Sell SA et al., 2006]. Synthetic polymers e.g PLA, nylon, PGA and nitrocellulose polydioxanone (PDS) can be electro-spun separately or in tandem [Sell SA et al., 2006]. In general, pore diameter and fibres increase as the starting polymer concentration increases with higher mandrel rotational speeds [Ayres CE et al., 2006, 2007].

A variety of post-electrospinning processing techniques can modify scaffold properties, making them more bio-accessible for cell growth and proliferation; for example, different cross-linkage [Barnes CP et al., 2007b], high surface area and a high porosity to volume ratio, and is favorable for cell attachment [Ma Z et al., 2005]. Self assembly, phase separation, and electro-spinning can be used successfully to produce nano-fibers similar to the natural range present in the native ECM (50–500 nm) [Barnes CP et al., 2007b]. This technique is non-toxic, simple and inexpensive. However, there are some limitations both in producing larger fibres and the availability of organic solvents that can be used in the electro-spinning process.

### *Advanced Scaffold Fabrication Methods - Rapid Prototyping (RP) Techniques*

Rapid prototyping (RP) is an advanced scaffold fabrication method that requires computer-aided design (CAD) data converted to an STL type file format. The name for this format is derived from the oldest of the RP technologies - stereolithography. The 3D scaffold model, designed with the computer program is converted into cross-sectional layers. Starting from the bottom and proceeding upwards, each layer is adhered to the previous layer to build up a solid model of the object presented on the computer screen. With this method, medical data obtained from CT or MRI images detailing the site of brain injury and the desired implant area can be used to create CAD models of scaffolds for brain restoration[Peltola SM et al., 2008]. With RP technologies, it may be possible to produce skeletons with more precise parameters, such as pore size, geometry, interconnectivity, porosity and geometric stability that would otherwise be impossible to create using "traditional" methods [Leong KF et al., 2003]. Furthermore, it is now conceivable that cells could be printed on the surfaces of such scaffolds [Mironov V, 2003], as well as the incorporation of different biological substrates into the prefabricated layer before the final assembly [Zhang H et al., 2005]. RP technique fall into three basic types: solid-based (fused deposition modelling), liquid-based (two-photon polymerization and stereolithography) and powder-based (3D printing and selective laser sintering) systems [Sun W et al., 2006; Weigel T et al., 2006; Ayres CE et al., 2010]. Although these techniques have a lot of advantages, there are also some limitations, for example, some agents used in SLA photopolymers are cytotoxic for transplanted cells and the fabrication process requires temperatures that exceed the viable limit for human cells. Researchers are trying to eliminate these barriers e.g. by completing fabrication prior to cell seeding. Furthermore, the original photopolymers are not biodegradable, however they can still be used in orthopaedics for cartilage regeneration, since most RP products are rather stiff and strong [Peltola SM et al., 2008].

### *Liquid-Based Technologies*

## 1.2.7. Stereolithography (SLA)

This process is based on the chemical reactions of photopolymerization [Dhariwala B et al., 2004] or cross-linking [Cooke MN et al., 2003] that occurs a photosensitive liquid polymer solution is exposed to UV laser radiation. The laser radiation induces a chemical reaction leading to the polymerization of the photosensitive material and causes the solidification of the polymer in the exposed area. The minimum thickness of the layer that can be generated in this method is as small as 0.005". Lee [Lee KW et al., 2007] described a technique called micro- stereolithography with higher resolution. The improved system utilizes an array of digital micro-mirrors instead of the conventional raster scanning laser to build scaffolds using polyethylene diacrylate as the crosslinking polymer. With this system, scaffolds can be manufactured to a size of approximately 20μm. The most frequently used photo-crosslinkable polymeric materials include methacrylated oligo(lactide-cocaprolactone), urethanes, polyglycerines and biopolymers such as hyaluronian, alignate or dextran.

### 1.2.8. Two-photon polymerization (2PP)

Belongs to the novel CAD/CAM technology and is similar to the method of stereolithography - laser radiation leading to polymerization of a photosensitive material. In stereolithography a UV laser, applied to the surface of the photosensitive material, can produce 2D patterns of polymerized material. To obtain a 3D structure, a layer-by-layer approach has to be applied.

The 2PP technique using a femtosecond laser allows for the fabrication of 3D photonic crystals with a high reproducibility confidence, an unprecedented resolution, and 3D structures [Claeyssens F et al., 2009].

*Powder-Based Methods*

### 1.2.9. Selective Laser Sintering (SLS)

This method is the similar to the SLA technique (infrared $CO_2$ laser beam), but the precursor material is solid e.g. wax, synthetic polymers polycarbonate [Curodeau A et al., 2000], polyamides [Giordano RA et al., 1996], PCL [Williams JM et al., 2005] or mixtures/coatings with polymers, such as poly(etheretherketone)/hydroxyapatite [Tan KH et al., 2005], ultra high molecular weight polyethylene or polyvinyl alcohol/hydroxyapatite [Rimell JT;Marquis PM, 2000].

The SLS machine consists of three chambers, two feed chambers with powdered material and a piston that moves the contents and one fabrication chamber. First, by a heating process, the powder is melted, then as a thin film it is transferred to the fabrication chamber. The laser starts the polymerization reaction fusing the powder in a pattern controlled by a computer program. When the scanning is complete, the fabrication chamber is adjusted and a new layer of powder is deposited for the next exposure. This technique is expensive because of the technology or a material involved and has some limitations such large size of formed skeletons (~400 μm). Modifications to the SLS system have been described, where PLLA/hydroxyapatite microspheres were used to produce porous bone scaffolds [Zhou WY et al., 2008].

*Three dimensional printing (3DP)* – The 3DP technique is very similar to the SLS system but the main difference between SLS and 3DP is that it uses a system similar to standard inkjet printer technology, where it deposits a liquid binder onto the power instead of using a laser. In the 3DP system, the melting process is omitted and broader range of materials can be applied.

The scaffolds created with this system have a weak structure and often need to be reinforced with an additional material. Wong and others investigated the PCL scaffold with various geometry (different types of grooves and channels) produced with this system in a cortical injury application [Wong W et al., 2010]. Wong observed that astrocyte elongation into the scaffold occurred more often in porous scaffolds with integrated channels containing microgrooves oriented in the desired direction of elongation.

*Solid-Based System*

### 1.2.10. Fused Deposition Modelling

In this system the fibres are formed from melted polymer in a temperature–controlled extruder. The fibres are deposited on a motor–driven table with x-y-z co-ordinates, forming layer after layer with computer controlled distance. As a result, the obtained 3D scaffolds have a precise porous morphology and 100% interconnectivity. After modification, instead of the filament, the polymer material can be formed into the pellets or granule shape similar to PCL scaffolds [Darling JT;Sun W, 2004]. The medical applications for this system are limited because the thermo-sensitive materials used are often slow to degrade [Byers BA et al., 2006], or are non-biodegradable. Such materials include acrylonitrile butadiene styrene (ABS) [Cai H et al., 2005] or polypropylene (PP) [Kalita SJ et al., 2004], whereas the use of biodegradable poly(lactic acid) (PLA) or PLGA in FDM is rarely reported [Hutmacher DW et al., 2001].

## 1.3. Computer-Aided Tissue Engineering Technique (CATE) - Scaffold Fabrication Supporting Processes

Apart from the main systems for scaffold preparation discussed above, computer intensive techniques are used to obtain the desired parameters in the fabrication process. These supportive methods described by Sun and colleagues [Semple JL et al., 2005; Sun W et al., 2002] can be divided into three groups [Cheah CM et al., 2004]:

- *Computer-aided tissue modelling* - requires 3D anatomical visualization with imaging-data acquisition, 3D reconstruction and CAD-based tissue modelling [Cheah CM et al., 2004]
- *Computer-aided* **tissue informatics** – requires computer-aided tissue characterization and the application for tissue identification at different tissue hierarchical levels [Sun W et al., 2002]
- *Computer-aided tissue scaffold design and manufacturing* - requires SFF of tissue scaffolds and bio-blueprint modelling [Sun W et al., 2002] - for 3D organs or cells printing [Mironov V et al., 2003].

## 1.4. Bio Functionalization of the Scaffolds

The control of stem cell fate in vitro is the associated with the construction of appropriate matrix microenvironments mimicking stem cell niche properties, enabling reciprocal interaction between cells and niche components. The scaffold material properties including chemical functionality, mechanical properties, as well as the presence of specific bioactive agents have been shown to be crucial in this process [Banerjee A et al., 2009; Lutolf MP et al., 2009; Recknor JB et al., 2006]. Transforming a bio-inert material into a biomimetic or even bio-active material requires its functionalization. This can be achieved by: 1] the changes of the surface chemistry and interfacial energy; 2] incorporation of ECM derived ligands; 3] incorporation of adhesion molecules; 4] tailoring mechanical properties and topography of the scaffold, 5] "smart" modifications by incorporation of bioactive agents into matrix materials and real-time manipulation of their physical and chemical properties.

### 1.4.1. Changes of the Surface Chemistry and Interfacial Energy

The common method employed to alter the surface chemistry of a biomaterial is plasma grafting [Chu PK, 2000]. The precision of this method in order to obtain localized domains ranges from several hundred angstroms to 10 mm. Bible et al.[2009] used plasma polymerized allylamine (ppAAm)-treated PLGA scaffold particles to enhance adhesion of neural stem cells to the particle surface.

Another method used to modify surface chemical properties is the hydrolytic degradation of ester bounds in polyesters biomaterials, resulting with the formation of carboxyl and hydroxyl residues at the surface. In this case, the cellular response is altered due to the increased hydrophilicity and decreased interfacial surface energy of the material [Jiao YP et al., 2007].

The PLGA surface is modified by base hydrolysis and aminolysis resulting in the formation of carboxyl or primary and secondary amines respectively [Croll TI et al., 2004]. Poly (hydroxyl butyrate (PHB) thin films were modified by plasma treatment using low-pressure ammonia. By enhancing hydrophilicity, further conjugation to protein via the introduced amine groups is possible [Nitschke M et al., 2002]. Photo-induced grafting is used to facilitate anchoring of monomers such as acrylic acid, vinyl acetate and acrylamide onto PLLA films and functional carboxyl, hydroxyl and amide groups on such biomaterials as hydroxyethyl methacrylate, methacrylic acid and acrylamide, respectively [Chu PK, 2000]. All these modifications were shown to influence cellular responses.

### 1.4.2. Incorporation of ECM Derived Ligands

The nano-sensing properties of the matrix substrate by the cellular components in the natural niche are performed through the transmembrane receptor proteins called integrins and their ligand domains of ECM proteins [Khang D et al., 2010]. The binding of the type specific integrins to their matrix ligands results in the activation of the intracellular cascade of events resulting in the expression of genes responsible for the cellular behaviour such as cell attachment, proliferation and differentiation. The ECM binding sites for the integrins are represented by well-defined cell-binding peptide sequences described by single letter amino acid nomenclature as: RGD and their synergistic domain PHSRN (localized only 32 Å from RGD), YIGSR and IKVAV and GFOGER, for fibronectin, laminin and collagen respectively. All these peptide domains have been shown to exert important influence on the cell adhesion to the engineered surfaces, however they were found (especially RGD) to fail directing cellular fate [Ruoslahti E, 1996]. One of the reasons of such cellular behaviour is the lack of strict specificity of these peptides to the single ECM protein. To avoid this problem and to exert greater control over integrin specificity, synergistic peptides can be arranged into a pattern with the simple peptides [Benoit DS;Anseth KS, 2005]. Methods used to incorporate ECM active domains to the matrix material involve the transfer of the long chains during polymerization and a coupling reaction attaching the peptides to carboxyl groups on the polymer after polymerization [Fussell GW;Cooper SL, 2004] and lithographic patterning

[Carrico IS et al., 2007]. The artificial matrix systems with incorporated ECM-derived ligands, though possessing active domains for integrin binding, like the temporal control over their presentation to cells as observed in the native ECM and do not strictly influence cellular differentiation. To avoid this problem, the incorporation of ECM recombinant proteins and "smart" modifications of the artificial matrix have been employed by several research groups and will be discussed below.

### 1.4.3. Incorporation of Adhesion Molecules (AMs)

Neural biomaterials are often modified by physical adsorbing/coating, blending, electrostatic attachment and covalent attachment of AMs on their surfaces, reviewed by Rao [Rao SS; Winter JO, 2009]. AMs are the class of the biomolecules that provide clues to regenerating neurons that recapitulate the native brain environment, promoting central nervous system regeneration. They are represented by ECM proteins and polyamino acids. One example of such biomaterial-AM composites includes fibrin-based hybrid gel incorporated with laminin and fibronectin using fresh rat plasma as a cross-linking agent. This resulted in the specific differentiation of the spinal cord neural progenitors into cholinergic motor neurons [Liu J et al., 2010]. In addition to the incorporation of the ECM proteins, several groups have proposed matrix surface functionalization by engineered recombinant ECM proteins with the specific order of the various receptor binding peptide domains. Stem cell differentiation in 2D and 3D micro-environments was controlled through the regulation of fibronectin domain stability, where integrin specific cellular responses were induced by incorporating to the fibronectin repeats displaying both the PHSRN and RGD binding sites [Martino MM et al., 2009]. The deposit of bioactive molecules onto the internal surfaces of porous scaffolds required additional technical developments. Introduction of solvent and non-solvent solution to the scaffold material in a specific order results in the permanent entrapment of gelatin within the scaffold [Liu X et al., 2005]. Alternatively, using porogen-induced surface modification, gelatin molecules were physically trapped within the 3D scaffold during the casting procedure [Liu X et al., 2006]. Another method employs gelatin molecules to modify the internal surfaces of 3D scaffolds. This involves a electrostatic layer-by-layer self-assembly process.

### 1.4.4. Tailoring Mechanical Properties and Topography of the Matrix Material

Integrins are the main mechano tranducers in cells [Schwartz MA; DeSimone DW, 2008]. It was previously shown that the change in the nano-topography of the ECM proteins using micro and nano-scale patterning technologies are capable of controlling integrin cluster size via the design and creation of tandem repeats of ECM fragments and/or peptides [Khang D et al., 2010; Stabenfeldt SE, 2010] and tailoring geometry of 2D ECM-based bioactive domains [Buzanska L et al., 2009; 2010] influence cellular fate and can direct neuronal outgrowth. However, in an attempt to understand cellular responses to environmental mechanical cues, current efforts to pattern 3D hydrogels in real time and via non-cell destructive means must continue to progress. To investigate how matrix mechanics, affect neural progenitor cells differentiation in 3D culture hyaluronic acid (HA) hydrogels with tuneable mechanical properties were fabricated. This was achieved by modifying the polymeric sugar with varying numbers of photo-crosslinks with methacrylate groups. An investigation of bulk hydrogel compressive moduli and native rat tissue enabled the development of an artificial matrix resembling the mechanical properties of neonatal brain and adult spinal cord. Neural progenitor cells encapsulated in such scaffolds were shown to differentiate into neurons and astrocytes respectively [Seidlits SK et al., 2010]. Recently, the influence of the topology of chitosan biomaterials on the differentiation and proliferation of neural stem cells have been also demonstrated. Chitosan films promoted astrocytic differentiation of NSCs, while chitosan multi-microtubule conduits and chitosan porous scaffolds significantly increased in neuronal differentiation [Wang G et al., 2010]. It was also demonstrated that nano scale ridge/groove pattern arrays of the polyurethane acrylate (PUA) mould can induce the differentiation of hESCs into a neuronal lineage without the use any differentiation-inducing agents [Lee MR et al., 2010].

### 1.4.5. "Smart" Modifications by Incorporation of Bioactive Agents Into Matrix Materials and Real-Time Manipulation of Their Physical and Chemical Properties

Micro- and nanotechnologies have been employed to fabricate 2D and 3D systems that are physiologically appropriate and capable of exerting a level of control over cell fate. Micro channel-patterned polydimethyl siloxane (PDMS) was investigated for its potential to induce neuron responses before and after functionalization with covalently immobilized NGF. PDMS micro topography itself increased axon initiation in 68% while NGF only in 28 % of embryonic hippocampal neurons [Gomez N et al., 2007]. However NGF additionally stimulated axonal elongating. This suggests that both 3D topography and surface functionalization with growth factors play an important role in cell fate control, though their modes of action are different. Increasing complexity into emerging 2D and 3D systems using modern approaches of spatial patterning are applied to obtain biomimetic matrix systems. This is achieved via modelling cellular microenvironment with active, smart modifications on demand, enabling real time-control of the material functional domains [Grayson WL et al., 2009]. Controlling the protein mobility and release within and from, this nanostructured scaffolding system is the important approach in building up the biomimetic artificial environment. Self-assembling peptides are proving promising platform for such control due to the programmability of their amino acid sequence which allows controlling and fine-tuning nanofiber properties at the molecular level. Recently, RADA16-I self-assembling, nanofiber forming peptides with neutral, net positive or negative charges located at the C-terminus have been engineered to facilitate slow and sustained release of active cytokines such as βFGF, VEGF and BDNF. Mobility of the incorporated cytokines and the final kinetics of their release were depended upon the charge induced interactions between the protein and peptide nano fibres and physical hindrances of the scaffold. Functional release of active cytokine (βFGF) from such system was observed up to three weeks when tested as the ability to influence on the adult neural stem cells differentiation [Gelain F et al., 2010]. The incorporation of epidermal growth factor (EGF) into a material composed of a synthetic polymer matrix was reported to increase stem cell survival and spreading [Fan VH et al., 2007]. Leipzig et al. [2011] developed a protein-biomaterial complex that allows the stable, rapid and homogenous linking of a growth factor (in that case recombinant fusion protein with pro-neural rat interferon-g rIFN-g) to a photo-crosslinkable material. Neural stem progenitor cells photo-encapsulated in biotin - rIFN-g immobilized methacrylamidechitosan

(MAC) hydrogel scaffolds were shown to differentiate predominantly into neuronal lineage. All the methods mentioned above allow the incorporation of bioactive agents into matrix materials with the real-time manipulation of their physical and chemical properties.

## 1.5. Bioprinting

The three dimensional bioprinting is referred to as the advanced technology assigned to deposit simultaneously the living cells with proteins (ECM components), biomaterials (hydrogels), biochemical factors or drugs into solid, gel or liquid substrate which in theory, can create artificial tissue or even a whole organ [Tasoglu S;Demirci U, 2013] Four, the most commonly used bioprinting technologies include inkjet-based printing [Nakamura M et al., 2005; Boland ED et al., 2006], laser printing [Nahmias Y et al., 2005], acoustic cell encapsulation [Fang Y et al., 2012] and valve-based printing [Moon S et al., 2010].

Based on the computer templates of desired organ 3D printer creates so called 'bio-paper' composed of biomaterial and 'bio-ink' of the cells, formed as small aggregates (spheroids). The problem to be solved in this field is small density of printed cells and their low survival level during the printing process (cell damage caused by the high speed of printing, high shear stress when the cells are ejected).The cells as well as the biomaterial have to be in the liquid phase running the printing process, however have to solid very quickly to perform a three dimensional structure while maintaining connectivity between cells or spheroids. These properties have to be preserved without biochemical changes in the biomaterial and without damage to the cells, what is very challenging [Carvalho JL et al., 2013]

Biologically active macromolecules (growth factors such as fibroblast growth factor-2 (FGF2), ciliary neurotrophic factor (CNTF), and foetal bovine serum (FBS) bioprinted on a polyacrylamide- based hydrogel have been shown to direct the differentiation of neural stem cells into glial or neuronal lineages [Ilkhanizadeh S et al., 2007].

Bioprinting is currently considered to be the leading edge technology, providing precision and control over the cellular microenvironment while building up artificial tissues and organs. In the future bioprinting technology is likely to be applied for neuro-restorative applications in clinical settings.

## 1.6. Tissue Engineering in Application for Nervous System Diseases or Damages

Bible directly injected plasma scaffolds into the injured brain, which acted as an artificial skeleton for neural stem cells. They showed that neuro-scaffolds integrated within the host tissue and created with endogenous neural progenitors a primitive neural tissue [Bible E et al., 2009]. Collagen scaffolds efficiently improved cell survival, differentiation and neurite outgrowth in the transplantation area, and resulted in better neural functional recovery in the rat TBI model [Guan J et al., 2013]. The scaffolds seeded with neural stem cells (NSCs) and SCs facilitated axonal regeneration and myelination and motor functional recovery in hemisected rat spinal cord [Xia L et al., 2013].Single-walled and multi-walled Carbon nanotubes (CNTs) have been used to direct the differentiation of progenitor/stem cells toward specific neurons and to enhance axon regeneration and synaptogenesis for the effective treatment of CNS injuries [Bokara KK1 et al., 2013]. Natural biological scaffold consisting of collagen, engineered bFGF, and NS/PCs could promote NS/PCs proliferation for nervous system repair [Ma F et al., 2014]. Combined Platelet-rich plasma (PRP) and BMSCs-overexpressed BDNF could promote functional recovery after SCI through enhancing migration of astrocytes into the transplants and axonal remyelination in a rat spinal cord hemi section model [Zhao T et al., 2013a]. Fibrin scaffolds containing ectomesenchymal stem cells also could improve the behavioural and histological recovery in a rat model of spinal cord injury [Liu J et al., 2013]. Agar-based bridges as biocompatible candidates provided guide cues in spinal cord injury repair, but neurites within the bridges were mostly peripheral sensory fibres and no central axons crossing from the spinal tissue to bridges [Martín-López E et al., 2013]. Poly ε-caprolactone (PCL) had similar effect on regenerating axons with autologous nerve grafting in a rat sciatic nerve injury model [Reid AJ1et al., 2013].Aligned seamless 3D electro spun collagen/PLGA nerve guides could promote axon regeneration, myelination, action potential propagation, neuromuscular transmission, and functional recovery in rat sciatic nerve defect model [Ouyang Y et al., 2013].

## 1.7. Conclusion

The exploration of scaffolds for tissue engineering is complex and has to be tissue specific, regarding structure, ECM components and function. It is still it is not clear what defines an optimal scaffold/cell or scaffold/neotissue construct. Thus, only the further inclusion of different scientific branches and multidisciplinary cooperation will enable further successful development of tissue restoration. The formation and design of scaffolds are an essential part of this progression for tissue engineeringregarding clinical its application for nervous system diseases and damages.

**Acknowledgment:** The above work was supported by polish National Science Centre grant No 05728/B/N24/2011/01.

# 2. Bioengineering

*Ying Li and Hongyun Huang*

Centre of Neurorestoratology, Beijing Rehabilitation Hospital, Capital Medical University, China

Bioengineering is the biological or medical application of engineering principles or engineering equipment – also called biomedical engineering, which can include genetic engineering or therapy and cell engineering. Both gene therapy and cell engineering can be used to restore lost functions for diseases in CNS by delivering therapeutic DNA into a patient's cells to treat disease. Three main approaches have been considered - replacing a mutated gene that causes disease with a healthy copy; inactivating, or “knocking out,” a mutated gene that is functioning improperly; introducing a new gene into the body to help fight a disease [http://ghr.nlm.nih.gov/handbook/therapy/genetherapy]. Gene therapy utilizes the delivery of DNA into cells, which can be accomplished by viral vectors and non-viral methods.

## 2.1. Neurorestorative Application of Bioengineering

The neuro-restorative application of Bioengineering for CNS mainly contains four contents: neurotrophic factors, enzyme, gene silencing and antibodies.

## 2.2. Genetically engineering cells secreting neurotrophic factor

In 1988, Rosenberg MB reported that fibroblasts genetically modified to secrete NGF implanted into the brains of rats with the fimbria-fornix lesions, survived and produced sufficient NGF to prevent the degeneration of cholinergic neurons of which sprouted axon projections in the direction of the cellular source of NGF [Rosenberg MB et al., 1988]. The foetal or genetically engineering cells secreting nerve growth factor also could protect neurons at a specific target from excitotoxin-induced lesions [SchumacherJM et al., 1991; Frim DM et al., 1993]. In Alzheimer's model of rats, the age-related memory loss could be reversed by grafting engineered cells secreting NGF and improve the cognitive impairments [Chen KS;Gage FH, 1995]. The Administration of NGF by intracerebroventricular infusion or the transplantation of NGF-secreting cells to the basal forebrain improves spatial memory in aged animals [Klein RL et al., 2000]. Tuszynski implanted autologous fibroblasts genetically modified to express human NGF into the forebrain of patient with Alzheimer's disease. After a mean follow-up of six subjects after 22 months, no long-term adverse effects of NGF occurred and increases in cortical 18-fluorodeoxyglucose after treatment, impeded the rate of cognitive decline [Tuszynski MH et al., 2005].

Transplanting transferring BDNF gene cells into striate could protect the striatal neurons [Bemelmans AP et al., 1999; Frim DM et al., 1994; Galpern WR et al., 1996]. Transplanting fibroblasts genetically engineered to produce BDNF into a spinal cord could help axonal regeneration and significant recovery of forelimb usage [Liu Y et al., 1999]; could reverse chronic neuropathic pain after unilateral chronic constriction injury (CCI) of the sciatic nerve [Eaton MJ et al., 2002]; improve hind-limb function in the adult rats of injured spinal cord [Blits Bet al, 2003].

Ruitenberg combined olfactory ensheathing glia (OEG) implantation with neurotrophin gene therapy, which not only resulted in promoting axonal outgrowth but could also lead to enhance recovery after injury [Ruitenberg MJ et al., 2003]. The transfer of GDNF genes into the red nucleus following spinal axotomy could counteract atrophy in both the acute and chronic stages after injury [RuitenbergMJ et al., 2004]. After human mesenchymal stromal cells (hMSCs) were transplanted intomuscle of ALS rats,they could survive within the muscle, release GDNF, and significantly increase the number of neuromuscular connections and motor neuron cell bodies in the spinal cord at mid-stages of the disease,potentialy increasing the overall lifespan of experimental ALS rats[SuzukiM et al., 2008].GDNF gene therapy could also induce the Parkinson model animal to express greater dopamine levels in the striatum with the intention of improving behavioural recovery [Wang Let al.,2002].

## 2.3. Genetically engineering cells expressing enzymes

Intracerebral gene therapy has been investigated in an attempt to reverse various neurodegenerative diseases. For example, a faulty lysosomal arylsulfatase A gene leads to an accumulation of sulfatides in brain oligodendrocytes, resulting in metachromatic leukodystrophy (MLD) a lethal neurodegenerative disease. The administration of vectors containing a correct ARSA gene hasbeen shown to reduce sulfatides in mice [Kawabata K et al., 2006; Piguet Fet al., 2012; Sevin C et al., 2006]. Such treatment approaches may serve to significantly improve neurologic symptoms in several intracerebral neurodegenerative diseases [Matzner U et al., 2001;Colle MA et al., 2010].

## 2.4. Gene Silencing

Gene silencing is considered as a gene knockdown mechanism since the methods used to silence genes, such as RNA interference (RNAi), generally reduce the expression of a gene by at least 70% but do not completely eliminate it.

Various laboratories have conducted a large number of tests of CNS restoration with RNAi. The Nogo-66 receptor (NgR) may be related to the formation of tangles in AD, and NgRis believed to contribute to the inhibitory activities of axon regeneration after injury[Zhu HY et al.,2007].Nogo-A gene plays a central role in the inhibition of axonal regeneration after optic nerve injury[Su Y et al.,2006].

RNAi-mediated silencing of SOD1 allows long-term reduction in gene expression by intraspinal injection and substantially retards both the onset and the progression rate of the disease and protects against ALS in mouse model[Burton A,2005].Conversely,Towne found intravenous delivery of recombinant adeno-associated virus (rAAV) did not influence the course of ALS in familial models, providing compelling evidence that SOD1-mediated damage within skeletal muscles does not contribute to the death of motor neurons in ALS[Towne C et al., 2008].

## 2.5. Antibody

Nogo-A is a myelin-associated neurite outgrowth inhibitory protein that limits the recovery and plasticity after CNS injury. Intracerebral IN-1 by neutralization of myelin-associated neurite growth inhibitors could help massive sprouting at the lesion site, and fine axons and fascicles could increase to 7-11 mm caudal to the lesion within 2-3 weeks [SchnellL; Schwab ME, 1990]. Intrathecal anti-Nogo-A antibodies in the SCI model could improve the axonal regeneration and motor function recovery [Liebscher T et al., 2005; Atalay B et al.,2007; Freund Pet al., 2007]. Combined treatment with anti-Nogo-A and chondroitinase ABC is more effective than single treatments for enhancing functional recovery after spinal cord injury [Zhao RR et al., 2013b]. The infusion of Anti-Nogo antibodies 24 hours after an induced experimental stroke could potentially improve the behavioural outcome in rats [Wiessner C et al., 2003].

NgR plays a key role in the failure of axonal regeneration in the adult mammalian CNS.The anti-NgR1 antibodies neutralized CNS myelin-dependent inhibition of neurite outgrowth, promoted axonal regeneration, and promoted functional recovery after spinal cord injury [GrandPré T et al.,2002]. Immunization with recombinant NgR promoted axonal regeneration and recovery of function after spinal cord injury in rats [Yu P et al.,2008].

The basic researchers took the initiative to provide means of neutralizing the inhibitory effect of Nogo-A and demonstrated enhanced fiber growth, regeneration and functional recovery in both rodent and primate models [BuchliAD et al.,2007].

Until now most bioengineering tests for neurorestoration remain at the experimental phase. The improved and consistent manufacture of niche scaffolds, confidence in cell cues and the restoration of function in disease models are required to move experimental research into translational studies.

# 3. Encapsulation of Genetically Engineered Cells by Tissue Engineering and Bioengineering

***Osamu Kano and Hongyun Huang***

Encapsulated cell technology has the potential to treat many diseases. The controlled and continuous production and delivery of therapeutic agents to the host by immune-isolated cells is proposed as a valuable and cost-effective therapy. The encapsulation of cells with a semi-permeable membrane reduces surveillance by the immune system while permitting the beneficial exchange of small molecules and proteins. This method was first described by Chang TM 1964, and showed that artificial microcapsules of the same dimensions and properties could be produced in large numbers with relative ease. In addition, the enzymes and proteins loaded into such capsules maintained a viable biological activity in both *in-vitro* and *in-vivo* [Chang TM, 1964]. Since the publication of this key paper, numerous studies have been conducted to perfect the process of microencapsulation. It is now possible to determine the size of the capsule, the stability of the interface, and semi-permeable membrane. Encapsulated cells have four important features; capsule permeability, capsule mechanical properties, immune protection, and biocompatibility. As the therapeutic product (protein, peptide, or antibody) within a semipermeable membrane provides a physical barrier to mask the implant from immune surveillance at a local level without the need for systemic immunosuppression; this serves to achieve a successful implantation and therapeutic function [Acarregui A et al., 2012].

Sagot Y used polymer encapsulated cell lines that were genetically engineered to release CNTF for amyotrophic lateral sclerosis in the murine animal model [Sagot Y et al., 1995]. The results suggested a reduction of the progressive motor neuronopathy. Emerich DF implanted polymer-encapsulated fibroblasts that were genetically modified to secrete human CNTF for the monkey -- nonhuman primate model of Huntington's disease, in which human CNTF exerted a significant neuroprotective effect on striated cells. This prevented the retrograde atrophy of motor cortex neurons [Emerich DF et al., 1997]. A pilot clinical trial using implants of encapsulated genetically modified BHK cells was conducted on 6 patients with Huntington's disease. These encapsulated cells contained a modifiedCNTF gene, allowing the implanted capsules to secrete and deliver CNTF directly to their target site of implantation [Bachoud-Lévi AC et al., 2000]. This trial further demonstrated promising safety data, feasibility, and tolerability for these encapsulated cells after 2 years [Bloch J et al., 2004].

Studies of encapsulated cell transplantation have also shown some benefits in animal models of traumatic brain injury [Heile AM et al., 2009]. Encapsulated transduced cells with secreted arylsulfatase A (ARSA) have shown potential as a new therapeutic strategy for the treatment of MLD [Lagranha VL et al., 2008]. In a murine model of MLD, the subcutaneous implantation were retrieved after 1 month and were shown to release hARSA at rates similar to unencapsulated cells and contained well preserved myoblasts. This demonstrated that the encapsulation of genetically modified cells is able to maintain stable transgene expression and long-term cell viability *in-vivo* [Consiglio A et al., 2007].

Fjord-Larsen transplanted encapsulated cells that secreted NGF into the basal forebrains of Göttingen minipigs [Fjord-Larsen L et al., 2010], and later, Wahlberg et al transplanted NGF-producing, genetically engineered encapsulated human cells into the basal forebrain of patients with AD via stereotaxis. The implantation procedure in AD patients was reported as safe, well tolerated and proposed as a feasible treatment for the cognitive decline in patients with cerebral neurodegeneration. In patients at 12 months, persistent NGF secretion was still detected in half of the patients [Wahlberg LU et al., 2012; Eriksdotter-Jönhagen M et al., 2012].

Cells with higher NGF production have been reported to exhibit a greater potency in preclinical experimental models [Fjord-Larsen L et al., 2012], suggesting a viable treatment for neuro-regeneration.

# References


Acarregui, A; Murua, A; Pedraz, JL; Orive, G; Hernández, RM. A perspective on bioactive cell microencapsulation. *BioDrugs*. 2012;26(5):283-301.

Atalay, B; Bavbek, M; Cekinmez, M; Ozen, O; Nacar, A Karabay, G; Gulsen, S. Antibodies neutralizing Nogo-A increase pan-cadherin expression and motor recovery following spinal cord injury in rats. *Spinal Cord.* 2007;45(12):780-6

Ayres, C; Bowlin, GL; Henderson, SC et al. Modulation of anisotropy in electrospun tissue-engineering scaffolds: Analysis of fiber alignment by the fast Fourier transform. *Biomaterials.* 2006;27:5524-34.

Ayres, CE; Bowlin, GL; Pizinger, R et al. Incremental changes in anisotropy induce incremental changes in the material properties of electrospun scaffolds. *Acta Biomater.* 2007;3:651-61.

Ayres, CE; Jha, BS; Sell, SA et al. Nanotechnology in the design of soft tissue scaffolds: innovations in structure and function. *Wiley Interdiscip Rev Nanomed Nanobiotechnol.* 2010;2:20-34.

Bachoud-Lévi, AC; Déglon, N; Nguyen, JP; Bloch, J; Bourdet, C; Winkel, L; Rémy, P; Goddard, M; Lefaucheur, JP; Brugières, P; Baudic, S; Cesaro, P; Peschanski, M; Aebischer, P. Neuroprotective gene therapy for Huntington's disease using a polymer encapsulated BHK cell line engineered to secrete human CNTF. *Hum. Gene Ther.* 2000;11(12): 1723-9.

Banerjee, A; Arha, M; Choudhary, S et al. The influence of hydrogel modulus on the proliferation and differentiation of encapsulated neural stem cells. *Biomaterials.* 2009;30:4695-9.

Barnes, CP; Pemble, CW; Brand, DD et al. Cross-linking electrospun type II collagen tissue engineering scaffolds with carbodiimide in ethanol. *Tissue Eng.* 2007a;13:1593-605.

Barnes, CP; Sell, SA; Boland, ED et al. Nanofiber technology: designing the next generation of tissue engineering scaffolds. *Adv. Drug Deliv. Rev.* 2007b;59:1413-33.

Bemelmans, AP; Horellou, P; Pradier, L; Brunet, I; Colin, P; Mallet, J. Brain-derived neurotrophic factor-mediated protection of striatal neurons in an excitotoxic rat model of Huntington's disease, as demonstrated by adenoviral gene transfer. *Hum. Gene Ther.* 1999;10(18):2987-97.

Benoit, DS; Anseth, KS. The effect on osteoblast function of colocalized RGD and PHSRN epitopes on PEG surfaces. *Biomaterials.*2005;26:5209-20.

Bible, E; Chau, DY; Alexander, MR et al. The support of neural stem cells transplanted into stroke-induced brain cavities by PLGA particles. *Biomaterials.* 2009;30:2985-94.

Blits, B; Oudega, M; Boer, GJ; Bartlett Bunge, M; Verhaagen, J. Adeno-associated viral vector-mediated neurotrophin gene transfer in the injured adult rat spinal cord improves hind-limb function. *Neuroscience.* 2003;118(1):271-81.

Bloch, J; Bachoud-Lévi, AC; Déglon, N; Lefaucheur, JP; Winkel, L; Palfi, S; Nguyen, JP; Bourdet, C; Gaura, V; Remy, P; Brugières, P; Boisse, MF; Baudic, S; Cesaro, P; Hantraye, P; Aebischer, P; Peschanski, M. Neuroprotective gene therapy for Huntington's disease, using polymer-encapsulated cells engineered to secrete human ciliary neurotrophic factor: results of a phase I study. *Hum. Gene Ther.* 2004;15(10):968-75.

Bokara, KK1; Kim, JY; Lee, YI; Yun, K; Webster, TJ; Lee, JE.Biocompatability of carbon nanotubes with stem cells to treat CNS injuries. *Anat. Cell Biol.* 2013;46(2):85-92.

Boland, ED; Matthews, JA; Pawlowski, KJ et al. Electrospinning collagen and elastin: preliminary vascular tissue engineering. *Front Biosci.* 2004;9:1422-32.

Boland, T; Xu, T; Damon, B; Cui, X. Application of inkjet printing to tissueengineering. *Biotechnol. J.*2006;1: 910–917.

Borden, M; Attawia, M; Khan, Y et al. Tissue-engineered bone formation in vivo using a novel sintered polymeric microsphere matrix. *J. Bone Joint. Surg. Br.* 2004;86:1200-8.

Buchli, AD; Rouiller, E; Mueller, R; Dietz, V; Schwab, ME.Repair of the injured spinal cord. A joint approach of basic and clinical research. *Neurodegener Dis.* 2007;4(1):51-6

Burton, A. RNA interference protects against ALS in mouse model. *Lancet Neurol.* 2005;4(5):274-5.

Buzanska, L; Ruiz, A; Zychowicz, M et al. Patterned growth and differentiation of human cord blood-derived neural stem cells on bio-functionalized surfaces. *Acta Neurobiol. Exp.*(Wars ). 2009;69:24-36.

Buzanska, L; Zychowicz, M; Ruiz, A et al. Neural stem cells from human cord blood on bioengineered surfaces--novel approach to multiparameter bio-tests. *Toxicology.*2010; 270:35-42.

Byers, BA; Guldberg, RE; Hutmacher, DW et al. Effects of Runx2 genetic engineering and in vitro maturation of tissue-engineered constructs on the repair of critical size bone defects. *J. Biomed. Mater. Res.*A. 2006;76:646-55.

Cai, H; Azangwe, G; Shepherd, DE. Skin cell culture on an ear-shaped scaffold created by fused deposition modelling. *Biomed. Mater Eng.* 2005;15:375-80.

Cao, Y; Zhang, B; Croll, T et al. Engineering tissue tubes using novel multilayered scaffolds in the rat peritoneal cavity. *J. Biomed. Mater Res.* A. 2008;87:719-27.

Carrico, IS; Maskarinec, SA; Heilshorn, SC et al. Lithographic patterning of photoreactive cell-adhesive proteins. *J. Am. Chem. Soc.* 2007;129:4874-5.

Carvalho, JL; de Carvalho, PH; Gomes, DA; de Goes, AM. Innovative Strategies for Tissue Engineering. InTech.2014. Available from: http://dx.doi.org/10. 5772/53337.

Chang, TM. Semipermeable Microcapsules. *Science.* 1964;146:524-5.

Cheah, CM; Chua, CK; Leong, KF et al. Automatic algorithm for generating complex polyhedral scaffold structures for tissue engineering. *Tissue Eng.* 2004;10:595-610.

Chen, KS; Gage, FH. Somatic gene transfer of NGF to the aged brain: behavioral and morphological amelioration. *J. Neurosci.*1995;15(4):2819-25.

Chu, PK. Plasma-surface modification of biomaterials. Materials Science and Engineering. 2000; 36:143-206.

Claeyssens, F; Hasan, EA; Gaidukeviciute, A et al. Three-Dimensional Biodegradable Structures Fabricated by Two-Photon Polymerization. *Langmuir.* 2009;*25* (5):3219–3223.

Colle, MA Piguet, F; Bertrand, L; Raoul, S; Bieche, I; Dubreil, L; Sloothaak, D; Bouquet, C; Moullier, P; Aubourg, P; Cherel, Y; Cartier, N; Sevin, C. Efficient intracerebral delivery of AAV5 vector encoding human ARSA in non-human primate. *Hum. Mol. Genet.* 2010; 19 (1):147-58.

Consiglio, A; Martino, S; Dolcetta, D; Cusella, G; Conese, M; Marchesini, S; Benaglia, G; Wrabetz, L; Orlacchio, A; Déglon, N; Aebischer, P; Severini, GM;Bordignon, C. Metabolic correction in oligodendrocytes derived from metachromatic leukodystrophy mouse model by using encapsulated recombinant myoblasts. *J. Neurol. Sci.* 2007;255 (1-2):7-16.

Cooke, MN; Fisher, JP; Dean, D et al. Use of stereolithography to manufacture critical-sized 3D biodegradable scaffolds for bone ingrowth. *J. Biomed. Mater Res. B Appl. Biomater.* 2003;64:65-9.

Croll, TI; O'Connor, AJ; Stevens, GW et al. Controllable surface modification of poly(lactic-co-glycolic acid) (PLGA) by hydrolysis or aminolysis I: physical, chemical, and theoretical aspects. *Biomacromolecules.* 2004;5:463-73.

Curodeau, A; Sachs, E; Caldarise, S. Design and fabrication of cast orthopedic implants with freeform surface textures from 3-D printed ceramic shell. *J. Biomed. Mater Res.*2000; 53:525-35.

Darling, AL; Sun, W. 3D microtomographic characterization of precision extruded poly-epsilon-caprolactone scaffolds. *J. Biomed. Mater Res. B Appl. Biomater.* 2004;70:311-7.

Dhariwala, B; Hunt, E; Boland, T. Rapid prototyping of tissue-engineering constructs, using photopolymerizable hydrogels and stereolithography. *Tissue Eng.* 2004;10:1316-22.

Eaton, MJ; Blits, B; Ruitenberg, MJ; Verhaagen, J; Oudega, M. Amelioration of chronic neuropathic pain after partial nerve injury by adeno-associated viral (AAV) vector-mediated over-expression of BDNF in the rat spinal cord. *Gene Ther.* 2002;9 (20): 1387-95.

Emerich, DF; Winn, SR; Hantraye, PM; Peschanski, M; Chen, EY; Chu, Y; McDermott, P; Baetge, EE; Kordower, JH. Protective effect of encapsulated cells producing neurotrophic factor CNTF in a monkey model of Huntington's disease. *Nature.* 1997 ;386(6623):395-9.

Eriksdotter-Jönhagen, M; Linderoth, B; Lind, G; Aladellie, L; Almkvist, O; Andreasen, N; Blennow, K; Bogdanovic, N; Jelic, V; Kadir, A; Nordberg, A; Sundström, E; Wahlund, LO; Wall, A; Wiberg, M; Winblad, B; Seiger, A; Almqvist, P; Wahlberg, L. Encapsulated cell biodelivery of nerve growth factor to the Basal forebrain in patients with Alzheimer's disease. *Dement. Geriatr. Cogn. Disord.* 2012;33(1):18-28.

Fan, VH; Tamama, K; Au, A et al. Tethered epidermal growth factor provides a survival advantage to mesenchymal stem cells. *Stem. Cells.* 2007;25:1241-51.

Fang, Y; Frampton, JP; Raghavan, S; Sabahi-Kaviani, R; Luker, G; Deng, CX; Takayama, S et al. Rapid generation of multiplexed cell cocultures using acoustic droplet ejection followed by aqueous two-phaseexclusion patterning. *Tissue Eng.*2012; Part C: Methods 18, 647–657.

Fjord-Larsen, L; Kusk, P; Emerich, DF; Thans, C; Torp, M; Bintz, B; Tornøe, J; Johnsen, AH; Wahlberg, LU. Increased encapsuolated cell biodelivery of nerve growth factor in the brain by transposon-mediated gene transfer. *Gene Ther.* 2012;19:1010-7.

Fjord-Larsen, L; Kusk, P; Tornøe, J; Juliusson, B; Torp, M; Bjarkam, CR; Nielsen, MS; Handberg, A; Sørensen, JC; Wahlberg, LU. Long-term delivery of nerve growth factor by encapsulated cell biodelivery in the Göttingen minipig basal forebrain. *Mol. Ther.* 2010; 18(12):2164-72.

Freund, P; Wannier, T; Schmidlin, E; Bloch, J; Mir, A; Schwab, ME; Rouiller, EM. Anti-Nogo-A antibody treatment enhances sprouting of corticospinal axons rostral to a unilateral cervical spinal cord lesion in adult macaque monkey. *J. Comp. Neurol.* 2007; 502(4):644-59.

Frim, DM; Simpson, J; Uhler, TA; Short, MP; Bossi, SR; Breakefield, XO; Isacson, O. Striatal degeneration induced by mitochondrial blockade is prevented by biologically delivered NGF. *J. Neurosci. Res.*1993;35(4):452-8.

Frim, DM; Uhler, TA; Galpern, WR; Beal, MF, Breakefield, XO; Isacson, O. Implanted fibroblasts genetically engineered to produce brain-derived neurotrophic factor prevent 1-methyl-4-phenylpyridinium toxicity to dopaminergic neurons in the rat. *Proc. Natl. Acad. Sci. USA.*1994;91(11):5104-8.

Fromstein, JD; Zandstra, PW; Alperin, C et al. Seeding bioreactor-produced embryonic stem cell-derived cardiomyocytes on different porous, degradable, polyurethane scaffolds reveals the effect of scaffold architecture on cell morphology. *Tissue Eng. Part A.*2008;14:369-78.

Fussell, GW; Cooper, SL. Synthesis and characterization of acrylic terpolymers with RGD peptides for biomedical applications. *Biomaterials.*2004;25:2971-8.

Galpern, WR; Frim, DM; Tatter, SB; Altar, CA; Beal, MF; Isacson, O. Cell-mediated delivery of brain-derived neurotrophic factor enhances dopamine levels in an MPP+ rat model of substantia nigra degeneration. *Cell Transplant.*1996;5(2):225-32.

Gelain, F; Unsworth, LD; Zhang, S. Slow and sustained release of active cytokines from self-assembling peptide scaffolds. *J. Control. Release.*2010;145:231-9.

Genetics Home Reference. What is gene therapy? June 30, 2014. Available from: http://ghr.nlm.nih.gov/handbook/therapy/genetherapy.

Giordano, RA. Wu, BM. Borland, SW et al. Mechanical properties of dense polylactic acid structures fabricated by three dimensional printing. *J. Biomater. Sci. Polym. Ed.* 1996;8:63-75.

Gomez, N. Lu, Y. Chen, S et al. Immobilized nerve growth factor and microtopography have distinct effects on polarization versus axon elongation in hippocampal cells in culture. *Biomaterials.* 2007;28:271-84.

GrandPré, T; Li, S; Strittmatter, SM. Nogo-66 receptor antagonist peptide promotes axonal regeneration. *Nature.* 2002 ;417(6888):547-51.

Grayson, WL; Martens, TP; Eng, GM et al. Biomimetic approach to tissue engineering. *Semin. Cell Dev. Biol.* 2009;20:665-73.

Guan, J; Zhu, Z; Zhao, RC; Xiao, Z; Wu, C; Han, Q; Chen, L; Tong, W; Zhang, J; Han, Q; Gao, J; Feng, M; Bao, X; Dai, J; Wang, R. Transplantation of human mesenchymal stem cells loaded on collagen scaffolds for the treatment of traumatic brain injury in rats. *Biomaterials.* 2013;34(24):5937-46.

Harrington, DA; Cheng, EY; Guler, MO et al. Branched peptide-amphiphiles as self-assembling coatings for tissue engineering scaffolds. *J. Biomed. Mater Res. A.*2006;78:157-67.

Heile, AM; Wallrapp, C; Klinge, PM; Samii, A; Kassem, M; Silverberg, G;Brinker, T. Cerebral transplantation of encapsulated mesenchymal stem cells improves cellular pathology after experimental traumatic brain injury. *Neurosci. Lett.* 2009;463: 176-181.

Holmes, TC; de LS, Su, X et al. Extensive neurite outgrowth and active synapse formation on self-assembling peptide scaffolds. *Proc. Natl. Acad. Sci. USA.* 2000;97: 6728-33.

Hosseinkhani, H; Hosseinkhani, M; Kobayashi, H. Proliferation and differentiation of mesenchymal stem cells using self-assembled peptide amphiphile nanofibers. *Biomed. Mater.*2006;1:8-15.

Huang, YX; Ren, J; Chen, C et al. Preparation and properties of poly(lactide-co-glycolide) (PLGA)/ nano-hydroxyapatite (NHA) scaffolds by thermally induced phase separation and rabbit MSCs culture on scaffolds. *J. Biomater. Appl.* 2008;22:409-32.

Hutmacher, DW; Schantz, T; Zein, I et al. Mechanical properties and cell cultural response of polycaprolactone scaffolds designed and fabricated via fused deposition modelling. *J. Biomed. Mater. Res.*2001;55:203-16.

Ilkhanizadeh, S; Teixeira, AI; Hermanson, O. Inkjet printing of macromolecules on hydrogels to steer neural stem cell differentiation. *Biomaterials* 2007 ;28(27):3936-43.

Jacobs, MA. Foam processing of poly(ethylene-co-vinyl acetate) rubber using supercritical carbon dioxide. Kemmere, M. F. and Keurentjes, *J. T. F. Polymer.* 2004; 45:7539.

Jiao, YP; Cui, FZ. Surface modification of polyester biomaterials for tissue engineering. *Biomed. Mater.*2007;2:24-37.

Kalita, SJ; Bose, S; Hosick, HL et al. CaO--P2O5--Na2O-based sintering additives for hydroxyapatite (HAp) ceramics. *Biomaterials.* 2004;25:2331-9.

Kawabata, K; Migita, M; Mochizuki, H; Miyake, K; Igarashi, T; Fukunaga, Y; Shimada, T. Ex vivo cell-mediated gene therapy for metachromatic leukodystrophy using neurospheres. *Brain Res.* 2006;1094(1):13-23.

Khang, D; Carpenter, J; Chun, YW et al. Nanotechnology for regenerative medicine. *Biomed. Microdevices.* 2010;12:575-87.

Kisiday, J; Jin, M; Kurz, B et al. Self-assembling peptide hydrogel fosters chondrocyte extracellular matrix production and cell division: implications for cartilage tissue repair. *Proc. Natl. Acad. Sci. USA*. 2002;99:9996-10001.

Klein, RL; Hirko, AC; Meyers, CA; Grimes, JR; Muzyczka, N; Meyer, EM. NGF gene transfer to intrinsic basal forebrain neurons increases cholinergic cell size and protects from age-related, spatial memory deficits in middle-aged rats. *Brain Res.* 2000;875(1-2):144-5.

Lagranha, VL; Baldo, G; de Carvalho, TG; Burin, M;Saraiva-Pereira, ML; Matte, U; Giugliani, R. In vitro correction of ARSA deficiency in human skin fibroblasts from metachromatic leukodystrophy patients after treatment with microencapsulated recombinant cells. *Metab. Brain Dis.* 2008;23:469-84.

Leach, JB; Achyuta, AK; Murthy, SK. Bridging the Divide between Neuroprosthetic Design, Tissue Engineering and Neurobiology. *Front Neuroengineering*. 2010;2:18.

Lee, KW; Wang, S; Fox, BC et al. Poly(propylene fumarate) bone tissue engineering scaffold fabrication using stereolithography: effects of resin formulations and laser parameters. *Biomacromolecules*. 2007;8:1077-84.

Lee, MR; Kwon, KW; Jung, H et al. Direct differentiation of human embryonic stem cells into selective neurons on nanoscale ridge/groove pattern arrays. *Biomaterials.*2010; 31:4360-6.

Leipzig, ND; Wylie, RG; Kim, H et al. Differentiation of neural stem cells in three-dimensional growth factor-immobilized chitosan hydrogel scaffolds. *Biomaterials.* 2011;32:57-64.

Leong, KF; Cheah, CM; Chua, CK. Solid freeform fabrication of three-dimensional scaffolds for engineering replacement tissues and organs. *Biomaterials.* 2003;24:2363-78.

Liebscher, T; Schnell, L; Schnell, D; Scholl, J; Schneider, R; Gullo, M; Fouad, K; Mir, A; Rausch, M; Kindler, D; Hamers, FP; Schwab, ME. Nogo-A antibody improves regeneration and locomotion of spinal cord-injured rats. *Ann. Neurol.* 2005;58(5):706-19.

Liu, J; Zhang; Z; Gong; A et al. Neuronal progenitor cells seeded in fibrin gel differentiate into ChAT-positive neuron. *In Vitro Cell Dev. Biol. Anim.* 2010;46:738-45.

Liu, J; Chen, Q; Zhang, Z; Zheng, Y; Sun, X; Cao, X; Gong, A; Cui, Y He, Q; Jiang, P. Fibrin scaffolds containing ectomesenchymal stem cells enhance behavioural and histological improvement in a rat model of spinal cord injury. *Cells Tissues Organs. 2013*;198(1):35-46.

Liu, X; Won, Y; Ma, PX. Porogen-induced surface modification of nano-fibrous poly (l-lactic acid) scaffolds for tissue engineering. *Biomaterials.*2006;27(21):3980-7.

Liu, X; Won, Y; Ma, PX. Surface modification of interconnected porous scaffolds. *J. Biomed. Mater. Res. A.*2005;74(1):84-91.

Liu, Y; Kim, D; Himes, BT; Chow, SY; Schallert, T; Murray, M; Tessler, A; Fischer, I. Transplants of fibroblasts genetically modified to express BDNF promote regeneration of adult rat rubrospinal axons and recovery of forelimb function. *J. Neurosci.* 1999; 19(11):4370-87.

Lutolf, MP; Gilbert, PM; Blau, HM. Designing materials to direct stem-cell fate. *Nature.* 2009;462:433-41.

Lutolf, MP; Hubbell, JA. Synthetic biomaterials as instructive extracellular microenvironments for morphogenesis in tissue engineering. *Nat. Biotechnol.* 2005;23: 47-55.

Ma, F; Xiao, Z; Chen, B; Hou, X; Han, J; Zhao, Y; Dai, J; Xu, R. Accelerating proliferation of neural stem/progenitor cells in collagen sponges immobilized with engineered basic fibroblast growth factor for nervous system tissue engineering. *Biomacromolecules.* 2014;15(3):1062-8.

Ma, Z; Kotaki, M; Inai, R et al. Potential of nanofiber matrix as tissue-engineering scaffolds. *Tissue Eng.* 2005;11:101-9.

Martín-López, E; Darder, M; Ruiz-Hitzky, E; Nieto Sampedro, M. Agar-based bridges as biocompatible candidates to provide guide cues in spinal cord injury repair. *Biomed. Mater. Eng.* 2013;23(5):405-21.

Martino, MM; Mochizuki, M; Rothenfluh, DA et al. Controlling integrin specificity and stem cell differentiation in 2D and 3D environments through regulation of fibronectin domain stability. *Biomaterials.* 2009;30:1089-97.

Matthews, JA; Wnek, GE; Simpson, DG et al. Electrospinning of collagen nanofibers. *Biomacromolecules.*2002;3:232-8.

Matzner, U; Schestag, F; Hartmann, D; Lüllmann-Rauch, R; D'Hooge, R; De Deyn, PP; Gieselmann, V. Bone marrow stem cell gene therapy of arylsulfatase A-deficient mice, using an arylsulfatase A mutant that is hypersecreted from retrovirally transduced donor-type cells. *Hum. Gene Ther.* 2001;12(9):1021-33.

Mironov, V. Printing technology to produce living tissue. *Expert. Opin. Biol. Ther.*2003; 3:701-4.

Mironov, V; Boland, T; Trusk, T et al. Organ printing: computer-aided jet-based 3D tissue engineering. *Trends Biotechnol.* 2003;21:157-61.

Moon, S; Hasan, SK; Song, YS; Xu, F; Keles, HO; Manzur, F; Mikkilineni, S et al. Layer by layer three-dimensional tissue epitaxyby cell-laden hydrogel droplets. *Tissue Eng.*2010; Part C: Methods 16, 157–166.

Nahmias, Y; Schwartz, RE; Verfaillie, CM; Odde, DJ. Laser-guided direct writing for threedimensionaltissue engineering. *Biotechnol. Bioeng.*2005; 92: 129–136.

Nair, LS; Bhattacharyya, S; Bender, JD et al. Fabrication and optimization of methylphenoxy substituted polyphosphazene nanofibers for biomedical applications. *Biomacromolecules*2004;5:2212-20.

Nakamura, M; Kobayashi, A; Takagi, F; Watanabe, A; Hiruma, Y et al. Biocompatible inkjet printing technique fordesigned seeding of individual living cells. *Tissue Eng.*2005; 11: 1658–1666.

Newman, KD; McBurney, MW. Poly(D,L lactic-co-glycolic acid) microspheres as biodegradable microcarriers for pluripotent stem cells. *Biomaterials.* 2004;25:5763-71.

Nitschke, M; Schmack, G; Janke, A et al. Low pressure plasma treatment of poly (3-hydroxybutyrate): toward tailored polymer surfaces for tissue engineering scaffolds. *J. Biomed. Mater. Res.*2002;59(4):632-8.

Ouyang, Y; Huang, C; Zhu, Y; Fan, C; Ke, Q. Fabrication of seamless electrospun collagen/PLGA conduits whose walls comprise highly longitudinal aligned nanofibers for nerve regeneration. *J. Biomed. Nanotechnol.*2013;9(6):931-43.

Peltola, SM; Melchels, FP; Grijpma, DW et al. A review of rapid prototyping techniques for tissue engineering purposes. *Ann. Med.* 2008;40:268-80.

Phadke, A; Zhang, C; Hwang, Y et al. Templated mineralization of synthetic hydrogels for bone-like composite materials: role of matrix hydrophobicity. *Biomacromolecules.* 2010;11:2060-8.

Pham, QP; Sharma, U; Mikos, AG. Electrospun poly(epsilon-caprolactone) microfiber and multilayer nanofiber/microfiber scaffolds: characterization of scaffolds and measurement of cellular infiltration. *Biomacromolecules.* 2006;7:2796-805.

Piguet, F; Sondhi, D; Piraud, M; Fouquet, F; Hackett, NR; Ahouansou, O; Vanier, MT; Bieche, I; Aubourg, P; Crystal, RG; Cartier, N; Sevin, C. Correction of brain oligodendrocytes by AAVrh.10 intracerebral gene therapy in metachromatic leukodystrophy mice. *Hum. Gene Ther.* 2012;23(8):903-14.

Rao, SS; Winter, JO. Adhesion molecule-modified biomaterials for neural tissue engineering. *Front Neuroengineering.* 2009;2:6-9.

Recknor, JB; Sakaguchi, DS; Mallapragada, SK. Directed growth and selective differentiation of neural progenitor cells on micropatterned polymer substrates. *Biomaterials.* 2006;27:4098-108.

Reid, AJ1; de Luca, AC; Faroni, A; Downes, S; Sun, M; Terenghi, G; Kingham, PJ. Long term peripheral nerve regeneration using a novel PCL nerve conduit. *Neurosci. Lett.* 2013;544:125-30.

Ren, K; Wang, Y; Ji, J et al. Construction and deconstruction of PLL/DNA multilayered films for DNA delivery: effect of ionic strength. *Colloids Surf. B Biointerfaces.* 2005;46:63-9.

Rezwan, K; Chen, QZ; Blaker, JJ et al. Biodegradable and bioactive porous polymer/inorganic composite scaffolds for bone tissue engineering. *Biomaterials.* 2006;27:3413-31.

Rimell, JT; Marquis, PM. Selective laser sintering of ultra high molecular weight polyethylene for clinical applications. *J. Biomed. Mater. Res.* 2000;53:414-20.

Rosenberg, MB; Friedmann, T; Robertson, RC; Tuszynski, M; Wolff, JA; Breakefield, XO; Gage, FH. Grafting genetically modified cells to the damaged brain: restorative effects of NGF expression. *Science.* 1988;242(4885):1575-8.

Ruhe, PQ; Hedberg, EL; Padron, NT et al. Biocompatibility and degradation of poly(DL-lactic-co-glycolic acid)/calcium phosphate cement composites. *J. Biomed. Mater. Res. A.*2005;74:533-44.

Ruitenberg, MJ; Blits, B; Dijkhuizen, PA; te Beek, ET; Bakker, A; van Heerikhuize, JJ; Pool, CW; Hermens, WT; Boer, GJ; Verhaagen, J. Adeno-associated viral vector-mediated gene transfer of brain-derived neurotrophic factor reverses atrophy of rubrospinal neurons following both acute and chronic spinal cord injury. *Neurobiol. Dis.*2004;15(2):394-406.

Ruitenberg, MJ; Plant, GW; Hamers, FP; Wortel, J; Blits, B; Dijkhuizen, PA; Gispen, WH; Boer, GJ; Verhaagen, J. Ex vivo adenoviral vector-mediated neurotrophin gene transfer to olfactory ensheathing glia: effects on rubrospinal tract regeneration, lesion size, and functional recovery after implantation in the injured rat spinal cord. *J. Neurosci.* 2003;23(18):7045-58.

Ruoslahti, E. RGD and other recognition sequences for integrins. *Annu. Rev. Cell Dev. Biol.* 1996;12:697-715.:697-715.

Sagot, Y; Tan, SA; Baetge, E; Schmalbruch, H; Kato, AC; Aebischer, P. Polymer encapsulated cell lines genetically engineered to release ciliary neurotrophic factor can slow down progressive motor neuronopathy in the mouse. *Eur. J. Neurosci.* 1995;7(6):1313-22.

Schnell, L; Schwab, ME. Axonal regeneration in the rat spinal cord produced by an antibody against myelin-associated neurite growth inhibitors. *Nature.* 1990;343 (6255):269-72.

Schumacher, JM; Short, MP; Hyman, BT; Breakefield, XO; Isacson, O. Intracerebral implantation of nerve growth factor-producing fibroblasts protects striatum against neurotoxic levels of excitatory amino acids. *Neuroscience.* 1991;45(3):561-70

Schwartz, MA; DeSimone, DW. Cell adhesion receptors in mechanotransduction. *Curr. Opin. Cell Biol.*2008;20:551-6.

Seidlits, SK; Khaing, ZZ; Petersen, RR et al. The effects of hyaluronic acid hydrogels with tunable mechanical properties on neural progenitor cell differentiation. *Biomaterials.* 2010;31:3930-40.

Sell, SA; McClure, MJ; Barnes, CP et al. Electrospun polydioxanone-elastin blends: potential for bioresorbable vascular grafts. *Biomed. Mater.* 2006;1:72-80.

Semple, JL; Woolridge, N; Lumsden, CJ. In vitro, in vivo, in silico: computational systems in tissue engineering and regenerative medicine. *Tissue Eng.* 2005;11:341-56.

Sevin, C; Benraiss, A; Van Dam, D; Bonnin, D; Nagels, G; Verot, L; Laurendeau, I; Vidaud, M; Gieselmann, V; Vanier, M; De Deyn, PP; Aubourg, P; Cartier, N. Intracerebral adeno-associated virus-mediated gene transfer in rapidly progressive forms of metachromatic leukodystrophy. *Hum. Mol. Genet.* 2006;15(1):53-64.

Singh, L; Kumar, V; Ratner, BD. Generation of porous microcellular 85/15 poly (DL-lactide-co-glycolide) foams for biomedical applications. *Biomaterials.*2004;25:2611-7.

Stabenfeldt, SE. Engineering ECM Complexity into Biomaterials for Directing Cell Fate. *Tissue Engineering and Biomaterials.* 2010;2: 1-18.

Stendahl, JC; Wang, LJ; Chow, LW et al. Growth factor delivery from self-assembling nanofibers to facilitate islet transplantation. *Transplantation.* 2008;86:478-81.

Su, Y; Wang, F; Zhao, SG; Liu, P; Cui, H; Teng, Y. Axonal regeneration of retinal ganglion cells after optic nerve crush: experiment of Nogo-A knockout mice. *Zhonghua Yi Xue Za Zhi.* 2006;86(48):3409-13.

Sun, W; Lal, P. Recent development on computer aided tissue engineering--a review. *Comput Methods Programs Biomed.* 2002;67:85-103.

Sun, W; Yan, Y; Lin, F et al. Biomanufacturing: a US-China National Science Foundation-sponsored workshop. *Tissue Eng.* 2006;12:1169-81.

Suzuki, M; McHugh, J; Tork, C; Shelley, B; Hayes, A; Bellantuono, I; Aebischer, P; Svendsen, CN. Direct muscle delivery of GDNF with human mesenchymal stem cells improves motor neuron survival and function in a rat model of familial ALS. *Mol. Ther.* 2008;16(12):2002-10.

Tan, KH; Chua, CK; Leong, KF et al. Selective laser sintering of biocompatible polymers for applications in tissue engineering. *Biomed. Mater Eng.* 2005;15:113-24.

Tasoglu, S;Demirci, U. Bioprinting for stem cell research, *Trends in Biotechnology.* 2013; 31(1): 10-19.

Teo, EY; Ong, SY; Chong, MS et al. Polycaprolactone-based fused deposition modeled mesh for delivery of antibacterial agents to infected wounds. *Biomaterials.* 2011; 32:279-87.

Towne, C; Raoul, C; Schneider, BL; Aebischer, P. Systemic AAV6 delivery mediating RNA interference against SOD1: neuromuscular transduction does not alter disease progression in fALS mice. *Mol. Ther.*2008;16(6):1018-25.

Tuszynski, MH; Thal, L; Pay, M; Salmon, DP; U, HS; Bakay, R; Patel, P; Blesch, A; Vahlsing, HL; Ho, G; Tong, G; Potkin, SG; Fallon, J; Hansen, L; Mufson, EJ; Kordower, JH; Gall, C; Conner, J. A phase 1 clinical trial of nerve growth factor gene therapy for Alzheimer disease. *Nat. Med.* 2005;11(5):551-5.

Vasita, R; Katti, DS. Nanofibers and their applications in tissue engineering. *Int. J. Nanomedicine.* 2006;1(1):15-30.

Wahlberg, LU; Lind, G; Almqvist, PM; Kusk, P; Tornøe, J; Juliusson, B; Söderman, M; Selldén, E; Seiger, Å; Eriksdotter-Jönhagen, M; Linderoth, B. Targeted delivery of nerve growth factor via encapsulated cell biodelivery in Alzheimer disease: a technology platform for restorative neurosurgery. *J. Neurosurg.*2012;117(2):340-7.

Walker, PA; Aroom, KR; Jimenez, F et al. Advances in progenitor cell therapy using scaffolding constructs for central nervous system injury. *Stem. Cell Rev.* 2009;5:283-300.

Wang, G; Ao, Q; Gong, K et al. The effect of topology of chitosan biomaterials on the differentiation and proliferation of neural stem cells. *Acta Biomater.*2010;6:3630-9.

Wang, L; Muramatsu, S; Lu, Y; Ikeguchi, K; Fujimoto, K; Okada, T; Mizukami, H; Hanazono, Y; Kume, A; Urano, F; Ichinose, H; Nagatsu, T; Nakano, I; Ozawa, K. Delayed delivery of AAV-GDNF prevents nigral neurodegeneration and promotes functional recovery in a rat model of Parkinson's disease. *Gene Ther.*2002;9(6):381-9.

Wei, G; Ma, PX. Structure and properties of nano-hydroxyapatite/polymer composite scaffolds for bone tissue engineering. *Biomaterials.* 2004;25:4749-57.

Weigel, T; Schinkel, G; Lendlein, A. Design and preparation of polymeric scaffolds for tissue engineering. *Expert. Rev. Med. Devices.* 2006;3:835-51.

Wiessner, C; Bareyre, FM; Allegrini, PR; Mir, AK; Frentzel, S; Zurini, M; Schnell, L; Oertle, T; Schwab, ME. Anti-Nogo-A antibody infusion 24 hours after experimental stroke improved behavioural outcome and corticospinal plasticity in normotensive and spontaneously hypertensive rats. *J. Cereb Blood Flow Metab.* 2003;23(2):154-6.

Williams, DF. Definitions in Biomaterials, Progress in Biomedical Engineering. Vol 4. Amsterdam, *Elsevier Scientific.*1987; p24.

Williams, JM; Adewunmi, A; Schek, RM et al. Bone tissue engineering using polycaprolactone scaffolds fabricated via selective laser sintering. *Biomaterials.* 2005;26:4817-27.

Wong, W; Fletcher, DF; Traini, D et al. Particle aerosolisation and break-up in dry powder inhalers 1: evaluation and modelling of venturi effects for agglomerated systems. *Pharm. Res.* 2010;27:1367-76.

Xia, L; Wan, H; Hao, SY; Li, DZ; Chen, G; Gao, CC; Li, JH; Yang, F; Wang, SG; Liu, S. Co-transplantation of neural stem cells and Schwann cells within poly (L-lactic-co-glycolic acid) scaffolds facilitates axonal regeneration in hemisected rat spinal cord. *Chin. Med. J.*(Engl). 2013;126(5):909-17.

Yoon, JJ; Park, TG. Degradation behaviors of biodegradable macroporous scaffolds prepared by gas foaming of effervescent salts. *J. Biomed. Mater Res.*2001;55:401-8.

Yu, P; Huang, L; Zou, J; Yu, Z; Wang, Y; Wang, X; Xu, L; Liu, X; Xu, XM; Lu, PH. Immunization with recombinant Nogo-66 receptor (NgR) promotes axonal regeneration and recovery of function after spinal cord injury in rats. *Neurobiol. Dis.* 2008;32 (3):535-42.

Zhang, H; Hutmacher, DW; Chollet, F et al. Microrobotics and MEMS-based fabrication techniques for scaffold-based tissue engineering. *Macromol. Biosci.* 2005;5:477-89.

Zhang, S. Fabrication of novel biomaterials through molecular self-assembly. *Nat. Biotechnol.*2003;21:1171-8.

Zhang, Z; Melanie, J; Gupte, MJ; Ma, PX.Biomaterials and stem cells for tissue engineering Expert Opin. *Biol. Ther.*2013; 13(4).

Zhao, RR; Andrews, MR; Wang, D; Warren, P; Gullo, M; Schnell, L; Schwab, ME; Fawcett, JW. Combination treatment with anti-Nogo-A and chondroitinase ABC is more effective than single treatments at enhancing functional recovery after spinal cord injury. *Eur. J. Neurosci.* 2013b;38(6):2946-61.

Zhao, T; Yan, W; Xu, K; Qi, Y; Dai, X; Shi,Z. Combined treatment with platelet-rich plasma and brain-derived neurotrophic factor-overexpressing bone marrow stromal cells supports axonal remyelination in a rat spinal cord hemi-section model. *Cytotherapy.* 2013a;15(7):792-804.

Zhou, WY; Lee, SH; Wang, M et al. Selective laser sintering of porous tissue engineering scaffolds from poly(L: -lactide)/carbonated hydroxyapatite nanocomposite microspheres. *J. Mater. Sci. Mater. Med.* 2008;19:2535-40.

Zhu, HY; Guo, HF; Hou, HL; Liu, YJ; Sheng, SL; Zhou, JN. Increased expression of the Nogo receptor in the hippocampus and its relation to the neuropathology in Alzheimer's disease. *Hum. Pathol.* 2007;38(3):426-34.

In: Neurorestoratology, volume 1
Editors: H. Huang, G. Raisman, P. R. Sanberg et al.
ISBN: 978-1-63463-599-8


*Chapter 9*

# Neurorestorative Surgery

***Hongyun Huang****
Beijing Rehabilitation Hospital of Capital Medical University
Beijing Hongtianji Neuroscience Academy, China

## 1. Cordotomy or Myelotomy

Following spinal cord injury, the resulting spinal cord swelling and any sustained external pressure may block normal cerebrospinal fluid flow and further increase spinal cord edema. Dura decompression may limit the level of secondary injury in human and animal spinal cord injury (Perkins PG et al., 1988; Smith JS et al., 2010). Cordotomy or myelotomy and early debridement of necrosis may be beneficial to prevent complete paralysis by stopping further expansion of secondary injury, reducing the pressure of spared tissue and cerebrospinal fluids, preserving the spared spinal cord tissue, and delaying the glial cell death in experimental studies (Campbell JB et al., 1973; Freeman LW et al., 1953; Isu T et al., 1990; Kalderon N et al., 2007; Larson RE and Plaa GL, 1965; Warden P et al., 2001). The procedure is described by Freeman: "This incision was made longitudinally into the mid-dorsal region of the spinal cord and extended for the entire length of the laminectomy, through approximately one-half of the thickness of the spinal cord."

Clinical myelotomy could improve neurological functions in patients with spinal cord injury (Tachibana S et al., 1984; Zhu H et al., 2008). The procedure is to do posterior longitudinal myelotomy and remove hematoma and necrotic tissue of the central gray of the spinal cord by using a microsurgical technique (Tachibana S et al., 1984).

* Email: hongyunh@gmail.com.

# 2. Neurotization or Nerve Bridging

Neurotization or nerve bridging have being practiced in clinics for chronic SCI since Carlsson CA started this procedure in 1967, in which T12 nerve roots above the lesion were transected and anastomosed bilaterally to the S2 and S3 ventral and dorsal roots emerging from the injured cord area (Carlsson CA and Sundin T, 1967; 1980). Then this procedure was used or improved, such as taking a peripheral nerve from above the injury site and bridging it to a peripheral nerve to innervate a paralyzed muscle below the injury site (Lin H et al., 2008; Livshits A et al., 2004; Tubbs RS et al., 2008; von Wild KR and Brunelli GA, 2003; Xiao CG et al., 2003; Yang ML et al., 2011; Zhang S et al., 2003). Procedures by neurotization or nerve bridging could restore some neurological functions, such as, breathing ability, urine control, and arm or leg strength.

## References

Campbell, JB; DeCrescito, V; Tomasula, JJ; Demopoulos, HB; Flamm, ES; Ransohoff, J. Experimental treatment of spinal cord contusion in the cat. *Surg. Neurol.* 1973;1(2):102-6.

Carlsson, CA; Sundin, T. Reconstruction of afferent and efferent nervous pathways to the urinary bladder in two paraplegic patients. *Spine (Phila Pa 1976).* 1980;5(1):37-41.

Carlsson, CA; Sundin, T. Reconstruction of efferent pathways to the urinary bladder in a paraplegic child. *Rev. Surg.* 1967;24(1):73-6.

Freeman, LW; Wright, TW. Experimental observations of concussion and contusion of the spinal cord. *Ann. Surg*. 1953;137(4):433-43.

Isu, T; Iwasaki, Y; Akino, M; Abe, H. Effect of mannitol administration and myelotomy on acute experimental spinal cord injury: investigation by spinal cord evoked potential. *No Shinkei Geka*. 1990;18(3):267-72.

Kalderon, N; Muruganandham, M; Koutcher, JA; Potuzak, M. Therapeutic strategy for acute spinal cord contusion injury: cell elimination combined with microsurgical intervention. *PLoS One*. 2007;2(6):e565.

Larson, RE; Plaa, GL. A correlation of the effects of cervical cordotomy, hypothermia and catecholamines on carbon tetrachloride-induced hepatic necrosis. *J. Pharmacol. Exp. Ther.* 1965;147:103-11.

Lin, H; Hou, CL; Zhong, G; Xie, Q; Wang, S. Reconstruction of reflex pathways to the atonic bladder after conus medullaris injury: preliminary clinical results. *Microsurgery.* 2008;28(6):429-35.

Livshits, A; Catz, A; Folman, Y; Witz, M; Livshits, V; Baskov, A; Gepstein, R. Reinnervation of the neurogenic bladder in the late period of the spinal cord trauma. *Spinal Cord.* 2004;42(4):211-7.

Perkins, PG; Deane, RH. Long-term follow-up of six patients with acute spinal injury following dural decompression. *Injury*. 1988;19:397-401.

Smith, JS; Anderson, R; Pham, T; Bhatia, N; Steward, O; Gupta, R. Role of early surgical decompression of the intradural space after cervical spinal cord injury in an animal model. *J. Bone Joint Surg. Am.* 2010;92(5):1206-14.

Tachibana, S; Okada, K; Ohwada, T; Yada, K. Posterior longitudinal myelotomy as a surgical treatment of acute cervical spinal cord injury. *No Shinkei Geka.* 1984;12(2):183-8.

Tubbs, RS; Pearson, B; Loukas, M; Shokouhi, G; Shoja, MM; Oakes, WJ. Phrenic nerve neurotization utilizing the spinal accessory nerve: technical note with potential application in patients with high cervical quadriplegia. *Childs Nerv. Syst.* 2008;24(11):1341-4.

von Wild, KR; Brunelli, GA. Restoration of locomotion in paraplegics with aid of autologous bypass grafts for direct neurotisation of muscles by upper motor neurons--the future: surgery of the spinal cord? *Acta Neurochir. Suppl.* 2003;87:107-12.

Warden, P; Bamber, NI; Li, H; Esposito, A; Ahmad, KA; Hsu, CY; Xu, XM. Delayed glial cell death following wallerian degeneration in white matter tracts after spinal cord dorsal column cordotomy in adult rats. *Exp. Neurol.* 2001;168(2):213-24.

Xiao, CG; Du, MX; Dai, C; Li, B; Nitti, VW; de Groat, WC. An artificial somatic-central nervous system-autonomic reflex pathway for controllable micturition after spinal cord injury: preliminary results in 15 patients. *J. Urol.* 2003;170(4 Pt 1):1237-41.

Yang, ML; Li, JJ; Zhang, SC; Du, LJ; Gao, F; Li, J; Wang, YM; Gong, HM; Cheng, L. Functional restoration of the paralyzed diaphragm in high cervical quadriplegia via phrenic nerve neurotization utilizing the functional spinal accessory nerve. *J. Neurosurg. Spine.* 2011;15(2):190-4.

Zhang, S; Johnston, L; Zhang, Z; Ma, Y; Hu, Y; Wang, J; Huang, P; Wang, S. Restoration of stepping-forward and ambulatory function in patients with paraplegia: rerouting of vascularized intercostal nerves to lumbar nerve roots using selected interfascicular anastomosis. *Surg. Technol Int.* 2003;11:244-8.

Zhu, H; Feng, YP; Young, W; You, SW; Shen, XF; Liu, YS; Ju, G. Early neurosurgical intervention of spinal cord contusion: an analysis of 30 cases. *Chin. Med. J. (Engl).* 2008;121(24):2473-8.

In: Neurorestoratology, volume 1
Editors: H. Huang, G. Raisman, P. R. Sanberg et al.
ISBN: 978-1-63463-599-8


*Chapter 10*

# Alternative Therapies Combined with Cell Therapy

***Laurance Johnston**, Ph.D.**
Consulting Scientist, Paralyzed Veterans of America & Icelandic SCI Project, Albuquerque, NM, US

## Abstract

Over the past decade, many function-restoring cell-transplantation programs have emerged throughout the world for numerous disorders. Clearly, in the 21st century, such programs are going to play an ever-increasing role in restoring function lost by disability, disease, or the entropy of aging. In the case of SCI, cell-transplantation procedures and results vary substantially between programs. For these nascent programs, "the devil will be in the details." For example, cells from numerous sources (e.g., blood, bone marrow, olfactory tissue, fetal tissue, etc) have been transplanted via several routes, including into the spinal cord or fluid, intravenously, or intramuscularly. Donor cells often are not selected based on the theoretical best regenerative potential but their relative isolation ease. Likewise, it's a lot easier and safer, but perhaps not as effective, to inject cells into a muscle, blood, or spinal fluid than surgically accessing the spinal cord.

Adding to this plethora of details, effects of the cell therapy can be positively or even negatively influenced by numerous therapies. Because the lessons of history indicate that breakthroughs are catalyzed by pulling together seemingly disparate pieces of the puzzle, we should consider the augmentative neurorestorative potential of such therapies.

## 1. Acupuncture

Traditional Chinese Medicine (TCM) believes that a life-force energy qi permeates all living things through meridian channels punctuated by acupuncture points. As a rough

* Email: LauranceJohnston@msn.com.

analogy, view the meridians as a pipeline through which the energy flows, the acupuncture points as periodically placed, flow-controlling valves, and the acupuncture needles as the socket wrench that opens the valves. Stimulating these points can promote health- and regeneration-enhancing qi flow.

In his book "Life Force, The Scientific Basis," physicist Dr. Claude Swanson reviews the science that supports this ancient healing tradition (Swanson, 2010). For example, studies have shown that acupuncture points and meridians do, indeed, have anatomical and physiological correlates. For example, acupuncture points correspond to small (~ 1 mm) skin areas of greatly reduced electrical resistance. The meridian pathways closely match up to "Bonhan ducts," which contain an abundance of biophoton-emitting DNA (perhaps one reflection of qi energy). Swanson states that a key component contained within these ducts "may be undifferentiated cells (adult stem cells) which flow to regions of growth and injury where they specialize into the needed type of cell, and provide the building blocks for tissue repair."

Studies indicate that acupuncture may restore some function after SCI (Paola & Arnold, 2003; Gao et al., 1996; Wang, 1992; Cheng et al., 1998; Wong et al., 2003; Honjo et al., 1998; Nayak et al., 2001; Dyson-Hudson et al., 2001; Dyson-Hudson et al., 2008; Rapson et al., 2003). It has been suggested that acupuncture 1) reduces the levels of proteins and cells (e.g., astrocytes) fostering injury-site scar formation, 2) decreases the creation of damage-perpetuating free-radicals, 3) lessens spinal cord atrophy after injury, 4) reduces stress as measured by the production of cortisol, 5) raises the levels of various regeneration-enhancing molecules, 6) increases blood flow to the area of injury, and 7) releases neuroprotective, opioid-mimicking molecules (Dorsher & McIntosh, 2011).

In addition, studies demonstrate that acupuncture influences the effects of cell therapy in animal models of several neurological disorders (Wang et al., 2006; Tang et al., 2005; Yang et al., 2005; Ding et al., 2009; Yan et al., 2011; Sun et al., 2009): Based on studies in rats with completely transected spinal cord, Dr Y. Ding and colleagues concluded that electroacupuncture promotes the survival and differentiation of transplanted cells (Ding et al., 2009). Cell transplantation combined with electroacupuncture "could promote axonal regeneration and partial locomotor recovery in the transected spinal cord in rats and indicate a promising avenue of spinal cord injury" treatment. The same investigators concluded that 1) electroacupuncture promotes the differentiation of cells and regeneration of nerve fibers in the injured spinal cord through the induction of neural growth factors, and 2) the combination of electroacupuncture and cell transplantation can improve partial function of paralyzed hind limbs (Yan et al., 2011). Dr. Sun Z et al., demonstrated that treatment with electroacupuncture combined with bone-marrow-derived stromal cell transplantation restored more function than either treatment by itself (Sun et al., 2009). According to Dr. Charles Shang, the acupuncture system and stem cells are closely linked through an "organizing center network" composed of under-differentiated, electromagnetically sensitive cells (Shang, 2001 & 2009). This network is created early in embryogenesis before the formation of other body systems (e.g., spinal cord) and has the potential to influence these later-formed systems throughout life. Under this model, acupuncture has extensive growth-control effects and can trigger network stem cells into action. As a crude analogy, view the acupuncture-sensitive "organizing center network" as a behind-the-lines' general ready to send in "green" reserve troops (i.e., stem cells) who will evolve into the front-line combatants replacing those who have fallen from the attacks of disease, trauma, and aging. In the case of transplanted stem cells, Shang speculates that they can be recruited into a new network for repair and regeneration (Shang, 2006).

## 2. Laser Therapy

Evidence indicates that laser therapy promotes functional recovery for a variety of neurological disorders. In the case of SCI, studies suggest that laser therapy has a quick neuroprotective effect, preserves injured nerve functional activity, decreases injury-site scar tissue, lessens degeneration in corresponding motor neurons of the spinal cord, and increases axonal growth and myelinization. In cell cultures, it accelerates neuronal cell migration, cell growth, fiber sprouting, and neurite budding (Anders, 2009; Gigo-Benato et al., 2005; Snyder et al., 2002; Shin et al., 2003; Rochkind, 2009; Rochkind et al., 2009).

Dr. Shimon Rochkind and colleagues examined the effects of embryonic spinal-cord-cell transplantation and laser therapy on recovery after SCI in rats (Rochkind, 2002). Results indicated that the best recovery of limb function and gait performance, electrophysiological conduction, and histological parameters occurred after cell implantation and laser radiation.

Dr. Kimberly Byrnes et al., showed that laser irradiation alters gene expression of OECs, a regeneratively endowed cell that has been transplanted into many individuals with neurological disorders (Byrnes, 2005). This alteration enhances the expression of key growth factors and extracellular matrix proteins that support neuronal regeneration. Her findings support the use of laser therapy in combination with OEC transplantation.

This research is particularly relevant because numerous individuals with SCI have attempted to maximize restored function after cell transplantation using laser-based therapies (e.g., Bohbot, 2008; Jacques, 2005), especially the Laserpuncture therapy developed by Dr. Albert Bohbot. Bohbot has treated numerous individuals with SCI, who have been the transplantation recipients of a variety of cell types from different programs throughout the world. In a recent article, Bohbot evaluated the impact of Laserpuncture on electromyographic parameters of three individuals with SCI who underwent OEC transplantation (Bohbot, 2010). Results suggested that the Laserpuncture/cell-transplantation-combination therapy restored some voluntary muscle activity.

Sidebar:

Laserponcture (Albert Bohbot)
Bohbot A, Director of the Laboratoire de Recherches sur le Laserponcture®, 3 Rue du Monument – Porte 13 – Auterive 31190 France

Laserponcture® combines two fundamental theories, acupuncture which has a 5,000-year-tradition, and various works on laser (Jame-Collet, 2001), the nerve impulse, DNA and its restructuring through the use of laser. In this field, significant experimental work has been done, namely by Peter P. Gariaev who discusses, in his article entitled "The DNA-wave Biocomputer", the quantum nonlocality direct relation "(i) to laser radiations from chromosomes, (ii) to the ability of the chromosome to gyrate the polarization plane of its own radiated and occluded photons and (iii) to the suspected ability of chromosomes, to transform their own genetic-sign laser radiations into broadband genetic-sign radio waves. In the latter case, the polarizations of chromosome laser photons are connected nonlocally and coherently to polarizations of radio waves" [Gariaev]. The machine, Laserponctor, is a multihead laser. Each of the ten heads is computer piloted and delivers a program with a pre-defined specific frequency and power. They are fixed on the skin and stimulate points located on the different meridians. The session lasts twenty minutes. Also a PROCOMP5™ with softwares BIOGRAPH INFINITI5® and REHAB SUITE™, and sensors MYOSCAN-PRO™ EMG (SA9401M-50) are used to record muscle activity.

# 3. Omental Transposition

Omental transposition procedures have been used to treat various nervous-system disorders, including SCI, stroke, cerebral palsy, Alzheimer's disease, and Parkinson's disease (Johnston, 2001; Goldsmith, 2000; Agner et al., 2001). The omentum is a highly vascular, fatty tissue approximately 14-inches long and 10-inches wide that hangs like an apron over the intestines and lower abdomen area. For SCI, the omentum is surgically tailored to create a pedicle of sufficient length and intact circulation so it can be attached to the cord's injury site (like cutting a square handkerchief into a long necktie).

Although historically the omentum has been viewed as an inert tissue bereft of significant biological function, scientists are now discovering that it is a physiologically dynamic tissue, possessing 1) regeneration-supporting angiogenic factors, 2) an extensive waste-disposing and edema-absorbing lymphatic system, and 3) various immune cells, growth factors, and other agents that may foster the healing of an injured nervous system. Regarding its angiogenic properties, Dr. Ignacio García-Gómez et al., have shown that human omentum contains stem cells, which synthesize key, blood-flow-enhancing growth factors (Garcia-Gomez et al., 2005).

# 4. Hyperbaric Oxygen

With hyperbaric oxygen (HBO) therapy, patients are put in chambers pressurized at 2-3 atmospheres containing up to 100% oxygen. Studies suggest that HBO is beneficial for treating a variety of neurological disorders in which blood-flow-related oxygenation is compromised, including SCI (Young, 2005; Yeo, 1978; Yeo, 1984; Jones et al., 1978; Gamache et al., 1981; Elinkii et al., 1984; Asamoto et al., 2000). The premise is that HBO will force oxygen into injured, oxygen-deprived CNS tissue.

Numerous animal studies suggest that HBO influences the expression of stem cells, including 1) promoting differentiation and proliferation into neurons (Chen et al., 2010; Yang et al., 2008), 2) enhancing migration to areas of injury (Wang et al., 2009), 3) suppressing stem-cell apoptosis (Pan et al., 2009), and 4) inducing stem-cell growth factors (Shyu et al., 2008) In humans, Dr. Stephen Thom et al., has shown that HBO stimulates the bone-marrow production of stromal cells (Thom et al., 2006). Specifically, stromal cells doubled in the circulation after a single two-hour, two-atmosphere HBO session, and after 20 treatments, increased eight-fold.

# 5. Psychoneuroimmunology

Psychoneuroimmunology is a scientific term to describe how our emotions, attitudes, and consciousness influence health. From a holistic mind-body-spirit view, the most powerful healing comes from adopting a health-enhancing consciousness, whose overarching influence transforms the physical. Long before stem cells became a blip on modern science's radar, the influence of consciousness on their expression was discussed in the Life and Teachings of the Masters of the Far East (Spalding, 1996):

1) "As the cell divides and creates a new cell, our thought is implanted upon it…In the first cell, all is perfect. That cell was first known as the Christ cell." (i.e., the anointed cell) "It is always just as young as ever it was. It never takes on old age. It is the primal spark of life. When we implant in it our thoughts of limitation or old age, or any condition outside of perfection, the body responds. Cells born from the first cell take on its image. Originally it is the image and likeness of God. It is perfect in every way. But it becomes the form we carry in our minds…if we carry the image of perfection always, what will it do for these cells? It will build perfection." (Vol. 6, Page 78)
2) "The moment a cell divides itself from the parent cell, and the instant before it divides itself, it takes on the exact image of the parent. As it goes out, it comes under the influence of this imperfection that we think for ourselves. What happens? We see the vibrations of the cell lowered, and in some instances when it attaches itself to the organ where it belongs, it is a dead thing…The very thought influence of imperfection influences that cell until it dies. The vibrations go so low that the dynamic influence flows out." (Vol. 6, Page 92)

A moving anecdotal example of how a shift in consciousness may have augmented functional return after embryonic stem-cell transplantation is discussed in a recently published article by the author (Johnston and Boxtel, 2010).

Scientists have proposed many physiological mechanisms by which emotions, attitudes, and overall consciousness can potentially transform our health and influence cells. Basically, under emerging epigenetic principles, we are not merely a hardwired manifestation of our genetic DNA as once thought. The genes we express and, as a result, who we become is influenced by diverse factors, including consciousness.

For example, Dr. Bruce Lipton hypothesizes that our consciousness affects DNA expression through electromagnetically induced shifts in the structure of proteins embedded in our cell membranes (Lipton, 2005). As shown in Menninger Clinic experiments, individuals are able to shift consciousness in a way that can alter the body's electromagnetic dynamics. Lipton hypothesizes that this alteration changes the physical configuration of membrane proteins, in turn, affecting communication between the outside and inside of cells. Roughly speaking, this consciousness-driven energy is like a radio signal triggering the garage door to open. This opening initiates a cascade of physiological events which regulate gene expression and, in turn, cell fate. Scientists, indeed, have shown that the subtlest of energies can affect stem-cell expression or viability. For example, these cells are exceptionally sensitive to cosmic radiation (Encinas et al., 2008).

## Summary

The author has funded many scientists considered at the forefront in the U.S. As such, it was eye opening to observe how many function-restoring contributions or insights have come out of not the U.S. but China in one form or another. For example, 1) in spite of their ancient origins, TCM has considerable contemporary relevance to Neurorestoratology; 2) the country is at the forefront of developing and implementing state-of-the-art, cell-transplantation strategies with real-world relevance; and 3) Chinese scientists have the open-minded willingness to integrate the ancient with the modern to provide a more expanded healing spectrum. Clearly, if the world's oldest healing tradition, acupuncture, can influence the most state-of-the-art therapy (i.e., cell therapy), we should pay attention, or the promising therapeutic potential of this nascent technology may be compromised.

# References

Agner C, Yeomans D, Dujovny M. The neurochemical basis for the applications of the greater omentum in neurosurgery. *Neurol. Res.* 2001; 23(1): 7-15.

Anders JJ. The Potential of light therapy for central nervous system injury and disease. Photo *Med. Laser Surg.*2009; 27(3): 379-380.

Ao Q, Sun X-H, Wang AJ, Fu PF, Gong K, Zuo HC, Gong YD, Zhang XF. Protective effects of extract of Ginkgo biloba (EGB 761) on nerve cells after spinal cord injury in rats. *Spinal Cord.* 2006; 44: 662-667.

Asamoto S, Sugiyama H, Doi H, Iida M, Nagao T, Matsumoto K. Hyperbaric oxygen (HBO) therapy for acute traumatic cervical spinal cord injury. *Spinal Cord.* 2000; 38(9): 538-540.

Bohbot A. Olfactory ensheathing glia transplantation combined with LASERPONCTURE in human spinal cord injury: Results measured by electromyography monitoring. *Cell Transplant.* 2010; 19(2): 179-184.

Byrnes KR, Waynant RW, Ilev, IK. Light promotes regeneration and functional recovery and alters the immune response after spinal cord injury. *Lasers Surg. Med.* 2005;36(3):171-185.

Byrnes KR, Wu X, Waynant RW, Ilev IK, Anders JJ. Low power irradiation alters gene expression of olfactory ensheathing cells. *Lasers Surg. Med.*2005; 37(2): 161-171.

Chen A, Wang H, Zhang J, Wu X, Liao J, Li H, Cai W, Luo X, Ju G. BYHWD rescues axotomized neurons and promotes functional recovery after spinal cord injury in rats. *J. Ethnopharmacol.* 2008; 117(3): 451-456.

Chen CF, Yang YJ, Wang QH, Yao Y, Li M. Effect of hyperbaric oxygen administered at different pressures and different exposure time on differentiation of neural stem cells in vitro. *Zhongguo Dang Dai Er Ke Za Zhi.* 2010; 12(5): 368-372.

Cheng PT, Wong MK, Chang PL. A therapeutic trial of acupuncture in neurogenic bladder of spinal cord injured patients – a preliminary report. *Spinal Cord.* 1998; 36(7): 476-480.

Ding Y, Yan Q, Ruan JW, Zhang YQ, Li Y, Dong H, Zeng YS. Electro-acupuncture promotes survival, differentiation of the bone marow mesenchymal stem cells as well as functional recovery in the spinal cord-transected rats. *BMC Neurosci.*2009; 10: 35.

Dorsher PT, McIntosh PM. Acupuncture's effects in treating the sequelae of acute and chronic spinal cord injuries: a review of allopathic and traditional Chinese medicine literature. *Evid. Based Complement Alternat Med.* 2011;2011:428108.

Drapeau C. Triple-blind randomized placebo-controlled study of the effect of StemEnhance on bone marrow stem cell mobilization. Nov 24, 2009. Available from: http://img.exigo.com/public/1595/websites/62/images/summaryoftripleblindstudyv2.pdf.

Dyson-Hudson TA, Kadar P, LaFountain M, Emmons R, Kirschblum SC, Tulsky D, Koaroff E. Acupuncture for chronic pain in persons with spinal cord injury: a small-scale clinical trial. *Arch. Phys. Med. Rehabil.* 2008; 89(1): 1276-1283.

Dyson-Hudson TA, Shiflett SC, Kirshblum SC, Bowen JE, Druin EL. Acupuncture and trager psychophysical integration in the treatment of wheelchair user's shoulder pain in individuals with spinal cord injury. *Arch. Phys. Med. Rehabil.* 2001; 82(8): 1038-1046.

Elinskii MP, Rafikov AM, Baibus GN. Therapeutic use of hyperbaric oxygenation in lesions of the spinal cord. *Zh Neropatol Psikhiatry Im S S Korsakova*. 1984; 84(5): 682-687.

Encinas JM, Vazquez ME, Switzer RC, Chamberland DW, Nick H, Levine HG, Scarpa PJ, Enikolopov G, Steindler DA. Quiescent adult neural stem cells are exceptionally sensitive to cosmic radiation. *Expl. Neurol.* 2008; 210(1): 274-279.

Fan L, Wang K, Cheng B. Effects of buying huanwu decoction on apoptosis of nervous cells and expressions of Bci-2 and bax in the spinal cord of ischemia-reprusion injury ion rabbits. *J. Tradit. Chin. Med.* 2006; 26(2): 153-156.

Gao X, Gao C, Gao J, Han C, Han F, Han B, Han L. Acupuncture treatment of complete traumatic paraplegia; Analysis of 261 Cases. *J. Traditional Chinese Medicine*. 1996; 16(2): 134-137.

Garcia-Gomez I, Goldsmith HS, Angulo J, Prados A, López-Hervás P, Cuevas B, Dujovny M, Cuevas P. Angiogenic capacity of human omental stem cells. *Neurol. Res.* 2005; 27(8): 807-811.

Gariaev PP, Birshtein BI, Iarochenko AM. The DNA-wave Biocomputer. June 30, 2014. Available at: http://www.laserponcture.net/anglais/gariaev.pdf.

Gigo-Benato D, Geuna S, Rochkind S. Phototherapy for enhancing peripheral nerve repair: A review of the literature. *Muscle Nerve*. 2005; 31(6): 694-701.

Goldsmith HS (editor). The Omentum Application to Brain and Spinal Cord. Wilton, CT: Forefront Publishing; 2000.

Honjo H, Kitakoji H, Kawakita K, Saitoh M, Ukimota O, Kojima M, Watanabe H, Aramaki S. Acupuncture for urinary incontinence in patients with chronic spinal cord injury. A preliminary report. *Nippon Hinyokika Gakkai Zasshi*. 1998; 89(7): 665-669.

Jacques E. Stem cell treatment for paralyzed patients. Program, ICS 39th North American Federation Congress, Acapulco, Mexico, June 15-18, 2005.

Jame-Collet C. Du dermatome au pibu, le lien: le laserponcture - Application clinique au travers de la para et de la tétraplégie. DUMETRAC. Université de Médecine Paris-Nord, Faculté Léonard de Vinci, U.F.R. Santé, Médecine, *Biologie*. 2001. PhD thesis

Gamache FW, Roy AM, Drucker TB, Cowley RA. The clinical application of hyperbaric oxygen therapy in spinal cord injury: A preliminary report. *Surg. Neurol.* 1981; 15(2): 85-87.

Johnston L. Boxtel A. Stem-Cell Consciousness: The Divine Ground of Healing, Townsend Letter: *The Examiner of Alternative Medicine*.2010 June; 50-55.

Johnston L. The omentum momentum. PN/Paraplegia News.2001 March; 48-52.

Jones RF, Unsworth IP, Marosszeky JE. Hyperbaric oxygen and acute spinal cord injuries in humans. *Med. J.* 1978 Aug; 2(12): 573-575.

Lipton B. The Biology of Belief. Santa Rosa, CA: Mountain of Love/Elite Books; 2005.

Nayak S, Shiflett SC, Schoenberg NE, Agostinelli S, Kirshblum S, Averill A, Cotter AC. Is acupuncture effective in treating chronic pain after spinal cord injury? *Arch. Phys. Med. Rehabil.* 2001; 82(11): 1578-1586.

Pan HC, Chin CS, Yang DY, Ho SP, Chen CJ, Hwang SM, Chang MH, Cheng FC. Human amniotic fluid mesenchymal stem cells in combination with hyperbaric oxygen augment peripheral nerve regeneration. *Neurochem. Res.*2009. 34(7) 1304-1316.

Paola FA, Arnold M, Acupuncture and spinal cord medicine. *J Spinal Cord Medicine*. 2003; 26(1): 12-20.

Prasad GC, Khanna RP, Prakash V, Udupa KN. Effect of lajjawanti (mimosa pudica Linn.) on regeneration of nerve. *Jur. Res. Ind. Med.* 1975; 10(4): 37-44.

Rapson LM, Wells N, Pepper J, Majid N, Boon H. Acupuncture as a promising treatment for below-level central neuropathic pain: a retrospective study. *J. Spinal Cord Med.* 2003; 26(1): 21-26.

Rochkind S, El-Ani D, Nevo Z, Shahar A. Increase of neuronal sprouting and migration using 780 nm laser phototherapy as a procedure for cell therapy. *Lasers Surg. Med.* 2009; 41(4): 277-281.

Rochkind S, Shahar A, Amon M, Nevo Z. Transplantation of embryonal spinal cord nerve cells cultured on biodegradable microcarriers followed by low power laser irradiation for the treatment of traumatic paraplegia in rats. *Neurol. Res.* 2002; 24(4): 355-360.

Rochkind S. Phototherapy in peripheral nerve regeneration: From basic science to clinical study. *Neurosurg Focus*. 2009; 26(2): E8.

Shang C. Electrophysiology of growth control and acupuncture. *Life Sci.* 2001; 68(12): 1333-1342.

Shang C, *Harvard Medical School* (personal communication, June 10, 2006).

Shang C. Prospective tests on biological models of acupuncture. Evid Based Complement *Alternat Med.* 2009; 6(1): 31-39.

Shen LH, Zhang JT. Ginsenoside Rg1 promotes proliferation of hippocampal progenitor cells. *Neurol. Res.* 2004; 26(4): 422-428.

Shin DH, Lee E, Hyun JK, Lee SJ, Chang YP, Kim JW, Choi YS, Kwon BS. Growth-associated protein-43 is elevated in the injured rat sciatic nerve after low power laser irradiation. *Neurosci. Lett.* 2003; 344(2): 71-74.

Shyu KG, Hung HF, Wang BW, Chang H. Hyperbaric oxygen induces placental growth factor expression in bone marrow-derived mesenchymal stem cells. *Life Sci.* 2008; 83(1-2): 65-73.

Snyder SK, Byrnes KR, Borke RC, Sanchez A, Anders JJ. Quantification of calcitonin gene-related peptide mRNA and neuronal cell death in facial motor nuclei following axotomy and 633 nm low power laser treatment. *Lasers Surg. Med.* 2002; 31(3): 216-222.

Spalding BT. Life and Teachings of the Masters of the Far East, Volume VI. Marina del Rey, CA: DeVorss & Company; 1996.

Sun J-H, Gao Y-M, Yang L, Wang X, Bao LH, Liu WJ, Yew D. Effects of buyyang huanwu decoction on neurite outgrowth and differentiation of neuroepithelial stem cells. *Chin. J. Physiol.* 2007; 50(4): 151-156.

Sun Z, Li X, Su Z, Wu M. Electroacupuncture-enhanced differentiation of bone marrow stromal cells into neuronal cells. *J. Sport Rehabil.* 2009; 18(3): 398-406.

Swanson C. Life Force, The Scientific Basis: Breakthrough Physics of Energy Medicine, Healing, Chi and Quantum Physics. Tucson, AZ: Poseidia Press; 2010.

Tang Y, Yin HY, Zeng F, Yu SG. Pondering in-situ induction of endogenous neural stem cells in hippocampus of rats with Alzheimer disease by acupuncture. *Zhing Xi Yi Jie He Xue Bao.* 2005. 3(5); 351-354.

Thom SR, Bhopale VM, Velazquez OC, et al. Stem cell mobilization by hyperbaric oxygen. *Am. J. Physiol. Heart & Circ. Physiol.* 2006; 290(4): 1378-1386.

Tohda C. Overcoming several neurodegenerative diseases by traditional medicines: the development of therapeutic medicines and unraveling pathophysiological mechanisms. *Yakugaku Zasshi.* 2008; 128(8): 1159-1167.

Wang HJ. A survey of the treatment of traumatic paraplegia by traditional Chinese medicine, *J Chin Med.* 1992; 12(4): 296-303.

Wang WC, Ma J, Wang H. Effects of Shuanggu Yitong needling method on proliferation and differentiation of nerve stem cells in the Parkinson's disease model rat. *Zhingguo Zhen Jiu.* 2006; 26(4): 277-288.

Wang XL, Yang YJ, Xie M, Yu XH, Wang QH. Hyperbaric oxygen promotes the migration and differentiation of endogenous neural stem cells in neonatal rats with hypoxic ischemia brain damage. *Zhongguo Dang Dai Er Ke Za Zhi.* 2009; 11(9): 749-752.

Wong AM, Leong CP, Su TY, Yu SW, Tsai WC, Chen CP. Clinical trial of acupuncture for patients with spinal cord injury. *Am. J. Phys. Med. Rehabil.* 2003; 82(1): 21-27.

Yan Q, Ruan JW, Ding Y, Li WJ, Li Y, Zeng YS. Electro-acupuncture promotes differentiation of mesenchymal stem cells, regeneration of nerve fibers and partial functional recovery after spinal cord injury. 2011 Jan;63(1-2):151-6.

Yang C, Li B, Liu TS, Zhao DM, HU FA. Effect of electroacupuncture on proliferation of astrocytes after spinal cord injury. *Zhongguo Zhen Jiu.* 2005; 25(8): 569-572.

Yang YJ, Wang XL, Yu XH, Wang X, Xie M, Liu CT. Hyperbaric oxygen induces endogenous neural stem cells to proliferate and differentiate in hypoxic-ischemia brain damage in neonatal rats. *Undersea Hyperb Med.* 2008; 35(2): 113-129.

Yeo J. Preliminary report on ten patients with spinal cord injuries treated with hyperbaric oxygen. *Med. J. Aust.* 1978: 2(12): 572-573.

Yeo JD. The use of hyperbaric oxygen to modify the effects of recent contusion injury to the spinal cord. *Cent. Nerv. Syst. Trauma*, 1984; 1(2): 161-165.

Young W. Hyperbaric oxygenation therapy. July 17, 2005. Available from: http://sci.rutgers.edu/index.php?page=viewarticle&afile=23_October_2001@HBOT2001.htm

Yune TY, Lee JY, Cui CM, Kim HC, Oh TH. Neuroprotective effect of Scutellaria bicalensis on spinal cord injury in rats. *J. Neurochem.* 2009; 110(4): 1276-1287.

In: Neurorestoratology, volume 1
Editors: H. Huang, G. Raisman, P. R. Sanberg et al.
ISBN: 978-1-63463-599-8


*Chapter 11*

# Neurorehabilitation

***Hongyun Huang****
Beijing Rehabilitation Hospital of Capital Medical University
Beijing Hongtianji Neuroscience Academy, China

Neurorehabilitation is a specialty of neuroscience, which deals with the study and application of complex medical processes aiming at recovery from nervous system injury and compensating for functional alterations. Neurorehabilitation therapies include occupational therapy, physical therapy, psychological therapy, speech and language therapy and more, which focus on daily function and community re-integration (http://en.wikipedia.org/wiki/Neurorehabilitation). As the most important alternative or complementary neurorestorative strategy, Neurorehabilitation can enhance more functional recovery after neurorestorative treatment.

Single behavior therapy cannot cure the disability but it plays an important role in a patient's function improvement. Physical therapy can be a significant compensation to the recovery of neural deficits. A preclinical study proves that task-specific training can enhance the effect after OEC transplantation (Kubasak MD et al., 2008). Constraint-Induced Movement therapy has also proved beneficial in improving the function of disabled limbs (Taub E et al., 1993). Our results also demonstrate that patients with sufficient rehabilitation (or active-movement target enhancement neurorehabilitation therapy, AMTENT) achieved more benefits after OEC therapy. Even patients with insufficient rehabilitation after OEC therapy also had some functional recovery and improve their quality of life, but further analysis found that some of their functional improvement had a close relationship to daily life, such as, sitting and the ability to turn their body over (Huang HY et al., 2012). This means that no matter whether they do rehabilitation training or not, daily life activities are similar to some of the rehabilitation training exercises.

Good neurorehabilitation can improve patients' quality of life, and avoid extra complications from origin injury or disability. Hence, all patients need to be encouraged to do AMTENT to enhance their effects of neurorestoration after neurorestorative treatment.

* Email: hongyunh@gmail.com.

# References

Huang, HY; Xi, HT; Chen, L; Zhang, F; Liu, YC. Long-term outcome of olfactory ensheathing cell therapy for patients with complete chronic spinal cord injury. *Cell Transplant.* 2012; 21:S23–S31.

Kubasak, MD; Jindrich, DL; Zhong, H; Takeoka, A; McFarland, KC; Muñoz-Quiles, C; Roy, RR; Edgerton, VR; Ramón-Cueto, A; Phelps, PE.OEG implantation and step training enhance hindlimb-stepping ability in adult spinal transected rats. *Brain.* 2008;131 (Pt 1):264-76.

Taub, E; Miller, NE; Novack, TA; Cook, EW III; Fleming, WC; Nepomuceno, CS; Connell, JS; Crago, JE. Technique to improve chronic motor deficit after stroke. *Archives of Physical Medicine and Rehabilitation.* 1993;74:347-354.

In: Neurorestoratology, volume 1
Editors: H. Huang, G. Raisman, P. R. Sanberg et al.
ISBN: 978-1-63463-599-8


# Postscript

***Hongyun Huang****
Beijing Rehabilitation Hospital of Capital Medical University and
Beijing Hongtianji Neuroscience Academy, China

When there is life there is hope. The sketch of ***Neurorestoratology*** took four years and is finally completed now. I would like to express my gratitude to all authors and editorial team for their hard work, and feel like having something more to say. I had a dream when I was a resident of neurosurgeon, that is, to let patients with incurable neural damages or diseases or their sequela to recover their functions.

Remember in 2001, our team was very surprised to firstly find in the world that patients with chronic complete spinal cord injury had functional recovery in a few days after olfactory ensheathing cell transplantation. It was like the apple which hit Newton's head. We wondered if it was an accidental phenomenon or a true fact. Hereafter, more studies by us and other physicians showed similar results. Hence we can firmly declare that this discovery is a true fact, that neurological damages or diseases can be partially restored. This overthrew my old concept, same with most neuroscientists, neurologists and neurosurgeons, that patients with sequela of neural damages or diseases have no chance to recover their functions. From this discovery we deduced it as ***CNS Neurorestorable theory***. However, at that time, we didn't know where the theoretic basis was, or which law it should abide by.

Prior to this discovery, I held the same viewpoint with majority of colleagues in this field, that is, neurological function recovery come from the mechanism of neuroregeneration. However, further studies showed that neuromodulation, neuroprotection, neuroplasticity, neurogenesis, etc. also played a role in restoring functions in different situations. Unfortunately all those mechanisms for different insults were studied and viewed in isolation at that time. Like Darwin who formerly entertained and then objected that "each species has been independently created". We believe that the right way is to put all related factors as a whole. When the entire neural insults with whatever causing the restoration were generalized as a whole process, which we called ***neurorestorative process***, we surprisingly find that each mechanism is just a part of the whole and plays a role in different stages. And all mechanisms are the basis of ***CNS Neurorestorable theory.***

* Cell phone: 86-13910116608 Email: hongyunh@gmail.com.

From the ***neurorestorative process***, one interventional strategy will exert a role through one or more neurorestorative mechanisms, but may not have enough ability to restore functions; also more strategies or combination have shown ability to enhance the neurorestorative extent based on our or many colleagues' studies. Furthermore, cell therapy is currently the most important neurorestorative strategy. Therefore we recommend cell-based comprehensive neurorestorative strategies as main methods for patients with neurological diseases or damages. Even though we are not sure which kind of combination is the best one, we should keep looking for better or more effective combination.

More importantly, from this ***neurorestorative process***, we revealed ***Neurorestorative law: more or less self-restoring always occurs by nature while facing insults, further active (appropriate) medical intervention can better restore functions or /and structures***. Obviously this law is applicable for all nervous activity in physiological and pathophysiological states. Self-restoring by nature may not be enough when facing strong insults, it is necessary to give active or appropriate intervention to better restore functions and improve quality of life. So the exploration by this law is forever and endless, including time of period, neurorestorative extent, mechanisms and strategies.

Considering many disciplines involving neurorestorative studies as their frontier edges, which focus on a common cross point- neurorestoration, we strongly felt that a new discipline should be put forward, and it should take the responsibility to solve all issues related to neurorestorative studies. Thus ***Neurrorestoratology*** was created, and fortunately we got extensive support and response in this field.

Because of new perspectives by ***CNS Neurorestorable theory, Neurorestorative Process*** and ***Neurorestorative Law***, more optimistic, positive, comprehensive neurorestorative strategies and mechanisms have been presented in neuroscience or clinical disciplines related with neurorestoration. We are happy to see clearly that patients with incurable neural damage or diseases or their sequela are no longer as helpless, and already have a chance to restore some functions and improve their quality of life.

It's our honour to play a role in pushing the new discipline development, helping people form new perspectives, and see great changes in many viewpoints of neuroscience or clinical disciplines related to neurorestoration.

"DREAMS
Hold fast to dreams
For if dreams die
Life is a broken winged bird
That cannot fly.
Hold fast to dreams
For when dreams go
Life is a barren field
Frozen with snow.
Langston Hughes"

Gladly, most neuroscientists, physicians in clinical disciplines related with neurorestoration or more others are happy seeing that my and also their (I believe so) dream has partially come true.

# Index

## A

## B



## C

## D

## E

## F



## G



## H

## I

## J



## K



## L



## M

## N

## O



## P

## Q



## R

## S

## T

## U



## V

## W



## X



## Z